PEDIATRICS - LABORATORY AND CLINICAL RESEARCH

REVIEWS IN PEDIATRIC EXERCISE SCIENCE

PEDIATRICS - LABORATORY AND CLINICAL RESEARCH

Additional books in this series can be found on Nova's website under the Series tab.

Additional E-books in this series can be found on Nova's website under the E-book tab.

SPORTS AND ATHLETICS PREPARATION, PERFORMANCE, AND PSYCHOLOGY

Additional books in this series can be found on Nova's website under the Series tab.

Additional E-books in this series can be found on Nova's website under the E-book tab.

PEDIATRICS - LABORATORY AND CLINICAL RESEARCH

REVIEWS IN PEDIATRIC EXERCISE SCIENCE

MICHAEL DUNCAN
EDITOR

Nova Science Publishers, Inc.
New York

For permission to use material from this book please contact us:
Telephone 631-231-7269; Fax 631-231-8175
Web Site: http://www.novapublishers.com

Additional color graphics may be available in the e-book version of this book.

Library of Congress Cataloging-in-Publication Data

Reviews in pediatric exercise science / editor, Michael Duncan.
p. cm.
Includes bibliographical references and index.
ISBN 978-1-61470-978-7 (hardcover)
1. Exercise for children. 2. Exercise therapy for children. I. Duncan, Michael.
RJ133.R48 2011
613.7'1083--dc23

2011030129

Published by Nova Science Publishers, Inc. † New York

Contents

Preface		**vii**
List of Contributors		**xix**
Chapter I	**Physical Activity, Play and the Pre-School Years** *Mareesa O'Dwyer, Zoe Knowles, Nicola Ridgers and Gareth Stratton*	**1**
Chapter II	**Physical Education and Sport, and Positive Attitudes towards Physical Activity** *Lorayne A. Woodfield*	**13**
Chapter III	**Promoting Cardiovascular Health in the Primary School Curriculum** *Moira N. McPherson, Kimberly Boardman, William J. Montelpare and Carlos E. Zerpa*	**27**
Chapter IV	**Breakfast, Metabolism, Health and Cognitive Function in Young People** *Keith Tolfrey, Julia K. Zakrzewski, Simon B. Cooper and Mary E. Nevill*	**43**
Chapter V	**Environmental Correlates of Physical Activity in Children and Adolescents** *Stacey Hargreaves, Michael J. Duncan and Samantha Birch*	**67**
Chapter VI	**Body Image Perception and its Relationship with Nutritional Status in Childhood and Adolescence** *Edio Luiz Petroski, Andreia Pelegrini and Diego Augusto Santos Silva*	**87**
Chapter VII	**The Efficacy of Exercise in Enhancing Children's Reading Ability** *Esther Curley, Michael J. Duncan and Samantha Birch*	**97**
Chapter VIII	**The Relationship between Fundamental Movement Skills and Physical Activity in Primary School Children: A Short Review** *Luke C. Baker, Samantha Birch and Michael J. Duncan*	**115**

Chapter IX	**Physical Activity Patterns in Children from Different Ethnic Backgrounds** *Emma Lisa Jane Eyre and Krystyna Anna Matyka*	**125**
Chapter X	**Heart Rate Variability, Weight Status and Physical Activity in Children: A Short Review** *Craig Franklin, Samantha Birch and Michael J. Duncan*	**147**
Chapter XI	**Thermoregulation in Children and Adolescents** *Michael J. Price*	**161**
Chapter XII	**Injuries in Sport among Children and Adolescents** *Sheila Leddington Wright and Andrew King*	**181**
Chapter XIII	**Sprinting and Plyometric Ability in Youths: The Effect of Natural Development and Training** *Michael G. Hughes, Rhodri Lloyd and Robert Meyers*	**201**
Chapter XIV	**Methods of Monitoring Training in Adolescent Soccer Players** *Matt Rains, Mark Noon and Doug Thake*	**217**
Index		**241**

Preface

Research relating to the exercising child and adolescent has expanded considerably over the last decade or two. This accelerating volume of research output covers a wide range of topics with both an academic and practical focus. Such topics range from studies on the effect of physical activity interventions on sedentary behavior in obese children to talent identification in young athletes. With such an array of cross disciplinary research being generated related to pediatric exercise science, there is a need for a periodic summarization and reflection on the scope of information available. This book presents a range of literature reviews in the field of pediatric exercise science that provides a bridge between scientific practice and the pediatric exercise practitioner.

Chapter I - It is well documented that regular physical activity among young children may contribute to social development (Sawyers 1994), psychological welfare (Ekelund et al. 2004), improvements in fundamental motor skill development (Cliff et al. 2009), maintenance of bone health (Janz et al. 2010), prevention of cardiovascular disease (Anderssen et al. 2007) and protection against excess weight gain (Abbott et al. 2004). Despite this evidence base, pre-school aged children are not accumulating enough physical activity to accrue health benefits of being active (Reilly 2010; Tucker 2008; Oliver et al. 2007). For the purpose of this chapter pre-school children in the United Kingdom (UK) are defined as those attending 15 hours of 'voucher' funded pre-school education (playgroups, day-care or school based nursery) or in the first compulsory school year in which they turn 5 years old.

From 1989 to 1998, there was a highly significant increase in weight and body mass index for boys and girls from the age of infancy to pre-school (Bundred et al. 2001). This problem still remains with overweight prevalence among pre-school children ranging from 12-32% in Western European countries (Cattaneo et al. 2010). Physical activity is an important behavior for pre-school children as it sets a foundation for facilitating and maintaining a healthy and active life through to adulthood (Cragg et al. 2006; Campbell et al. 2001). Unfortunately, limited data exist on the physical activity levels of pre-school children but a recent study in Australia reported that 44% and 21% of Australian pre-school aged children are not meeting the recommended daily physical activity guidelines on weekdays and weekend days, respectively (Okely et al. 2009). A similar issue is apparent in the UK, with only 40% of pre-school children achieving the recommended daily guidelines for MVPA during weekdays and weekend days (O'Dwyer et al. 2011). One of the reasons for these worryingly low levels of activity may be explained by the perceptions held by teachers and parents. These significant others assume that pre-school children are very active and spend most of their time continually running around thus believing that they engage in sufficient amounts activity (Sallis et al. 1988). However, research has suggested that prolonged screen time, fewer siblings to play with and safety concerns among parents regarding play spaces have resulted in increased sedentary behavior (Burdette et al. 2005).

The aim of this chapter is to inform the reader about the different types of play that exist among pre-school children as well as describe importance of play, specifically active play. The reader will be introduced to the recommendations for physical activity for this population. Lastly, this chapter aims to provide a summary of interventions aimed at increasing physical activity which have been conducted in pre-school settings.

Chapter II - The aim of this chapter is to consider the role that physical education and sporting activities can play in the promotion of positive attitudes towards physical activity and healthy lifestyles. Although it is claimed that attitude is one of the most researched areas of social psychology (Olson and Zanna, 1993, cited in Biddle and Mutrie, 2008), literature investigating young people's attitudes toward physical education is limited. Lifestyle development has been an aim of physical education for many years and is explicitly stated in national curricula (please see Bailey, 2009 for a review of the benefits and aims of physical education), yet the life expectancy of the youth of today is predicted to be lower than their parents due to the largest increases in obesity occurring during childhood (Olshansky et al., 2005).

It has been widely published that young people who participate in physical activity will accrue health benefits including improved coronary heart disease risk profile, improved mental health, and reduced risk of osteoporosis, and it has also been stated that young people may have improved academic performance (Strong et al., 2005). However, the evidence base for the benefits of physical activity in young people is inconclusive (Patrick et al., 2004; Twisk, 2001). The findings of the seminal Amsterdam Growth Study conducted over a period of 15 years concluded that activity levels after the adolescent period is "of utmost importance" to physical fitness (Kemper and van Mechelen, 1995: 186). More recently, the work of Guerra et al. (2006) found that between the ages of 8-15 years, boys classified as less active were more likely to be obese than those classified as more active whilst no such association was found amongst girls of the same age. Indeed, research has made conflicting findings namely that obesity in girls is linked to low levels of physical activity but no relationship was found amongst boys (Mota et al., 2002). Therefore, the nature of any associations between physical activity and health in youth is complex.

Patterns of health-related behaviours are often acquired and established during childhood and adolescence (Kelder et al., 1994) and research conducted by Janz et al. (2002) proposed that sedentary activity and vigorous activity are moderately stable variables that track from late childhood into middle adolescence even though this is a period of substantial psychological and biological development. However, the current evidence base to support the tracking of physical activity throughout the life course is limited as relatively few longitudinal studies have been conducted in the area due to the methodological demands of such study designs (Ben-Shlomo and Kuh, 2002). That said, research has found that other health status variables do track into young adulthood with overweight children more likely to become overweight adults (Deshmukh-Taskar et al., 2006) and, among males, "an elevated BMI in childhood predicated the risk of hypertension in young adulthood" (Field et al., 2005: 163). Young people are at the same risk of sedentary lifestyles as adults either during their childhood or when they themselves become adults. Exposure to physically inactive pursuits such as watching television, and using personal computers and games consoles has the potential to occupy a large proportion of leisure time and research suggests that young people who watch more than four hours of television per day are 40% more likely to be classified as overweight (Eisenmann et al., 2002). Consequently, many children are failing to attain the activity level recommendations which are thought necessary to confer health benefits in later life due to sedentary activity. Current recommendations for young people's activity are internationally accepted to be one hour of moderate and vigorous intensity activity over the course of the day (NICE, 2009). Thus, there is a real need for beginning the prevention of these adult diseases during childhood and adolescence.

Flodmark and collagues. (2006) reported that the prevention of obesity among children and adolescents is possible through school-based programmes that combine physical activity and healthy diet promotion. In recognition of the complex nature of young people's physical activity levels, one intervention study considered a range of approaches to increasing activity including: daily physical education classes, short activity breaks during academic lessons, activities during school breaks and before and after school, physical activity homework, active transport to and from school, and initiatives to encourage families of the school children to become more active (Zahner et al., 2006). Thus, physical activity interventions in youth populations may need to go beyond the classroom, or indeed the school, to be effective. That said, schools are ideal settings in which to educate young people about the benefits of leading a physically active life due to the fact that schools provide access to virtually all children for 40-45 percent of their waking day (Fox and Harris, 2003).

Chapter III - Cardiovascular disease is one of the leading causes of death worldwide (Institute of Medicine, 2010). Yet more important is the number of individuals affected by the progressive characteristics of the disease. Dai, Bancej, Bienek, Walsh, Stewart, and Wielgosz (2009) reported that about four percent of the total population of Canada is living with heart disease and one out of every three adult deaths in Canada can be attributed to some form of cardiovascular disease. Conditions such as obesity, hypertension, and diabetes, are known contributing factors to cardiovascular disease, and as such increase the prevalence of cardiovascular disease, globally.

The impact of cardiovascular disease on death rate and loss of quality of life years remaining is so profound that Donatelle (2009) suggested if all forms of cardiovascular disease were eliminated, the life expectancy in the United States could increase by seven years. In 2008 it was estimated that the economic burden of cardiovascular disease in the United States was more than 448.5 billion dollars (Rosamond et al., 2008). This estimated cost is attributed to several factors, such as, the cost of physician and nursing services, in-hospital care charges, as well as nursing home services, medications and various home health care needs. In addition to the direct medical costs of cardiovascular disease related illnesses, the financial burdens within a society are also impacted by the loss of productivity due to illness, absenteeism-replacement workers, health insurance increases, family hardship, and decreased quality of life years remaining.

One condition that reduces cardiovascular health is atherosclerosis. Atherosclerosis involves the thickening of the walls of the arteries and loss of elasticity as a result of atheroma plaque accumulation. Over time, a reduction in blood flow could result in a myocardial infarction, also known as a heart attack. In addition to the build-up of plaque, the potential accumulation of blood can result in the artery becoming weak and rupturing. There is an increased recognition that the atherosclerotic process can start in children as early as six months of age (Harrell, McMurray, Gansky, Bangdiwala, and Bradley, 1999).

A direct effect of atherosclerotic plaque development is the reduction of oxygenated blood supply to the myocardium. The resulting ischemic condition may cause a variety of degrees of chest pain also known as angina pectoris. Congestive heart failure occurs when the heart muscle is overworked or damaged and does not have the capacity to continue to circulate blood normally throughout the body. If the heart is weakened there will be a reduction in the driving pressure required to push blood throughout the arterial system. A decrease in arterial driving pressure will eventually reduce the pressure that moves the blood returning through the veins, and thereby lead to congestion in the body tissues. As a result, the heart muscle can hypertrophy, or become larger, and therefore decrease its efficiency. The decreased efficiency of the myocardium can limit blood flow throughout the body, and as a result, blood can accumulate in the lower extremities or the lungs (Kavey, Daniels, Lauer, Atkins, Hayman, and Taubert, 2003).

It is crucial that children be introduced to the controllable risk factors for cardiovascular disease and the potential health implications of poor heart health behaviours, at an early age. For example, congestive heart failure is a result of previous harm done to the heart muscle, yet the condition can be avoided if care is taken at a young age. Since children who are overweight often carry the risk factors of cardiovascular disease into adulthood, an increased number of adults are at risk of dying from cardiovascular disease or incurring co-morbidities such as adult onset diabetes, hypertension or chronic obstructive pulmonary disease (Veugelers and Fitzgerald, 2005; Sin, Anthonisen, Soriano, and Agusti, 2006, Fuster and Kelly, 2010).

Cardiovascular disease risk factors can be categorized into factors that can be controlled and factors that cannot be controlled. Among the factors that we cannot control are: heredity, age, sex and race. The factors that can be controlled include tobacco avoidance (smoking), frequency, intensity and duration of quality daily physical activity, stress, and the dietary consumption of saturated fats and cholesterol. These factors are controlled by behaviour choices that if attended to in the pre-pubescent years can change the risk for cardiovascular disease as well as many other health related problems.

The health consequences of a poor lifestyle, leading to progressive cardiovascular disease, are a heavy burden to the health care system and as such primary prevention through health education and illness awareness for primary school aged children is critical (Kavey, et al., 2003). Children may have the ability to improve their health status by consciously maintaining a healthy diet while adopting a lifestyle that includes daily physical activity and avoiding exposure to tobacco products (Donatelle, 2009).

Cardiovascular disease risk factors can be reduced through a variety of intervention strategies. School health interventions that focus on cardiovascular health provide a great opportunity to enhance the future health and well-being of children because they involve children during critical periods of growth and maturation (Veugelers and Fitzgerald, 2005).

The objective of this chapter is to discuss research that has examined the effectiveness of cardiovascular health intervention programs that have incorporated knowledge from the study of physical education and exercise science, and have been delivered in the primary school classroom. A second objective is to describe strategies for success in overcoming challenges to changing health behaviours.

Chapter IV - The often cited phrase 'breakfast is the most important meal of the day' may have been largely anecdotal and lacking empirical evidence originally, particularly where children and adolescents (young people) are concerned. However, this chapter will provide a critical overview of the literature that supports carers of young people who have gone great lengths to convince their charges of the virtues of breakfast; thus, demonstrating this practice has more substance than mere anecdote. The chapter is divided into two distinct halves; the first focusing on the link between breakfast consumption and young people's physical health – with a specific emphasis on breakfast composition, ready to eat cereals and breakfast glycaemic index (GI). The second half reviews how this first meal of the day might be a very important factor when examining cognitive function in young people – the focus is on the effects of breakfast consumption and composition on various components of cognitive function. Many of the studies in this section use chronological age to define maturation; whilst we recognise that this does not provide a valid indication of maturation, we have used the authors' definitions of children and adolescents if they failed to provide a recognised measure of maturation (e.g., secondary sexual characteristics, wrist-hand x-ray, peak height velocity). Sometimes we refer to adult-based studies when they provide the necessary foundation for other research that includes children and/or adolescents or to highlight areas that are particularly lacking in empirical findings from young people. Most of the terminology in the chapter should be familiar to the reader and should not require any specialised knowledge of the 'breakfast literature'; however, for clarity – breakfast skipping is defined as a habitual choice in free-living conditions (e.g., a child who chooses, for whatever reason, not to eat breakfast). In contrast, breakfast omission refers to an experimental manipulation that a study participant has consented to comply with when asked (e.g., it could include an adolescent who normally eats breakfast on a regular basis, but has completed some measurements after an overnight fast as part of an experimental study). Although the chapter cannot be considered an exhaustive, systematic review of the literature, we have made every effort to avoid any obvious bias in our presentation of the evidence and hope that it provides a platform for future research with young people in the specific areas that are critically reviewed below. Finally, despite numerous benefits relating to health and cognitive function, breakfast consumption has declined in young people and also declines from childhood to adolescents (Rampersaud, Pereira, Girard, Adams, and Metzl, 2005). Consequently, strategies to promote the regular consumption of a healthy breakfast in young people are warranted.

Chapter V - Physical activity when taken regularly is a health enhancing behaviour and reduces the risk for many chronic diseases. In children, future health benefits are also obtained by engaging in physical activity, such as a strong heart, healthy joints, strong bones and good mental health. Despite this, many children are not reaching their recommended levels of physical activity and overweight and obesity levels are increasing in children (Ferreira et al, 2006). Physical activity is the most important recommendation for a healthy lifestyle throughout the lifespan and if children are taught healthy habits in their early years may positively influence their health in adulthood (Strong et al, 2005). As the physical activity behaviours learnt in childhood is likely to continue into adulthood (Kjonniksen et al, 2008), it is important to address the deficit of physical activity to improve current and future health benefits (Craig and Mindell, 2008).

As levels of overweight have risen and physical activity declined worldwide, investigators have attempted to find the reasons for the increase in obesity in children and adolescents, and also the decrease in physical activity (van Sluijs et al, 2008; Giles-Corti,

2009; Schofield et al, 2009, Jones et al, 2010). They have found no single theory that explains all of the factors that contribute with genetic factors, socio-cultural variables and environmental factors all thought to contribute. As a change to the gene pool is unlikely to have taken place across the time span in which overweight and obesity has risen, it is likely that socio-cultural and environmental variables play a key part in level of overweight and obesity in children (Giles-Corti, 2009; Schofield et al, 2009, Jones et al, 2010). As a result, research is now needed to understand the interaction between environmental factors and physical activity and obesity in children and young people (Booth et al, 2005). The purpose of this review is to provide an overview of current research assessing the environmental correlates of physical activity in children and adolescents (Booth et al, 2005).

Chapter VI - Along the years, bodily beauty ideals have undergone some changes, given the concern with physical appearance increasingly evident in contemporary society, which leads people to worry excessively about it.

Body image perception can be defined as the individual's accuracy of judging his own body size, shape and weight in relation to its proportion, while body image dissatisfaction is defined as the negative assessment of one's own body, being usually diagnosed through patterns of body silhouettes and questionnaires, which focus concerns about weight, shape and body fat (Smolak, 2001).

In recent years, thinness has been promoted as a standard of female beauty and images shown by the media, considered ideal, have become progressively thinner. Body shape changes end up by leading to significant increased body image dissatisfaction among women.

Thus, the proportion of people who are dissatisfied with their physical appearance has increased in recent decades, with smaller proportions in western countries.

In relation to nutritional status, although subjects with normal body weight can be dissatisfied with their body image, overweight students are the most susceptible. In recent years, the obesity prevalence increased significantly in developed and developing countries, which worsens the body image dissatisfaction among children and adolescents.

In this sense, body image dissatisfaction has aroused great interest among researchers, mainly due to the close relationship between this and eating disorders (anorexia and bulimia). Adolescent girls dissatisfied with their body image often adopt abnormal eating behaviors and inadequate weight control practices, such as the use of diuretics, laxatives, self-induced vomiting, and exhausting physical activity. Thus, body image dissatisfaction in adolescence has been identified as the most important risk factor for developing eating disorders such as anorexia and bulimia (Alves, Vasconcelos, Calvo, and Neves, 2008).

Eating disorders (anorexia nervosa and bulimia nervosa) are characterized by a morbid fear of gaining weight, obsessive concern with food, persistent desire for becoming thin and body image distortion, causing biological and psychological damage and increased morbidity and mortality.

Thus, this chapter aims to present the topic body image perception and its relationship with nutritional status and eating disorders in childhood and adolescence.

Chapter VII - Evidence to support the positive health benefits of physical activity abounds. Research demonstrates a dose-response relationship, in that as physical activity levels increase so do the associated health gains (Janssen, and LeBlanc, 2010). Physical inactivity on the other hand increases a person's risk of suffering non-communicable diseases, such as cardiovascular disease, diabetes and cancer (World Health Organisation 2010). In view of these risks, children's physical activity levels give reason for concern, as only 32% of boys and 24% of girls in England were reported to have achieved recommended guidelines in 2008 (The NHS Information Centre, 2010). Unfortunately given the self-reported nature of this data, young people's inactivity levels may be somewhat higher than testified (Basterfield, *et al.,* 2008).

To date, the main objectives driving Government plans to increase physical activity levels, appear to have been focused around reducing individual health costs of inactivity and the economic burden to society and the National Health Service (Department of Health, 2009). It seems that academic gains are a less prominent motivating factor behind the promotion of physical activity, yet studies indicate that exercise can enhance the health of the brain and facilitate learning (Cotman, Berchtold, and Christie, 2007). The effects of physical activity on school children's academic performance however, remain unclear, due to studies drawing mixed results (Taras, 2005).

Educational attainment is the strongest predictor of adult life outcomes/chances (National Literacy Trust, NLT, 2005). For instance, individuals with low literacy skills are more likely to experience social exclusion, be unemployed by the time they reach 30 years of age (NLT, 2010) or find themselves turning to youth offending (Audit Commission, 2004). Data from longitudinal studies, such as the National Child Development Study (Centre for Longitudinal Studies, CLS, 2008), depict how education can mould young people's direction in life. For instance poor educational attainment has been found to be the strongest risk factor associated with young pregnancy; as well as playing a key role in disadvantage, low wages, and unemployment (CLS, 2008). Such data underscores the importance of promoting good literacy skills. Statistics show that one in six people in the UK experience poor literacy (NLT, 2010), and one in three children, aged between 6 and 16 years, are identified with special educational needs (SEN) (Department for Children, Schools, and Families, DCSF, 2010). The prospect of a child with SEN and reaching national expectations, five A-C grades at GCSE level (General Certificate of Secondary Education in the UK), is low if they come from a low income family (DCSF, 2010). Only 7.5% of children dealing with the combined challenge of SEN and disadvantage, managed to achieve national expectations in 2009 (DCSF, 2010).

A review conducted by the Office for Standards in Education, Children's Services and Skills (Ofsted, 2010), into the best teaching practices in England, found that systematic phonic teaching lay behind the success of 12 outstanding schools boasting high standards of reading. However, the view of effective reading tuition did not reference the contribution that physical activity may have upon a child's academic or literacy attainment. School administrators and parents may harbour fears that increased time allotted to physical activity may reduce more valuable time that could be spent in the classroom improving performance in core subject areas. This issue has been acknowledged by a number of studies, which have found that despite a failure to always observe significant academic improvement as a result of physical activity, academic performance was not compromised (Ahamed, *et al* 2007, Carlson *et al* 2008, and Trudeau, and Shephard, 2008).

Berg (2010) presents a review of empirical findings in an attempt to raise the profile of physical education (PE) in schools. His review includes a number of studies to support anatomical and physiological changes in the brain following bouts of exercise. For instance, animal studies have shown that the production of brain-derived neurotrophic factor (BDNF) increases in the hippocampus, as a result of several days of running. BDNF is a neurotrophic factor or protein, proposed to enhance the survival and growth of neurons in the brain, whilst the hippocampus plays a part in spatial memory (Kolb, and Whishaw 2011) and learning

(Vayman, Ying, and Gomez-Pinilla, 2003). Berg (2010) is encouraged by animal studies which have found a link between increased BDNF in rats and their ability to solve mazes quicker, as such findings may benefit cognitive functioning and learning in humans. An investigation into the link between exercise-induced cognitive enhancement and BDNF action, discovered that by blocking BDNF in rats, former exercise-induced improvements in learning was eliminated (Vayman, Ying, and Gomez-Pinilla, 2004). Although a number studies have demonstrated that synaptic-plasticity changes in the brain are enhanced by exercise, and that BDNF is utilised in exercise to improve learning acquisition and memory retention (Berg, 2010, Vayman, Ying, and Gomez-Pinilla, 2004, and Vayman, Ying, and Gomez-Pinilla, 2003), further research is needed to clarify the type, frequency and amount of exercise needed in order for significant benefits to be experienced (Cotman, Berchtold, and Christie, 2007). In addition, a call has been made for animal studies to increase their relevance to humans, since human studies tend to analyse the completion of tasks co-ordinated by the forebrain, whilst animal studies usually assess hippocampus-dependent learning (Cotman, Berchtold, and Christie, 2007).

Chapter VIII - Declines in Physical activity (PA) and increasing obesity levels in children have encouraged increasing interest in understanding children's PA behaviour. Currently in the United Kingdom (UK), an estimated 1 in 3 children in the age range of 4-11 are overweight (NCMP, 2010). Existing research in this field has related these statistics with the lack of PA children engage in (Gorely *et al.*, 2004; Mackett and Paskins, 2008) and the rise in sedentary behaviours such as video gaming or sustained periods watching television (Salmon *et al.* 2005).

PA tracking has identified a substantial decrease from childhood to adolescence (Malina *et al..* 1990; Telama *et al..* 1996). This is primarily related to movement skill refinement and the ability to move efficiently and perform these skills competently (Okely, Chey and Booth. 2001; Timmons *et al.*, 2007). Movement skills track at low-moderate levels during childhood, so greater motor proficiency may be predictive of later PA (Pate and Kann, 2002).

The mastery of fundamental movement skills (FMS) is a potential correlate of the involvement of children's PA participation (Welk, 1999). These movement skills form the prerequisites for sport competence and other forms of PA (Gallahue and Ozmun, 2002; Barnett et al., 2009), therefore acquiring these skills during early childhood may increase the likelihood for longer term PA. Young children who are equipped with movement skills are more likely to be successful in PA and will be able to seek greater opportunities to be physically active (Sallis *et al.*, 2002; Fisher *et al.*, 2005). Conversely, children without these skills lack the confidence in their ability and may therefore be more likely to drop out of sport, games and physical activity in the future (Gallahue and Ozmun, 2002).

With this in mind, the development of FMS in children could be important for PA promotion and the enhancement of public health. However, despite suggestions that the development of FMS in children leads to increased PA (Gallahue and Ozmun, 2002), few studies have actually examined the relationship between these two variables in primary and pre-school children since the majority of research has focussed on using older children and adolescents (McKenzie *et al.*, 2002; Wrotniak *et al.*, 2006). Such a focus on older children and adolescents arguably has little effect in improving PA habits as it may be too late for those children who have not yet already gained prerequisite mastery in the FMS to do so for wider activity benefit. Furthermore, during early childhood, the developing neuromuscular systems are at optimal readiness to learn these basic movement skills (Gallahue and Ozmun,

2003; Lubans el al., 2010). Prior research has also relied heavily on using subjective measures and non validated instruments such as self report measures (Fisher et al. 2005) to assess PA and its relationship with FMS (Duncan *et al.*, 2007), therefore future research may benefit from using objective measures of PA (Morgan *et al.* 2008). This short review will focus on the previous literature examining FMS and PA and various correlates of the two such as age, gender and weight status.

Chapter IX - Patterns of cardiovascular and metabolic disease vary in ethnic groups. British South Asian adults have an increased risk of type 2 diabetes mellitus which is associated with increased cardiovascular disease (CVD) death rates (Mckeigue, Shah and Marmot, 1991; Balarajan, 1996; Bhopal, Unwin, White, Yallop, Walker, and Alberti , 1999). People from Afro Caribbean descent experience lower CVD mortality rates but are at higher risk of type 2 diabetes mellitus and hypertension compared to White Europeans (Cruickshank, Cooper, Burnett, Macduff and Drubra, 1991; Chaturvedi, Mckeigue and Marmot, 1994; Cappucio, Cook, Atkinson and Strazullo, 1997; Lane, Beevers and Hip, 2002; Thom et al, 2006).

Growing evidence suggests that early markers of metabolic disease risk emerge in childhood which is strongly related to ethnicity and obesity (Berenson, Srinivasan, Bao, Newman, Tracy and Wattigney 1998; Ehtisthan, Barrett, and Shaw, 2000; Whincup , Gilg, Owen, Odoki, Alberti and Cook, 2002; Whincup, Owen, Orfei, McKay and Cook, 2007). Higher levels of fasting insulin are evident in South Asian and Black children compared to white children (Whincup et al, 2010). Insulin levels have been found to track well into adulthood and are positively related to measures of obesity, systolic and diastolic blood pressure, triglyceride and cholesterol levels. Children from ethnic minorities have also been found to have differences in body composition which have been demonstrated in the neonatal period suggesting that some of this risk is likely to be inherited rather than related to lifestyle (Yajnik et al, 2002).

Physical inactivity is identified as the fourth leading modifiable risk factor for global mortality (WHO, 2010). The metabolic benefits of physical activity are well described both in adults and children (Powell, Thompson, Caspersen, and Kendrick, 1987; Strazzullo et al, 1988; Berlin and Coldwitz, 1990; Brage et al, 2004). Studies have shown low levels of objectively measured activity in childhood to be associated with increased adiposity and insulin resistance (Ekelund et al, 2004; Ekelund, Neovius, Linné, Brage, Wareham and Rössner, 2005; Sardinha et al 2008; Wittmeir, Mollard, and Kriellaars, 2008; Riddoch et al, 2007). However, little is known about differences in physical activity patterns between ethnic groups and the possible contribution to CVD risk.

The aim of this review is to examine the objective evidence of patterns of physical activity in children from differing ethnic backgrounds.

Chapter X - Heart Rate Variability (HRV) is defined as an index of tonic autonomic activity (Blom et al., 2009) which in layman's terms is the fluctuations between consecutive heart beats. These fluctuations represent the changing levels of the activity of sympathetic and parasympathetic nerves, known collectively as the autonomic nerves, and modulate the intrinsic sinus node firing rate (Yutaka et al., 1989). The normal rhythm of the heart is controlled by the membrane processes of the sinoatrial node (SA node) which are controlled by the divisions of the sympathetic and parasympathetic nerves of the autonomic system (ANS) (Berntson et al., 1997). At rest the parasympathetic nerve systems dominates the heart rate (Goldberger et al., 2001). HRV is a non-invasive tool that measures the autonomic control of the heart (Leicht, Sinclair, and Spinks 2008), and has considerable potential to assess the role of autonomic system fluctuations in normal individuals and in patients with cardiovascular disorders (Task Force, 1996).

Reduced beat-to-beat variability is a predictor of mortality and arrhythmic complications and is found in individuals with a variety of cardiac abnormalities (Bigger et al., 2007). The risk of mortality has been proposed to be significantly greater in individuals with HRV less than 50ms (Kleiger et al., 1987; Martin et al., 1987). A reduced HRV positively correlates with obesity (Nagai et al., 2004), poor aerobic fitness (Aubert et al., 2001), low habitual physical activity (Blom et al., 2009), and increasing age (Silvetti et al., 2001), as well as racial differences (Reed et al 2006). However, although the literature on HRV contains is considerable, it has predominantly focused on the adult population while little research exists for children.

HRV measures are split into two categories; time domain indices, and frequency domain indices. There are two main groups of time domain variable measures (Stein and Kleiger, 1999). The first of which include; mean R-R intervals (the differences between successive R-R intervals) and SDRR (average standard deviation of all R-R intervals), which are known to reflect the circadian rhythms and therefore total variability (Stein and Kleiger, 1999). The second group includes pNN50 (the percentage of adjacent cycles that are >50 ms apart) and RMSSD (the root mean square of successive differences) which have been found to reflect vagal modulation of the SA node and correlate strongly with the high frequency (HF) power band (Pagani et al., 1986).

The frequency domain indices represent power density of HRV and provide information on the distribution of power as a frequency band; formed of both the high frequency band and the low frequency band. The HF (above 15Hz) frequency reflects respiratory mediated HRV, while LF (0.04 to 0.15Hz) is modulated by both the sympathetic and parasympathetic nervous systems (Stein and Kleiger, 1999). In addition to HF and LF, frequency domain measures also include very low frequency (VLF) and ultra-low frequency (ULF), although the underlying physiological mechanisms involved are less distinguished than HF and LF (Task Force, 1996).

Chapter XI - The ability to undertake prolonged exercise in the heat has long been of interest to physiologists. Of the many limiting factors to exercise performance, body temperature responses in both cool and hot conditions in particular have been the subject of considerable interest. Research in this area has examined the underlying concepts of heat balance within the body with wide ranging applications from marathon running (Pugh et al., 1967) and other athletic performances (Marsh and Sleivert, 1999; Myler et al., 1989) to the effects of protective clothing on vocational and military operations (Giesbrecht et al., 2007, Cheung and McLellan, 1998; House et al., 1997). More recent research has focussed upon methods to improve the ability to work in the heat such as cooling techniques (Marino, 2000), cool fluid (Lee et al., 2007) and 'slushie' ingestion (Ross et al., 2010) and populations with thermal dysfunction (Price, 2006).

Of the populations traditionally considered to be at risk of increased heat injury, research examining thermoregulation in children has received considerable interest (Falk and Dotan, 2011; Naughton and Carlson, 2008; Rowland 2008). Previous research studies have generally reported differences in thermoregulatory responses between children and adults as a result of the greater body surface area (BSA) to body mass ratio in children when compared to adults, maturational difference in exercise economy and lower sweat rates in children when compared to adults, with children thus relying more on dry heat exchange for heat dissipation (Falk and Dotan, 2011; Rowland, 2008; Shibasaki et al., 1997). These differences also imply that children absorb more heat from the environment as well as demonstrating a reduced heat loss potential which may compromise heat tolerance while exercising in thermally stressful environments (Rivera-Brown et al., 2006).

In a recent review Rowland (2008) revisited the area of thermoregulation in children during exercise in the heat. It was noted that previous literature had not used appropriate child-adult comparisons, failed to match subjects by relative exercise intensity or had involved extremes of ambient temperature. With such factors in mind it was concluded that the current literature failed to indicate differences in thermoregulatory responses between adults and children. Furthermore, it was noted that there was no convincing evidence that children were at any greater risk than adults of exercising in the heat, a view that was similarly taken by Naughton and Carlson (2008). The current review will consider the comments of Rowland (2008) in considering thermoregulatory responses from an absolute and relative exercise intensity perspective as well as considering heat injury and prevention in the paediatric population, exercise performance in the heat and thermal factors at exhaustion in children, thermoregulatory aspects of specific clinical subgroups within the paediatric population and future research directions. Where possible, existing data from studies of adult thermoregulation will be briefly reviewed in order to provide context from which the associated responses from the paediatric literature can be compared.

Chapter XII - Sporting injuries occur among children and adolescents just as among adults, but there are important differences in the rate of incidence, the nature of the injuries, and the recovery afterwards. This chapter will examine the evidence as it currently stands in relation to the incidence of different types of sporting injuries in young people, noting the lack of authoritative evidence for the UK. It will divide injuries into the acute and traumatic on the one hand – contusions, bruises, sprains, lacerations and fractures – and the overuse injuries on the other. Traumatic acute injuries have a definite onset and occur after large tensile, load or impact forces cause tissue failure or breakdown. In contrast, overuse injuries result from repetitive low loading, and often have no specific onset. Skeletally immature athletes are different from their adult counterparts mainly because of the different physiology and biomechanics in immature bone. These differences mean different points of weakness compared to those in the adult musculoskeletal system. Common overuse injuries in children include osteochondroses such as Osgood-Schlatter's syndrome, anterior knee problems, and bony problems such as fractures of the lumbar spine or spondylolisthesis. Although the literature is sparse, the chapter will review any evidence on the effectiveness of rehabilitation and prevention strategies in relation to these injuries. Some short case studies will illustrate how young athletes often react to injury and present to coaches, parents, and medical and sports injury professionals. The chapter will conclude with some points regarding assessment, and the roles of coaches and parents in detecting and preventing injuries, noting that it is necessary to take measures to confirm the presence or absence of less common pathologies that would need further investigation. Any pain in a young athlete that lasts more than a few weeks requires detailed assessment, investigation and analysis.

For the purposes of research and surveillance studies it is easiest to define young people in terms of age (for example under 18, or under 16), but it is more appropriate to define young people in terms of their physiological development. Adolescents before puberty have characteristic physiology that differs from that of adults, whereas under-18s who have completed puberty tend to incur injuries similar to those of adult sportsmen and women (Hawkins, and Metheny, 2001). Children may be defined as under-10s, but again it might be better to define them in terms of their development, as in the state of their bony growth, and epiphyseal distinction. For example, in this field of paediatric injuries Haywood and Boyce (1996) define children as 'all individuals prior to the age of skeletal maturity', although this could include some males up to the age of 25!

Chapter XIII - It is established that children and adolescents, defined here as individuals up to the age of 18 years (Faigenbaum et al., 2009), often perform activity in bursts of high intensity exercise interspersed with rest (Ratel, Bedu, Hennegrave, Doré, and Duché, 2004). Such intermittent activity is also characteristic of many sports (Glaister, 2005) and is likely to be crucial to competitive success in racket sports, court sports and field sports (Doré et al., 2005). Additionally, underlying components of high-intensity exercise performance such as strength, speed and stretch-shortening cycle characteristics are developed in childhood and become crucial determinants of exercise capacities in adulthood. The development of plyometric ability, sprint speed and strength tends to occur naturally as infants develop into adults but these aspects of physical performance are also increased by physical training. The purpose of this chapter is to discuss the development of aspects of explosiveness in children and adolescents (i.e., youths). The development of strength in this way has been reviewed elsewhere (Faigenbaum et al., 2009) so the focus here is to review the effects of maturation, development and training on sprinting and plyometric ability in youths.

Chapter XIV - The football playing adolescents of today are our stars of tomorrow. Adolescence is a transitional phase of physical and mental development, generally occurring between puberty and adulthood, often characterised as beginning and ending with the teenage stage (ages 13-19; Kent, 1998). During this time physical, physiological and psychological features, essential for success in soccer, alter with growth and evolve at varying rates (Williams and Reilly, 2000).

List of Contributors

Gareth Stratton
Lorayne A. Woodfield
Moira N. McPherson
Kimberly Boardman
William J. Montelpare
Carlos E. Zerpa
Keith Tolfrey
Julia K. Zakrzewski
Simon B. Cooper
Mary E. Nevill
Stacey Hargreaves
Michael J. Duncan
Samantha Birch
Edio Luiz Petroski
Andreia Pelegrini
Diego Augusto Santos Silva
Esther Curley
Michael J. Duncan
Samantha Birch
Luke C. Baker
Samantha Birch
Michael J. Duncan
Emma Lisa Jane Eyre
Krystyna Anna Matyka
Craig Franklin
Samantha Birch
Michael J. Duncan
Michael J. Price
Sheila Leddington Wright
Andrew King
Michael G Hughes
Rhodri Lloyd
Robert Meyers

Matt Rains
Mark Noon
Doug Thake

In: Reviews in Pediatric Exercise Science
Editor: Michael Duncan, pp. 1-12
ISBN: 978-1-61470-978-7

Chapter I

Physical Activity, Play and the Pre-School Years

***Mareesa O'Dwyer*[1], *Zoe Knowles*[1], *Nicola Ridgers*[2] *and Gareth Stratton*[1]**
[1] Liverpool John Moores University, UK.
[2] Deakin University, Australia.

Introduction

Importance of Physical Activity during Pre-School Years

It is well documented that regular physical activity among young children may contribute to social development (Sawyers 1994), psychological welfare (Ekelund et al. 2004), improvements in fundamental motor skill development (Cliff et al. 2009), maintenance of bone health (Janz et al. 2010), prevention of cardiovascular disease (Anderssen et al. 2007) and protection against excess weight gain (Abbott et al. 2004). Despite this evidence base, pre-school aged children are not accumulating enough physical activity to accrue health benefits of being active (Reilly 2010; Tucker 2008; Oliver et al. 2007). For the purpose of this chapter pre-school children in the United Kingdom (UK) are defined as those attending 15 hours of 'voucher' funded pre-school education (playgroups, day-care or school based nursery) or in the first compulsory school year in which they turn 5 years old.

From 1989 to 1998, there was a highly significant increase in weight and body mass index for boys and girls from the age of infancy to pre-school (Bundred et al. 2001). This problem still remains with overweight prevalence among pre-school children ranging from 12-32% in Western European countries (Cattaneo et al. 2010). Physical activity is an important behavior for pre-school children as it sets a foundation for facilitating and maintaining a healthy and active life through to adulthood (Cragg et al. 2006; Campbell et al. 2001). Unfortunately, limited data exist on the physical activity levels of pre-school children but a recent study in Australia reported that 44% and 21% of Australian pre-school aged children are not meeting the recommended daily physical activity guidelines on weekdays and weekend days, respectively (Okely et al. 2009). A similar issue is apparent in the UK, with only 40% of pre-school children achieving the recommended daily guidelines for MVPA during weekdays and weekend days (O'Dwyer et al. 2011). One of the reasons for these worryingly low levels of activity may be explained by the perceptions held by teachers and parents. These significant others assume that pre-school children are very active and spend most of their time continually running around thus believing that they engage in sufficient amounts activity (Sallis et al. 1988). However, research has suggested that prolonged screen time, fewer siblings to play with and safety concerns among parents regarding play spaces have resulted in increased sedentary behavior (Burdette et al. 2005).

The aim of this chapter is to inform the reader about the different types of play that exist among pre-school children as well as describe importance of play, specifically active play. The reader will be introduced to the recommendations for physical activity for this population. Lastly, this chapter aims to provide a summary of interventions aimed at increasing physical activity which have been conducted in pre-school settings.

Guidelines for Physical Activity

Up until July 2011 there were no specific physical activity guidelines for children under 5 years of age. Previously guidelines recommended that children and young people should accumulate at least 60 minutes of at least moderate intensity physical activity each day. At least twice a week this should include activities to improve bone health, muscle strength and flexibility (Department of Health 2004). Newly released recommendations from the Chief Medical Officers report (Department of Health 2011) state that infants who are not yet walking should be encouraged from birth to be physically active, particularly through floor-based play in safe environments. Children of pre-school age who are capable of walking unaided should be physically active daily for at least 3 hours. This type of activity should involve translocation of the trunk (movement of the trunk from one place to another). Children in their early years (from birth to school age) should also be discouraged from being sedentary. More specifically, no sedentary behavior should last for more than one hour at a time, except when the child is sleeping. This includes time restrained within a high chair, small playpen, car, pram or buggy, watching TV or other screen time, or any other sedentary behavior that limits opportunities to engage in physical activity.

The low levels of physical activity within the pre-school population are a public health concern and reinforce the necessity for interventions to be developed and implemented. One suitable setting for the delivery of interventions aiming to increase physical activity among this age group is the pre-school setting (Dowda et al. 2009). Childcare facilities have been identified as the strongest determinant of physical activity and accounted for nearly 50% of the variation in activity during the pre-school attending hours (Finn et al. 2002). It has been reported that in most countries in Western Europe, over 90% of pre-school children attend some form of childcare provision now, compared with less than 20% in the mid 1990's (Reilly et al. 2006). There are several reasons why these settings are appropriate. Firstly, services such as SureStart children's centre's in the UK and Head Start Programmes in the US provide comprehensive education, health, nutrition, and parent involvement services to a large number of children and their families for a substantial time of the day (Ward et al. 2010). Secondly, childcare facilities have an existing infrastructure (e.g. staff, equipment and space) which lends itself as a suitable environment for promoting physical activity (Story et al. 2006). Thirdly, staff in childcare settings have shown to be willing to assist in programmes which aim to increase children's activity levels (Cashmore et al. 2008). Lastly, theoretical models such as Bronfenbrenner's Ecological Model (1989) have proposed that childcare setting and the professionals working within them are important in terms of influencing lifestyle patterns and behaviors. This ecological model proposes that the classroom and teachers belong in the micro system [see figure 1]. It is in the micro system that the most direct interactions with social agents take place e.g. with parents, peers, and teachers, thus reinforcing the importance and suitability of the childcare setting in the promotion of physical activity.

Where Do Pre-School Children Get their Physical Activity from?

Children accumulate their physical activity in a variety of ways including through school, sports clubs, use of active travel, informal play, after school clubs and via adult organized activity with most children obtaining their activity from more than one setting (Department of Health 2004). This is potentially beneficial for children as taking part in different types of activity provides different health and social benefits (Department of Health, 2004). For pre-school children, the context of physical activity is often more playful and unstructured and the type of physical activity tends to be different. Pellegrini et al. (1998) identify three types of play, all with different functions. These are rhythmic stereotypies, exercise play and rough-and-tumble. These types of play are very much determined by age. Pre-school aged children are reported to take part in more exercise play and rough-and-tumble with exercise play peaking during the pre-school years, accounting for up to 20% of observed school recess behavior (Pelligrini et al. 1998).

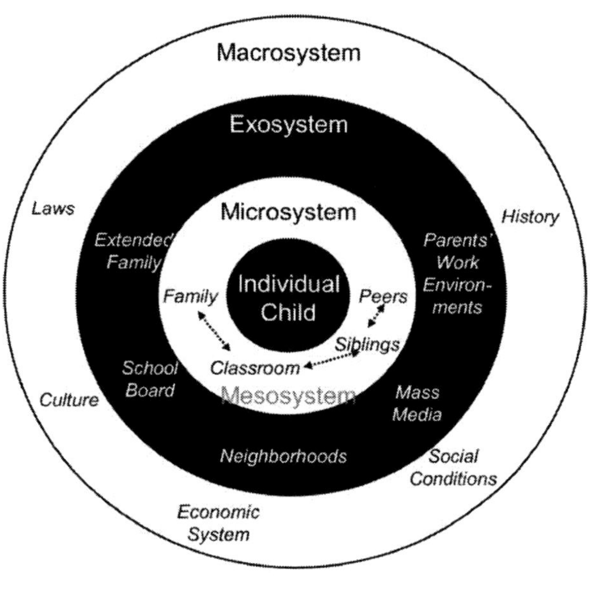

Figure 1. Ecological Model. Bronfenbrenner's Ecological Model describing the environmental influences on a child, with permission from Eisenmann et al. (2008) and Biomed Central (2008).

Play during late pre-school years (e.g. 5 years old) has been characterized by childhood development experts as being predominately rough-and-tumble in nature (Smith, 1982). This type of play refers to vigorous behavior such as wrestling, kicking, rolling around and tumbling. Often on the playground this can be mistaken for aggressive behavior yet it is its playful context that sets it apart from anti-social behaviors. Rough-and tumble-play is a male dominated area of physical activity (Pelligrini 1989). These gender differences are influenced by hormonal events centering around the effects of endogenous and exogenous androgens on neural organization and behavior (Meaney et al. 1985). Children's socialization interactions with their parents (Maccoby et al. 1986) have been shown to reinforce this gender difference, with fathers spending more time with their sons than their daughters (Parke et al. 1981) and this activity tending to be more vigorous (Carson et al. 1993). To date, the majority of physical activity research has focused on older children and is limited to sports clubs, adult organized activities during and after school and active travel (Veitch et al., 2007). This chapter aims to address a relatively neglected area of research in pre-school children and active play.

What is Play and why is It Important?

The word "*play*" is usually used to describe the activities of children from infancy until the early teenage years. It has been reported that observers often recognize play but struggle to put forward an all encompassing definition for the complicated phenomenon (Pellegrini et al., 1998). An abundance of child development literature exists in this area and it is accepted that not one operational definition is required or even sufficient (Martin et al., 1985) to explain the complexity of play. One of the most commonly agreed upon definitional criteria for play is that it does not appear to serve any purpose. More specifically, play has been defined as freely chosen, personally directed, and intrinsically motivated behaviour that actively engages the child (National Playing Fields Association, 2000). The global importance of play is noted in Article 31 of the United Nations Convention on the Rights of the Child (1989) which states "That every child has the right to rest and leisure, to engage in play and recreational activities appropriate to the age of the child and to participate freely in cultural life and the arts…".

The benefits of play are wide reaching and extend far beyond the health gains from physical activity (Brockman et al. 2011). Children who engage in play enjoy a range of benefits, including development of their imagination, increased dexterity and improved physical, emotional and cognitive strength (Ginsburg, 2007). More specifically, play is important for healthy brain development (Tamis-LeMonda et al. 2004), conquering fears (Pellegrini et al. 1998), enhancing confidence, encouraging group work, resolving issues and negotiating with each other (Erickson 1985). In contrast to passive games, unstructured free play has been suggested as a mechanism for building active healthy bodies through increased physical activity participation, which in turn is deemed important in the fight against childhood obesity (Burdette et al. 2005). Aside from the direct benefits play brings to the individual child, there are also benefits for the families of children and the communities they live in. The 2010 Playday Report (Gleave 2010) outlines how community play is important in fostering positive social relationships for adults and children, allowing children to explore their local environment and as well as constructing social and personal identities. Gleave

(2010) also reports that children who are given the freedom in their community and are perceived as valued members of that community are more likely to act positively and contribute towards their local neighbourhood. The economic benefit of play must not go unreported. A recent report compiled by Play England (2010) suggested that investing in staffed adventure playgrounds and after school clubs staffed with qualified play personnel generate positive net benefits and discontinuing such provision would result in more costs than are saved.

Different Types of Play

Play research dates back as far as 1932 when Parten classified play into six different categories. The first is *unoccupied play* where the child is relatively stationary and appears to be performing random movements with no apparent purpose. This is a relatively infrequent style of play. Second is *solitary play,* where the child is completely engrossed in playing and does not seem to notice other children. This type of play is most often seen in children between the ages of 2 and 3 years old. Third is *onlooker play,* where the child takes an interest in other children's play but does not join in. During this type of play the child may ask questions or just talk to other children, but the main activity is simply to watch. Fourth is *parallel play,* where the child mimics other children's play but does not actively engage with them. For example they may use the same toy side by side by not communicate with each other. Fifth is *associative play,* where the child is more interested in one another than the toys they are using. This is the first category of play that involves strong social interaction between the children while they play. Last is *cooperative play,* where some organisation enters children's play, and playing has some end goal and children often adopt roles and act as a group. Since Partens classification of play in 1932, there has been a vast amount of research specifically in the area of child development which attempts of define and categorize play. While these explanations vary hugely according to age and setting (Smith 1985) for the purpose of this chapter we will focus on 'active play' or 'physical activity play' (Pellegrini et al. 1998). Active play may involve symbolic activity or games with rules; this activity maybe part of a group or by oneself but the distinguishing features are a playful context, combined with activity that is significantly above resting metabolic rate (Simons-Morton et al. 1990). Due to the increased energy expenditure, this type of play is a more physically demanding and typically involves actions such as carrying, climbing, hide and seek and rough-and-tumble which helps develop and maintain muscular fitness and flexibility. Play is deemed important as it permits children to use their creativity while developing their imagination, dexterity, and physical, cognitive, and emotional strength (Tamis-LeMonda , Shannon, Cabrera et al. 2004). From infancy, children naturally use play to promote their own learning; they do not have to be persuaded into playing. A playful orientation appears to be part of childhood for the young of all mammals, of which human beings are a part.

Threats Facing Play

'At Least 5 a Week' (Department of Health 2004) outlines the many contemporary threats facing children's overall physical activity levels. They posit that there is now a greater use of cars transporting children which could easily be achieved via active travel. Parental reluctance to allow children to play outdoors may have increased through perceived dangers within the physical environment, such as heavy traffic and 'stranger danger'.

A study investigating play in the natural environment and children's perceptions, knowledge and experience of outdoor play (Ridgers et al. in 2012) identified a range of barriers suggested by the children in relation to the natural environment. The majority of barriers related to parents constraints that were closely linked to safety concerns such as fears of abduction, heavy road traffic and risk of injury. Other barriers included children not being allowed to play without an adult supervising and weather constraints. The Playday Report (Gleave 2010) emphasized the importance of children playing outside in their local neighbourhood and how this can foster positive social relationships for children and adults as well as give children the opportunity to explore their local environment. However, it is noted that over time there has been a breakdown in community cohesion, which has resulted in a decline in children's presence within the community as children feel unwelcome in public spaces due to either fears about their safety or concerns that they will cause trouble. Moreover, Davey (2008) suggests that fears about children's wellbeing and safety is a prominent factor contributing to the decline of children playing within their communities. Research conducted by Thomas and Thompson (2004) reported that streets were the most dangerous environment for children to play in. The majority of children felt that the only outdoor space they felt safe in was their own private garden. Parents of these children also felt the same. Another barrier to playing outside reported by Barnes (2007) related to children's access to public spaces. It was noted that although children had amenities such as parks and grassy areas nearby, their use of these spaces was limited. It was reported that these areas were poorly maintained or prone to anti-social behavior. Parents reported that their primary concern was smashed glass and drug paraphernalia. All of these issues present barriers which prevent children from being as active as they should be.

Interventions Aiming to Increase Physical Activity in the Pre-School Population

There is a growing body of evidence to illustrate the importance of play and play provision to children's mental and physical health (National Childrens Bureau 2009). Recently, this area of research has led to better play opportunities and changes in Government policy. A decade ago it was reported that there was a serious obesity problem among pre-school aged children and the main solution for this was to promote playtime and reduce screen time (Dietz 2001). Almost 10 years on, the situation remains the same with nearly a quarter (23.1%) of the reception children in the UK (age 4-5) classified as either overweight or obese (National Child Measurement Programme 2010). It's important to note that this state has not worsened suggesting that the investment in programmes and initiatives may have had a small but beneficial effect. Potentially serious health consequences exist which are associated with being overweight in childhood thus highlighting the need for population based interventions aimed at prevention rather than treatment (Reilly et al. 2003). Developing effective prevention and intervention programmes for the formative pre-school years is seen as an important step in combating the obesity problem (Wang et al. 2006). Despite the urgency to develop effective interventions aimed at pre-school children, a review by Van Sluijs et al. (2008) reported that interventions in this age group are rare.

A small scale literature search was conducted to source relevant evidence in PubMed, Google Scholar and Science Direct. The search period was from January 2005 – present day. The following search terms were used: pre-school, pre-school, early childhood, young children, physical activity, physical inactivity, sedentary behavior, active play, play, physical education and intervention. Each article was screened by reading the abstract and article where necessary. Reference lists from review articles (Hinkley et al. 2008; Olivier et al. 2007) were manually screened for relevant literature. Articles were only included if one of the aims of the study was to increase physical activity levels in pre-school children under the age of 6-years of age. Duplicate publications and studies published only in abstract were excluded. The literature search found 10 published articles (see Table 1) which included data on 3,293 children. Seven of the studies used accelerometry to measure PA, of these seven studies; two were protocol articles and did not include any results, three reported no changes in PA levels post-intervention and two reported positive changes in PA levels post-intervention. Two of the studies which used accelerometry also used direct observation to quantify PA levels. Pedometers and Actiheart monitors were used in two of the studies to measure PA; however both of these studies were protocol articles and consequently did not report any results. The one remaining article used self report; the results from this study suggest that structured physical activity increased post intervention.

It is clear that interventions in the pre-school population are receiving more attention from researchers, given the surge in publications in recent years. It is also likely that many studies are currently ongoing and have not yet been published in peer reviewed literature. However in comparison to older children, the evidence base still remains sparse. While the studies outlined in Table 1 varied in design, mode, and precise setting of intervention delivery, there were some common elements to their design. Many of the interventions employed a selection of intervention delivery types and the majority of this delivery was conducted within the school setting. While most of the studies employed the randomised control trial (RCT) design, the quality and reporting of some of the studies was not ideal. Many of the studies in this review showed no impact on PA levels, which is surprising given the low levels of PA among children attending pre-school (Tucker 2008) and the robust research design of many of the studies. There are a number of factors that may explain the lack of findings in these studies, including insufficient power to detect small but meaningful changes in PA, a notable observation among these studies was the lack of a parental component. It is suggested that during the formative pre-school years, parental involvement is extremely important in facilitating real and sustainable behavior change.

A limitation of some of the studies was the lack of reference to the theoretical framework which underpinned the intervention. Not reporting this withholds key information which may help other researchers when designing interventions aimed at increasing PA within this age group. Similarly, the cost effectiveness of the various interventions was not reported. This too may provide vital information about the economic feasibility of certain approaches to increasing PA.

The individual studies reviewed in Table 1 offer a mixed message about the effectiveness of interventions aimed at increasing levels of PA among the pre-school population.

Table 1. Interventions aimed at increasing physical activity in pre-school children. Table ordered by publication date (newest to oldest)

Study	Design; country	Participants; setting	Intervention	PA assessment	Results
O'Dwyer et al. (2011)	RCT United Kingdom	n=50 (4.5±0.6 years) Pre-school	Children: 6 weekly Active Play sessions during school time	Accelerometry	Protocol paper only – no results
De Bock et al. (2010)	RCT Germany	n=741 (pre-school) Pre-school	Children: state sponsored gym lessons Parents: focused intervention	Actiheart	Protocol paper only – no results
Finch et al. (2010)	RCT Australia	n=300 (3-5 years) Day care	Children: Daily FMS activities, increased movement based activities, increased verbal guidance during PA, less screen time, equipment provision. Staff: 6 hour training workshop	Pedometers	Protocol paper only – no results
Cardon et al. (2009)	RCT Belgium	n=583 (5.3±0.4 years) School playground	Children: playground markings and play equipment	Accelerometry	No significant change in PA
Williams et al. (2009)	Pilot observational study USA	n=270 (3-5 years) School classroom	Children: daily classroom activity (10 mins)	Self-report: teacher proxy	No direct measure of PA but structured PA increased by 47 min.
Harvey-Berino et al. (2009)	RCT USA	n=43 (22±8 months)	Parents: 16 week obesity prevention and parenting support programme	Accelerometry	No significant change in PA
Niederer et al. (2009)	RCT Switzerland	n=655 (4-6 years) School and gym	Staff: educational workshops Children: additional PA lessons (160 min per week) Parents: Information evening	Accelerometry Self report: parent proxy	Protocol paper only – no results
Trost et al. (2008)	RCT USA	n=42 (4.1 ± 0.7) Classroom	Children: 8-week move and learn program during curriculum time	Accelerometry Direct observation: OSRAP	INT children significantly increased their classroom MVPA Significant differences were also noted for classroom VPA over the final 2 weeks
Hannon and Brown (2008)	RCT USA	n=64 (3-5 years) School playground	Children: playground equipment	Accelerometry Direct observation: OSRAC-P	Boys and girls significantly increased light, moderate and vigorous activity and decreased sedentary time
Reilly et al. (2005)	RCT Scotland	n=545 (4.2±0.2 years) Nursery	Children: 24 weekly PA sessions (3X30mins) Parents: home education	Accelerometry	No significant change in PA

Key to symbols: PA = physical activity; RCT = randomised controlled trial; FMS = fundamental movement skills; OSRAP = Observational System; OSRAC-P = Observational System for Recording Physical Activity in Children-Preschool Version;INT = intervention; MVPA = moderate-to-vigorous physical activity; VPA = vigorous physical activity for Recording Activity in Preschoolers.

However, importantly they support the premise that parents and carers are receptive to intervention programmes. While this field of research is expanding, there still remains an urgent need to build on the work that has been conducted.

References

Abbott, R. A. and Davies, P. S. W. (1989). Ecological Systems Theory. *Annals of Child Development*, 6, 187-249.

Abbott, R. A. and Davies, P.S.W. (2004). Habitual physical activity and physical activity intensity: their relation to body composition in 5.0-10.5-y-old children. *European Journal of Clinical Nutrition*, 58, 285-291.

Anderssen, S. A., Cooper, A. R., Riddoch, C., Sardinha, L. B., Harro, M., Brage, S. and Andersen, L. B. (2007). Low cardiorespiratory fitness is a strong predictor for clustering of cardiovascular disease risk factors in children independent of country, age and sex. *European Journal of Cardiovascular Prevention and Rehabilitation,* 14(4), 526-31.

Barnes, J. (2007). *Down Our Way: The relevance of neighbourhoods for parenting and child development.* Chicester: Wiley.

Brockman, R., Fox, K.R. and Jago, R. (2011). What is the meaning and nature of active play for today's children in the UK? *International Journal of Behavioural Nutrition and Physical Activity*, 8. DOI:10.1186/1479-5868-8-15.

Bronfenbrenner, U. (1989). Ecological systems theory. *Annals of Child Development*, 6, 187-249.

Bundred, P., Kitchiner,D. and Buchan, I. (2001). Prevalence of overweight and obese children between 1989 and 1998: population based series of cross sectional studies. *British Medical Journal*, 322, 326-328.

Burdette, H. L. and Whitaker, R.C. (2005). Resurrecting free play in young children: looking beyond fitness and fatness to attention, affiliation, and affect. *Archives of Paediatrics and Adolescents Medicine,* 159(1), 46-50.

Burdette, H.L. and. Whitaker, R.C. (2005). A national study of neighborhood safety, outdoor play, television viewing, and obesity in pre-school children, *Pediatrics,* 116, 657–662.

Campbell, P. T., Katzmarzyk, P. T., Malina, R.M., Rao, D.C., Perusse, L. and Bouchard C. (2001). Prediction of physical activity and physical work capacity (PWC150) in young adulthood from childhood and adolescence with consideration of parental measures. *American Journal of Human Biology*, 13(2), 190-196.

Carson, J. L., Burks, V. S., and Parke, R. D. (1993). Parent-child physical play: Determinants and consequences. In K. MacDonald (Ed.), *Parent-child play: Descriptions and implication* (pp. 197-220). Albany, NY: State University of New York Press

Cashmore, A. W. and S. C. Jones (2008). Growing up active: a study into physical activity in long day care centers. *Journal of Research in Childhood Education*, 23(2), 179-182.

Cattaneo, A., Monasta, L., Stamatakis, E., Lioret, S., Castetbon, K., Frenken, F., ...Brug, J. (2010). Overweight and obesity in infants and pre-school children in the European Union: a review of existing data. *Obesity Reviews,* 11(5), 389-398.

Cliff, D. P., Okely, A.D., Smith, L.M. and McKeen, K. (2009). Relationships between fundamental movement skills and objectively measured physical activity in pre-school children. *Paediatric Exercise Science*, 21(4), 436-49.

Cragg, S. and Cameron, C. (2006). Physical Activity of Canadian Youth: An Analysis of 2002 Health Behaviour in School-Aged Children Data. Ottawa, ON: Canadian Fitness and Lifestyle Institute.

Davey, C. and Dimmock, S. (2008). *What do they know? Investigating the human rights concerns of children and young people living in England.* London: Children's Rights Alliance for England.

Department of Health (2004). At least five a week: Evidence of the impact of physical activity and its relationship to health: A report from the Chief Medical Officer. London: Department of Health.

Department of Health (2011). Start Active, Stay Active: A report on physical activity for health from the four home countries'. A report from the Chief Medical Officer. London: Department of Health.

Directgov (2011). Understanding the National Curriculum.Retrieved from Directgov website http://www.direct.gov.uk/en/Parents/Schoolslearninganddevelopment/ExamsTestsAndTheCurriculum/DG_4016665

Dowda, M., Brown, W. H., McIver, K.L., Pfeiffer, K.A., O'Neill, J.R. Addy, C.L. and Pate, R.R. (2009). Policies and characteristics of the pre-school environment and physical activity of young children. *Paediatrics*, 123(2), 261-266.

Eisenmann, J. C., Gentile, D.A., Welk, G.J., Callahan, R., Strickland, S., Walsh, M. and Walsh, D.A. (2008). SWITCH: rationale, design, and implementation of a community, school, and family-based intervention to modify behaviours related to childhood obesity. *BMC Public Health*, 8, 223.

Ekeland, E., Heian, F., Hagen, K.B., Abbott, J.M. and Nordheim, L. (2004). Exercise to improve self-esteem in children and young people. *Cochrane Database of Systematic Reviews.*

Erickson, R. J. (1985). Play contributes to the full emotional development of the child. *Education*, 105(3), 261-263.

Finn, K., Johannsen, N. and Specker, B. (2002). Factors associated with physical activity in pre-school children. *Journal of Paediatrics*, 140(1), 81-85.

Ginsburg, K. R. (2007). The importance of play in promoting healthy child development and maintaining strong parent-child bonds. *Pediatrics*, 119(1), 182-91.

Gleave, J. (2010). Community play: A literature review. London: Play England.

Hinckley , T., Crawford, D, Salmon, J., Okely, A.D. and Hesketh, K. (2008). Pre-school children and physical activity: a review of the correlates. *American Journal of Preventive Medicine*, 34, 435-441.

Janz, K. F., Letuchy, E.M., Eichenberger Gilmore, J.M., Burns, T.L., Torner, J.C. Willing, M.C. and Levy, S.M. (2010). Early Physical Activity Provides Sustained Bone Health Benefits Later in Childhood. *Medicine and Science in Sports and Exercise*, 42(6), 1072-1078.

Maccoby, E. E. (1986). *Social groupings in childhood: Their relationship to prosocial and antisocial behaviour in boys and girls*. New York: Academic Press.

Martin, P. and Caro, T. (1985). *On the function of play and its role in behavioural development*. New York: Academic Press

Meaney, M. J., Stewart, J. and Beatty, W.W. (1985). *Sex difference in social play*. New York: Academic Press.

National Playing Fields Association (2000). *What play provision should do for children?* London: National Playing Fields Association.

O'Dwyer, M.V., Foweather, L. Stratton, G. and Ridgers, N.D. (2011) Physical activity in non-overweight and overweight UK pre-school children: Preliminary findings and methods of the Active Play Project, *Science and Sports*, Doi : 10.1016/j. scispo. 2011.01. 006

Office of the United Nations High Commissioner for Human Rights (1989) Convention on the Rights of the Child, General Assembly Resolution 44/25 of 20th November 1989.

Okely, A. D., Trost, S.G., Steele, J.R., Cliff, D.P. and Karen, M. (2009). Adherence to physical activity and electronic media guidelines in Australian pre-school children. *Journal of Paediatrics and Child Health,* 45(2), 5-8.

Oliver, M., Schofield, G. M., Kolt, G.S. and Schluter, P.J. (2007). Pedometer accuracy in physical activity assessment of pre-school children. *Journal of Science in Medicine and Sport*, 10(5), 303-10.

Oliver, M., Schofield, G.M. and Kolt. (2007). Physical activity in pre-schoolers: understanding prevalence and measurement issues. *Sports Medicine*, 32, 1045 – 1070.

Parke, R. D. and Suomi, S.J. (1981). *Adult male infant relationships: Human and nonhuman primate evidence*. New York: Cambridge University Press.

Parten, M. B. (1932). Social participation among pre-school children. *The Journal of Abnormal and Social Psychology,* 27(3), 243-269.

Pellegrini, A. D. and Smith, P.K. (1998). Physical activity play: the nature and function of a neglected aspect of playing. *Child Development,* 69(3), 577-98.

Pellegrini, A. D. (1989). Elementary school children's rough-and-tumble play. *Early Childhood Research Quarterly,* 4(2), 245-260.

Play England (2010). An economic evaluation of play provision: 66.

Reilly, J. J. and Z. C. McDowell (2003). Physical activity interventions in the prevention and treatment of paediatric obesity: systematic review and critical appraisal. *Proceedings of the Nutrition Society,* 62(3), 611-619.

Reilly, J. J., Kelly, L., Montgomery, C., Williamson, A., Fisher, A., McColl, J.H., ... Grant, S. (2006). Physical activity to prevent obesity in young children: cluster randomised controlled trial. *British Medical Journal,* 333(7577), 1041-1044.

Reilly, J.J. (2010). Low levels of objectively measured physical activity in pre-schoolers in childcare. Medicine and Science in Sports and Exercise, DOI: 10.1249/MSS0b013e3181cea100

Ridgers, N.D., Knowles, Z. R. and Sawyers, J. (2012) Encouraging play in the natural environment: A child-focused case study of forest school, *Childrens Geographies.*

Sallis, J.F., Patterson, T.L., Buono, M.J., Atkins, C.J. and Nader, P.R. (1988) Aggregation of physical activity habits in Mexican-American and Anglo families, *Journal of Behavioral Medicine,* 11(1) 31-41.

Sawyers, J. K. (1994). The Preschool Playground: Developing Skills through Outdoor Play. *Journal of Physical Education, Recreation and Dance*, 65, 31-33.

Simons-Morton, B. G., O'Hara, N. M., Parcel, G.S., Hunang, I.W., Baronwski, T. and Wilson, B. (1990). Children's frequency of participation in moderate to vigorous physical activities. *Research Quarterly for Exercise and Sport,* 61(4), 307-314.

Smith, P. K. and Vollstedt, R. (1985). On defining play: An empirical study of the relationship between play and various play criteria. *Child Development*, 56(4), 1042-1050.

Smith, P. K. (1982). Does play matter? Functional and evolutionary aspects of animal and human play. *The Behavioural and Brain Sciences,* 5, 139-184.

Story, M., Kaphingst, K.M. and French, S. (2006). The role of child care settings in obesity prevention. *Future Child,* 16(1), 143-68.

Tamis-Le Monda, C. S., Shannon, J.D., Cabrera, N.J. and Lamb, M.E. (2004). Fathers and mothers at play with their 2- and 3-year-olds: contributions to language and cognitive development. *Child Development*, 75(6), 1806-1820.

Thomas, G. and G. Thompson (2004). A Child's Place: Why environment matters to children. London: Green Alliance and Demos.

Tucker, P. (2008). The physical activity levels of pre-school-aged children: A systematic review. *Early Childhood Research Quarterly*, 23, 547-558.

Veitch, J. (2007). Children's perceptions of the use of public open spaces for active free-play. *Children's Geographies*, 5(4), 409-422.

Ward D. S., Vaughan, A., McWilliams, C. and Hales, D. (2010). Interventions for Increasing Physical Activity at Child Care. *Medicine and Science in Sports and Exercise,* 42(3), 526-534.

In: Reviews in Pediatric Exercise Science
Editor: Michael Duncan, pp. 13-26
ISBN: 978-1-61470-978-7

Chapter II

Physical Education and Sport, and Positive Attitudes towards Physical Activity

Lorayne A. Woodfield
Newman University College, UK.

Introduction

The aim of this chapter is to consider the role that physical education and sporting activities can play in the promotion of positive attitudes towards physical activity and healthy lifestyles. Although it is claimed that attitude is one of the most researched areas of social psychology (Olson and Zanna, 1993, cited in Biddle and Mutrie, 2008), literature investigating young people's attitudes toward physical education is limited. Lifestyle development has been an aim of physical education for many years and is explicitly stated in national curricula (please see Bailey, 2009 for a review of the benefits and aims of physical education), yet the life expectancy of the youth of today is predicted to be lower than their parents due to the largest increases in obesity occurring during childhood (Olshansky et al., 2005).

It has been widely published that young people who participate in physical activity will accrue health benefits including improved coronary heart disease risk profile, improved mental health, and reduced risk of osteoporosis, and it has also been stated that young people may have improved academic performance (Strong et al., 2005). However, the evidence base for the benefits of physical activity in young people is inconclusive (Patrick et al., 2004; Twisk, 2001). The findings of the seminal Amsterdam Growth Study conducted over a period of 15 years concluded that activity levels after the adolescent period is "of utmost importance" to physical fitness (Kemper and van Mechelen, 1995: 186). More recently, the work of Guerra et al. (2006) found that between the ages of 8-15 years, boys classified as less active were more likely to be obese than those classified as more active whilst no such association was found amongst girls of the same age. Indeed, research has made conflicting findings namely that obesity in girls is linked to low levels of physical activity but no relationship was found amongst boys (Mota et al., 2002). Therefore, the nature of any associations between physical activity and health in youth is complex.

Patterns of health-related behaviours are often acquired and established during childhood and adolescence (Kelder et al., 1994) and research conducted by Janz et al. (2002) proposed that sedentary activity and vigorous activity are moderately stable variables that track from late childhood into middle adolescence even though this is a period of substantial psychological and biological development. However, the current evidence base to support the tracking of physical activity throughout the life course is limited as relatively few longitudinal studies have been conducted in the area due to the methodological demands of such study designs (Ben-Shlomo and Kuh, 2002). That said, research has found that other health status variables do track into young adulthood with overweight children more likely to become overweight adults (Deshmukh-Taskar et al., 2006) and, among males, "an elevated BMI in childhood predicated the risk of hypertension in young adulthood" (Field et al., 2005: 163). Young people are at the same risk of sedentary lifestyles as adults either during their childhood or when they themselves become adults. Exposure to physically inactive pursuits such as watching television, and using personal computers and games consoles has the potential to occupy a large proportion of leisure time and research suggests that young people who watch more than four hours of television per day are 40% more likely to be classified as overweight (Eisenmann et al., 2002). Consequently, many children are failing to attain the activity level recommendations which are thought necessary to confer health benefits in later life due to sedentary activity. Current recommendations for young people's activity are internationally accepted to be one hour of moderate and vigorous intensity activity over the course of the day (NICE, 2009). Thus, there is a real need for beginning the prevention of these adult diseases during childhood and adolescence.

Flodmark and collagues. (2006) reported that the prevention of obesity among children and adolescents is possible through school-based programmes that combine physical activity and healthy diet promotion. In recognition of the complex nature of young people's physical activity levels, one intervention study considered a range of approaches to increasing activity including: daily physical education classes, short activity breaks during academic lessons, activities during school breaks and before and after school, physical activity homework, active transport to and from school, and initiatives to encourage families of the school children to become more active (Zahner et al., 2006). Thus, physical activity interventions in youth populations may need to go beyond the classroom, or indeed the school, to be effective. That said, schools are ideal settings in which to educate young people about the benefits of leading a physically active life due to the fact that schools provide access to virtually all children for 40-45 percent of their waking day (Fox and Harris, 2003).

Attitude Theory: Why Developing Positive Attitudes to Physical Activity is Important

According to Eiser (1994) attitude is the most commonly used term in social psychology. Attitude is "a relatively enduring organisation of beliefs, feelings and behavioural tendencies towards socially significant objects, groups, events or symbols. A general feeling of evaluation – positive or negative – about some person, object or issue" (Hogg and Vaughan,

1998: 116). Attitudes are learned from experience or from other people (Doganis and Theodorakis, 1995). Furthermore, attitude has been defined more succinctly as a subjective evaluative experience which can be communicated (Eiser, 1994). Attitude is a hypothetical psychological construct which exits in theory but is not directly observable. Not only can attitudes be communicated, they can also predict future behaviour, therefore, our attitudes predispose us to act the way we do (Eiser, 1994). Thus, attitudes persist over time and are formed of a cluster of feelings, likes and dislikes (Hogg and Vaughan, 1998). However, it is important to acknowledge that attitudes are not permanent and can change or be changed (Eiser, 1994).

Attitudes are considered to be multi-dimensional. Rosenberg and Hovland (1960) proposed that attitude should be considered as a complex of three classes of components (a three-component model), and not as a single concept, comprising affective (feelings and emotions), belief (cognitive), and functional (behavioural) dimensions. Generally, both affective and cognitive dimensions encompass individual beliefs and values, and a normative component concerning the extent to which one wishes to comply with the beliefs of significant others (Biddle, 1994). Beliefs can be either positive or negative (Silverman and Subramaniam, 1999), therefore, if an individual holds a positive belief about an object such as physical activity a more favourable attitude follows and this will have some influence on behaviour (Biddle and Mutrie, 2008). These components are predictors of intentions and behaviours in physical activity. The three dimensions can sometimes cohere with each other and then sometimes not (Eiser, 1994).

The Theory of Reasoned Action (TRA) (Figure 1) (Ajzen and Fishbein, 1980) outlines that attitudes should not be expected to predict behaviour and that it is intention which should be predicted. The theory also proposes that intention is not only influenced by attitude; the extent to which an individual believes that the way in which he or she acts will gain approval or disapproval from significant others such as family, friends and in the context of young people, their teachers, also pays an important part. This is termed your subjective norm. Therefore, your subjective norm may pull you in one direction while your attitude may pull you in an opposing direction.

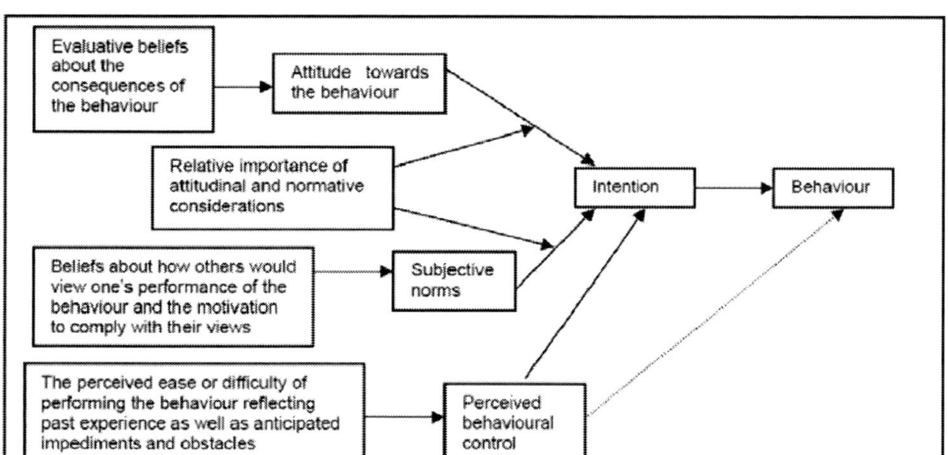

Figure 1. The theories of reasoned action (excluding perceived behavioural control) (Ajzen and Fishbein, 1980) and planned behaviour (including perceived behavioural control) (Ajzen, 1988).

It is important to recognise that the TRA has previously been criticised for a number of reasons. One such criticism is that theory is unable to predict behaviour when behavioural barriers may prevent participation in physical activity from being totally volitional (Biddle and Mutrie, 2008). For example, disposable income, distance to facilities, and familial responsibilities can impact upon an individual's behaviour and therefore their participation in physical activity or exercise. These behavioural barriers are applicable to both adult and child populations. Subsequently, the TRA was revised to include perceived behavioural control (Ajzen, 1988) which takes into account perceived obstacles to performing the behaviour. Thus, the Theory of Planned Behaviour (TPB) was proposed. The TPB acknowledges that some individuals will want to be physically active (therefore hold positive attitudes towards physical activity) but, because they feel that they cannot overcome certain behavioural barriers, will not become physically active.

Specifically referring to young people, Hagger and Chatzisarantis (2008) claim that young people are likely to enjoy participating in certain sporting activities that reflect their affective attitudes. Similarly, they may also hold positive beliefs about these pastimes because they see instrumental benefits to themselves (e.g., social benefits, improving health, developing skill). The behavioural dimension could show itself in young people planning to pursue these sporting activities in the future.

The Role of Schools in Promoting Physical Activity and Healthy Lifestyles

It has been suggested that insufficient levels of physical activity in childhood are also a likely result of 'out-dated' modified and traditional sports which are available in community settings (Naughton et al., 2006) which fail to acknowledge the diverse activity interests of young people. Schools provide arenas where physical activity and healthy lifestyles can be promoted as sport and physical activity are presented to almost all pupils (Cale and Harris, 2006; Carr et al., 1999). However, currently the school environment is failing to instil the significance of a physically active lifestyle for future health and well-being (Naughton et al., 2006) as statistics still suggest that the prevalence of overweight and obesity among young people continues to rise (Wardle et al., 2006). In the United Kingdom, this rise is in spite of statutory frameworks (e.g., National Curriculum for England Physical Education key process making informed choices about healthy, active lifestyles), UK Government recommendations (a minimum of two hours of physical education per week), and various strategies (e.g., The physical education and sport strategy for young people (PESSYP); British Heart Foundation 'Active School'). Collectively, these initiatives and guidelines aim to provide young people with the skills and opportunities to become "independently active for life" (Harris and Penney, 2000: 252). After reviewing the evidence base, Bailey (2009: 31) concluded that young people's social exclusion from physical education and sport "can be associated with a legacy of inactivity and associated ill-health in the years to come".

Although it has previously been suggested that young people in England are more active throughout the school day than during their domestic leisure time (Duncan et al., 2007), research findings are inconsistent and studies have found that physical activity undertaken outside of school hours is a key contributor to a child's overall level of physical activity (Cox et al., 2006). Research conducted in New Zealand using pedometers found that children in New Zealand completed more steps outside of school than during school (Cox et al., 2006). A more complex pattern of physical activity was observed by Mota et al. (2003) who used accelerometers to measure weekday moderate and vigorous physical activity patterns amongst Portuguese youth. Mota and colleagues found that boys engaged in more moderate and vigorous activity and were therefore more active after school (i.e. late afternoons and evenings) and girls were more active during school. Therefore, it can be argued that boys' and girls' physical activity patterns on school days differ and research findings which fail to distinguish between genders should be treated with caution.

Although it is acknowledged that young people's activity occurs in a variety of settings including physical education and school sport (Fox and Harris, 2003), physical education and the school environment alone cannot meet the physical activity needs of all young people (Cale and Harris, 2005). Nevertheless, there is an assumption that the primary goal of physical education is to promote lifelong physical activity (Corbin, 2002). Indeed, according to Green (2008: 100) the assumption is that "increasing people's knowledge and understanding is likely to lead to changes in their attitudes and, subsequently, and more importantly, their health-related behaviours".

Attitude towards Physical Education and Its Association with Physical Activity

Previous attitude research has reported that attitudes towards participation in physical activities outside of school can be attributed to students' attitudes towards physical education (Carlson, 1995; Portman, 1995; Ennis, 1996). Sleap and Warburton (1992) maintain that with reference to future participation in physical activity, positive attitudes to participation need to be fostered so that physical activity continues through adulthood. Moreover, a good attitude toward physical education is an important component in promoting an active lifestyle in young people (Silverman and Subramaniam, 1999). In the 1980s it was suggested that young people's attitudes are formed somewhere before 10 to 12 years of age (Pease and Andersen, 1986) and between 13 to 14 years of age (McIntosh and Albinson, 1982), the age when young people are in compulsory education. In addition, qualitative research conducted among British adolescents revealed that participation in community sport programmes was influenced by previous experiences in physical education (Coakley and White, 1992). Therefore, having positive attitudes towards physical education is important for the formation of future attitudes towards physical activity and exercise. Although, it is important to note that research has made findings to the contrary and a study conducted in the US reported that enjoyment of physical education is not an indicator of regular exercise (Ryan et al., 2009).

It has been advocated that in physical education, pupils should always be challenged if they display negative attitudes towards the subject (Rose, 1997). This acts as an attempt to somehow redress an instinctive love of physical activity that children are born with which is gradually eroded because of unpleasant experiences (Sleap and Warburton, 1996). Thus, it is the task of physical education not to turn children off physical education but to make it valued and enjoyed. Macfadyen (2000) highlights that even though physical education is a worthwhile and enjoyable experience for many pupils, physical education lessons can become an unpleasant ordeal for many others and therefore there are implications for later attitudes toward physical activity.

Research has also attempted to establish if choice of physical education activity (Prusak et al., 2004) and the nature of the activity (individual or team sports) (Hodges Kulinna et al., 2003) have any effect upon participation. The findings of Prusak et al. (2004) suggested that choice in physical education can indeed result in increased motivational levels and therefore the intention to adopt a physically active lifestyle throughout adolescence and adulthood. Students prefer to receive instruction in a wide range of activities during physical education classes although there appears to be a dislike of fitness activities (Rikard and Banville, 2006) and a preference for games-based activities (Barney and Deutsch, 2009). Therefore, what is taught during physical education lessons should be carefully considered by practitioners.

An experimental study found that an increased and specialised physical education programme during primary schooling did not encourage participants to adopt a more physically active lifestyle during adulthood than those who received standard physical education teaching (Trudeau et al., 1999). The experimental subjects who received a more positive and enthusiastic experience of physical education did not hold more positive attitudes toward physical activity as adults. The findings of this study therefore indicate that a specialised physical education programme has no effect upon attitudes towards physical activity. Sleap of Warburton (1992) suggest that daily physical education lessons are problematic as there is a danger that children could perceive physical activity as an unpleasant duty and a chore, thus developing negative attitudes and reducing possible adult participation in physical activity and sport. Subsequently, some children may already believe that physical activity as an unpleasant duty due to their experience of physical education.

Persistent negative feelings towards physical education can result in pupils feeling alienated. Work by Carlson (1995) discusses the three affective states associated with alienation (meaninglessness, powerlessness and isolation) and has provided their application to physical education. For example, some students do not see a purpose for physical education in their lives (meaninglessness), others do not feel that they have control over what happens during physical education lessons (powerlessness) and finally, some students feel either socially or emotionally isolated from their peers in physical education classes (isolation). As a result, it was advocated that a physical education approach which "includes all and alienates none" be developed (Carlson, 1995:475). However, it must be acknowledged that this would not be easily achieved due to the diverse needs and interests of young people. Furthermore, there are financial and time constraints in the preparation of prospective physical education teachers (Fox and Harris, 2003) which impacts upon teacher training in this area.

Studies conducted into adolescents' attitudes and beliefs about various components of physical education have made a variety of findings. Milosevic (1996) found eleven to sixteen year olds to hold certain beliefs about physical education activities. Participants deemed certain activities to be specifically for males or females whilst other activities were considered to be suitable for both genders. Furthermore, both boys and girls stated that boys have considerably more opportunities to take part in extra curricular sporting activities than girls. Milosevic (1996) therefore identified a need for broader co-educational activities in physical education throughout the 11-16 age range to arrest the decline in attitudes towards the subject. However, research by Arabaci (2009) found that although Turkish 15-17 year olds prefer co-educational physical education, 12-14 year olds preferred single-sex classes. As young people's preferences regarding single-sex physical education may vary for a number of reasons, it may be more appropriate to consider teaching both single-sex and co-educational physical education as experience of one system may negatively impact upon attitudes towards the subject.

Quite often a student's dislike of physical education stems from contextual factors and not from the physical activity itself (Williams and Bedward, 1999). Issues such as physical education uniform impact attitudes towards the subject; students find it unacceptable that they are expected to play outdoor games during the winter months wearing limited sports clothing. However, research conducted in Canada found that curriculum content and physical education teacher behaviour are considered the most important determinants of attitudes towards physical education (Luke and Sinclair, 1991). In support of this, Macfayden (2000) reported that 14–15 year olds identify various physical education teachers (both past and present) as the most influential figures in the formation of their attitudes toward physical activity. Therefore, teachers are highly influential in determining attitudes towards both physical education and physical activity and should therefore carefully consider both what they teach and their teaching behaviours to foster positive attitudes in their students.

Research indicates that boys hold more positive attitudes towards physical education and that their participation in both curricular and extra-curricular activity is looked upon as being compatible with prevailing notions of masculinity (Hopwood and Carrington, 1994). Research conducted in Turkey reported that, irrespective of whether they participate in sport (i.e. either school athletic clubs or amateur sports clubs outside school), boys hold significantly more favourable attitudes towards physical education than their female counterparts (Koca and Demirhan, 2004). More recently published work with Turkish school students also reported that 15-17 years old boys have more positive attitudes than their female counterparts, although no gender difference was found among 12-14 year olds (Arabaci, 2009). Fifteen and sixteen year old girls are twice as likely as boys to excuse themselves from physical education (Milosevic, 1996) and this dislike of physical activity looks as though it would continue after compulsory education. Interviews conducted by Williams and Bedward (1999) found a significant number of adolescent girls expressed a dislike of winter games whilst others considered team games to be the highlight of their physical education timetable. Similarly, in a qualitative study, interviews conducted among young women attending secondary schools showed that there was a general dislike of the subject and that many girls would attempt different strategies to avoid taking part, including the use of the same sick note for several weeks (Mulvihill, et al., 2000). Furthermore, Milosevic (1996) found that only 14% of girls were highly likely to continue with activities after leaving school compared with 42% of boys. Shropshire et al. (1997) recognised that adolescent girls are the group which is most at risk of losing interest thus engaging in less physical activity. Therefore, ways need to be found to arrest the fall in girls' enthusiasm for physical education from an early age.

Physical education in itself can develop a feeling of alienation for many young people although the problem may indeed be more of an issue for girls. Many students with extreme body images are more likely to be those who do not like physical education (Ryan, et al., 2009). As female pubertal development is accompanied by significant weight gain and fat deposits around the hips, thighs, buttocks and waist (Levine and Smolak, 2002) some adolescent girls are particularly sensitive to body-shape changes in terms of their perceived body image (Sharp, 1995). Levine and Smolak (2002: 75) suggest that as girls move through the stages of puberty in early adolescence there is an association between "increased body mass, a more negative body image, and higher levels of drive for thinness and dieting". Therefore, it can be suggested that these factors influence adolescents' attitudes towards physical education and potentially their physical activity intentions. Teachers and health practitioners need to develop physical education programmes which consider the issues surrounding body image particularly in adolescent girls.

Research conducted in Poland concluded that school sports clubs can "greatly improve" young people's attitudes towards physical education as it was found that those who are members of school sports clubs have more positive attitudes towards physical education than non-members especially in the behavioural component (Tomik, 2008). Furthermore, Tomik (2008) states that participation in school sports clubs significantly inhibited the worsening of attitude towards physical education with age. Encouraging more young people to attend extra-curricular activities, by offering programmes that they may find attractive, may help to arrest the age-related decline in positive attitudes towards physical education.

Measurement of Attitudes towards Physical Activity and Physical Education

Until relatively recently pupils' attitudes towards physical education were largely assessed by subjective means, and it was noted some years ago that there was a need for the objective measurement of attitudes towards curriculum physical education using reliable and valid instruments (Jones, 1988). This is due to the fact that open-ended response techniques make the quantification of data difficult and the comparison of attitudes between child population groups fraught with difficulties (Shropshire, 1997). A number of quantitative instruments have been designed that measure young people's attitudes towards physical activity. However, it has previously been reported that it is difficult for researchers to make decisions on the appropriateness of the research tool due to the fact that many studies do not fully outline the procedures used to establish reliability and validity (Silverman and Subramaniam, 1999).

In her review of literature regarding children's attitudes toward physical education, Shropshire (1997) reported that there was no single instrument available that was appropriate for the measurement of children's attitudes toward curriculum physical education. Shropshire felt that at that time, existing questionnaires were inadequate as questionnaires failed to deal with physical education specifically and focused on attitudes towards physical activity (e.g., Simon and Smoll, 1974) or sport outside of school (e.g., Wankel and Pabich, 1982). Furthermore, Shropshire considered it inappropriate to utilise a questionnaire designed for different population groups; (e.g., children of different age groups, or children in other countries). A questionnaire devised by Jones (1988), the Attitude towards Curriculum Physical Education (ATCPE) scale, was designed for use in British schools by teachers. The questionnaire was a 25 item Likert type scale assessing children's general attitudes towards curriculum physical education. According to Jones (1988), the scale possessed acceptable levels of test-retest reliability and internal consistency. However, Shropshire felt that the questionnaire was inappropriate for her study as it was designed for use with primary aged children as young as nine years, and the scale was too general as it did not have a factorial structure therefore failing to examine any underlying constructs (Shropshire, 1997). Thus, the Pre-Adolescent Attitude towards Physical Education Questionnaire (PAAPEQ, Shropshire, 1997) was developed specifically to provide a reliable and valid instrument which would successfully measure pre-adolescent British schoolchildren's attitudes towards physical education. The questionnaire was rated on a four point Likert type scale and was composed of 23 items in five factors (general interest, assessment, teacher, environmental adjustment and organisational choice). The PAAPEQ has been shown to possess high internal consistency (a=0.80) and high inter-item reliability ($p<0.001$) making it suitable for future research into the attitudes of pre-adolescent children towards school physical education.

Since the development of the PAAPEQ, further instruments to assess young people's attitude towards physical education have been created and validity and reliability established. For example, Subramaniam and Silverman (2000) created an instrument to assess attitudes towards physical education among North American school-aged youth, and the Attitude Towards PE Scale (Demirhan and Altay, 2001 cited in Koca Asci and Demirhan, 2005) designed for Turkish students. However, the validity and reliability of these questionnaires have been established amongst different populations with students attending different school systems and of different age ranges and therefore, the appropriateness of this method for use with all school-aged children can be questioned.

Over recent years attitude data has primarily been collected through the use of quantitative methods. However, a more qualitative approach has been advocated by some and interviewing as a research tool has been utilised as an alternative method to assess attitude towards physical education (Carlson, 1995). Additionally, a mixed methods approach has been taken whereby both quantitative and qualitative measures have been used (Rikard and Banville, 2006). Although researchers can employ a variety of methods to increase the validity of the data collected (e.g., member checking, including triangulation), interviewing has its own complexities. For example, when carrying out attitude research using interviews with younger children, an inability to verbalise responses can affect the validity and reliability of the responses provided (Silverman and Subramanian, 1999).

Conclusion

This review has aimed to highlight the importance of physical education in promoting positive attitudes towards physical activity and healthy lifestyles given existing concerns about the health and well-being of young people. However, literature is equivocal in supporting the notion that those who hold more positive attitudes towards physical education are those who are more recreationally active, and participate in more sport throughout childhood, adolescence and adulthood. Although attitude theory can be used to hypothesise the link between attitude towards physical education and physical activity behaviour, it would be naive to assume that ensuring that all young people receive positive physical education experiences will increase physical activity levels and therefore reduce obesity levels. However, promoting positive attitudes toward physical activity is an aim of physical education programmes internationally and therefore practitioners must endeavour to offer physical education lessons that engage students. This practice should hopefully avoid school-based activity contributing to the development of negative attitudes. Researchers can contribute to existing knowledge by developing new and appropriate instruments to measure young people's attitudes towards physical education. This body of knowledge may help in understanding the complex nature of attitudes towards physical education and contribute to targeting physical education interventions to arrest any decline in young people's attitudes.

References

Ajzen, I. (1988). *Attitudes, personality and behaviour.* Milton Keynes: Open University Press.

Ajzen, I. and Fishbein, M. (1980) *Understanding Attitudes and Predicting Social Behaviour.* New Jersey: Prentice Hall.

Arabaci, R. (2009). Attitudes toward physical education and class preferences of Turkish secondary and high school students. *Elementary Education Online*, 8(1): 2-8.

Bailey, R. (2009). Physical Education and Sport in Schools. In R. Bailey and D. Kirk (Ed.) *The Routledge Physical Education Reader*. London: Routledge, pp. 28-37.

Barney, D. and Deutsch, J. (2009). The effect of middle school physical education curriculum on student attitudes. *Asian Journal of Physical Education and Recreation*, 15(1): 12-20.

Ben-Shlomo, Y. and Kuh, D. (2002). A life course approach to chronic disease epidemiology: conceptual models. empirical challenges and interdisciplinary perspectives. *International Journal of Epidemiology*, 31: 285-293.

Biddle, S. (1994). What helps and hinders people being more physically active? In A.J. Killoran, P. Fentem and C. Caspersen (Eds.) Moving on: international perspectives on promoting physical activity. London: Health Education Authority, pp. 110-148.

Biddle, S.J.H. and Mutrie, N. (2008). Psychology of physical activity: determinants, well-being and interventions (2nd edn.) London: Routledge.

Cale, L. and Harris, J. (2005). Promoting physical activity within schools. In L. Cale and J. Harris (Eds.) *Exercise and young people: issues, implications and initiatives.* Basingstoke: Palgrave Macmillan, 162-190.

Cale, L. and Harris, J. (2005). Physical activity promotion interventions, initiatives, resources and contacts. In L. Cale and J. Harris (Eds.) *Exercise and young people: issues, implications and initiatives.* Basingstoke: Palgrave Macmillan, 232-270.

Carlson, T.B. (1995). We hate gym: student alienation from physical education. *Journal of Teaching Physical Education,* 14: 467-477.

Carr, S., Weigand, D.A., and Hussey, W. (1999). The relative influence of parents, teachers, and peers on children and adolescents' achievement and intrinsic motivation and perceived competence in physical education. *Journal of Sport Pedagogy*, 5(1): 28-50.

Coakley, J. and White, A. (1992). Making decisions: gender and sport participation among British adolescents. *Sociology of Sport Journal*, 9: 20-35.

Corbin, C.B. (2002). Physical activity for everyone: what every physical educator should know about promoting lifelong physical activity. *Journal of Teaching in Physical Education*, 21: 128-144.

Cox, M., Schofield, G., Greasley, N. and Kolt, G.S. (2006). Pedometer steps in primary school-aged children: a comparison of school-based and out-of-school activity. *Journal of Science and Medicine in Sport*, 9: 91-97.

Deshmukh-Taskar, P., Nicklas, T.A., Morales, M., Yang, S-J., Zakeri, I. and Berenson, G.S. (2006). Tracking of overweight status from childhood to young adulthood: the Bogalusa Heart Study. *European Journal of Clinical Nutrition*, 60: 48-57.

Doganis, G. and Theodorakis, Y. (1995). The influence of attitude on exercise participation. In S. J. H. Biddle (Ed.) *European Perspectives on Exercise and Sport Psychology.* London: Routledge, pp26-49.

Duncan, M. J., Al-Nakeeb, Y., Woodfield, L.A. and Lyons, M. (2007). Pedometer determined physical activity levels in primary school children from central England. *Preventative Medicine*, 44: 416-420.

Eisenmann, J.C., Bartee, R.T. and Wang, M.Q. (2002). Physical activity, TV viewing, and weight in U.S. youth: 1999 Youth Risk Behaviour Survey. *Obesity Research*, 10: 379-385.

Eiser, R.J. (1994). *Attitudes, chaos and the connectionist mind.* Oxford: Blackwell Publishers.

Ennis, C.D. (1996). Students' experiences of sport-based physical education: (more than) apologies are necessary. *Quest*, 48: 453-456.

Field, A.E., Cook, N.R., Gillman, M.W. (2005). Weight status in childhood as a predictor of becoming overweight or hypertensive in early adulthood. *Obesity Research*, 13(1): 163-169.

Flodmark, C-E., Marcus, C. and Britton, M. (2006). Interventions to prevent obesity in children and adolescents: a systematic literature review. *International Journal of Obesity*, 30: 579-589.

Fox, K. and Harris, J. (2003). Promoting physical activity through schools. In J. McKenna and C. Riddoch (eds.) *Perspectives on health and exercise.* Basingstoke: Palgrave MacMillan

Green, K. (2008) *Understanding physical education.* London: Sage.

Guerra, S., Teixeira-Pinto, A., Ribeiro, J.C., Ascensao, A., Magalhaes, J., Andersen, L.B., Duarte, J.A. and Mota, J. (2006). Relationship between physical activity and obesity in children and adolescents. *Journal of Sports Medicine and Physical Fitness*, 46: 79-83.

Hagger, M.S. and Chatzisarantis, N.L.D. (2008). Youth attitudes. In A.L. Smith and S.J.H. Biddle (Eds.) *Youth physical activity and sedentary behaviour: challenges and solutions.* Champaign, Il: Human Kinetics. pp.167-192.

Harris, J. and Penney, D. (2000). Gender issues in health-related exercise. *European Physical Education Review*, 6: 249-273.

Hodges Kulinna, P., Martin, J., Lai, Q., Kliber, A. and Reed, B. (2003). Student physical activity patterns: grade, gender, and activity influences. *Journal of Teaching in Physical Education*, 22: 298-310.

Hogg, M.A. and Vaughan, G.M. (1998). *Social psychology (Second Edition)* London: Prentice Hall.

Hopwood, T. and Carrington, B. (1994). Physical education and feminity. *Educational Research*, 36(3): 237-246.

Hovell, M.F., Sallis, J.F., Kolody, B. and McKenzie, T. (1999). Children's physical activity choices: a developmental analysis of gender, intensity levels and time. *Pediatric Exercise Science*, 11: 158-168.

Janz, K.F., Dawson, J.D. and Mahony, L.T. (2002). Increases in physical fitness during childhood improves cardiovascular health during adolescence: The Muscatine Study. *International Journal of Sports Medicine*, 23: S15-S21.

Jones, B.A. (1988) A scale to measure attitudes of school pupils towards their lessons in physical education. *Educational Studies,* 14: 51-63.

Kelder, S., Perry, C., Klepp, K. and Lythe, L. (1994). Longitudinal tracking of adolescent smoking, physical activity and food choices behaviour. *American Journal of Public Health*. 84: 1121-1126.

Kemper, H.C.G. and van Mechelen, W. (1995). Physical fitness and the relationship to physical activity. In H.C.G. Kemper (Ed.) *The Amsterdam Growth Study*. Champaign, Il: Human Kinetics, pp. 174-188.

Koca, C. and Demirhan, G. (2004). An examination of high school students' attitudes toward physical education with regard to sex and sport participation. *Perceptual and Motor Skills*, 98: 754-758.

Koca, C., Asci, F.H. and Demirhan, G. (2005). Attitudes toward physical education and class preferences of Turkish adolescents in terms of school gender composition. *Adolescence,* 40(158): 365-375.

Levine, M.P. and Smolak, L. (2002). Body image development in adolescence. In T. Cash and T. Pruzinsky (Eds.) *Body image: a handbook of theory, research, and clinical practice.* New York: Guilford, pp 74-82.

Luke, M.D. and Sinclair, G.D. (1991). Gender differences in adolescents' attitudes toward school physical education. *Journal of Teaching in Physical Education*, 11: 31-46.

Macfadyen, T. (2000). An analysis of the influence of secondary school physical education on young people's attitudes towards physical activity. *The Bulletin of Physical Education*, 35(3): 157-171.

McIntosh, D. K. and Albinson, A. (1982). Physical education in Ontario secondary schools: a follow-up study. *Canadian Association for Health Education and Recreation Journal*, 48: 14-17.

Milosevic, L. (1996). Pupils experience of P.E. questionnaire results. *The British Journal of Physical Education,* Spring: 16-20.

Mota, J. Santos, P., Guerra, S., Ribeiro, J.C. and Duarte, J.A. (2002). Differences of daily physical activity levels of children according to body mass index. *Pediatric Exercise Science*, 14: 442-452.

Mota, J., Santos, P., Guerra, S., Ribeiro, J.C. and Duarte, J.A. (2003). Patterns of daily physical activity during school days in children and adolescents. *American Journal of Human Biology*, 15: 547-553.

Mulivhill, C., Rivers, K. and Aggleton, P. (2000). *Physical activity 'at our time'. Qualitative research among young people aged 5 to 15 years and parents.* London: Health Education Authority.

National Institute for Health and Clinical Excellence (NICE) (2009). *Promoting physical activity, active play and sport for pre-school and school-age children and young people in family, pre-school, school and community settings.* London: National Institute for Health and Clinical Excellence. NICE public health guidance 17.

Naughton, G.A., Carlson, J.S. and Greene, D.A. (2006). A challenge to fitness testing in primary schools. *Journal of Science and Medicine in Sport*, 9: 40-45.

Olshansky, S.J., Passaro, D.J., Hershow, R.C., Layden, J., Carnes, B.A., Brody, J., Hayflick, L., Butler, R.N., Allison, D.B., and Ludwig, D.S. (2005). A Potential Decline in Life Expectancy in the United States in the 21st Century. *The New England Journal of Medicine.* 352(11): 1138-1145.

Patrick, K., Norman, G.J., Calfas, K.J., Sallis, J.F., Zabinski, M.F., Rupp, J. and Cella, J. (2004). Diet, Physical Activity, and Sedentary Behaviours as Risk Factors for Overweight in Adolescence. *Archives of Pediatric Adolescent Medicine*, 158: 385-390.

Pease, D. G. and Andersen, D. F. (1986). Longitudinal analysis of children's attitudes toward sport team involvement. *Journal of Sport Behaviour*, 9: 3-10.

Portman, P.T. (1995). Who is having fun in physical education classes? Experiences of six grade students in elementary and middle schools. *Journal of Teaching in Physical Education*, 14: 445-453.

Prusak, K.A., Treasure, D.C., Darst, P.W. and Pangrazi, R.P. (2004). The effects of choice on the motivation of adolescent girls in physical education. *Journal of Teaching in Physical Education,* 23: 19-29.

Rikard, G.L. and Banville, D. (2006). High school student attitudes about physical education. *Sport, Education and Society*, 11(4): 385-400.

Rose, C. (1997). Equal opportunities in physical education. *The Bulletin of Physical Education*, 33(1): 26-31.

Rosenberg, C.I. and Hovland, M.J. (Eds) (1960). *Attitude Organization and Change*: *An Analysis of Consistency among Attitude Components.* New Haven, Connecticut: Yale University Press.

Ryan, S., Todorovich, J.R., Bridges, F.S., and Mokgwathi, M.M. (2009). Body shape perceptions, attitudes toward physical education, and physical activity levels of middle school students. *International Journal of Fitness, 5(2):* 21-30.

Sharp, C. (1995). The health of the next generation: health through fitness and sport. *Journal of the Royal Society of Health*, February: 48-55.

Shropshire, J. (1997). *Psychosocial factors associated with children's physical activity levels pre and post transfer to secondary school.* Unpublished PhD thesis, University of Manchester.

Shropshire, J., Carroll, B, and Yim, S. (1997). Primary school children's attitudes to physical education: gender differences. *European Journal of Physical Education*, 2: 23-38.

Silverman, S. and Subramaniam, P.R. (1999). Student attitude toward physical education and physical activity: a review of measurement issues and outcomes. *Journal of Teaching in Physical Education,* 19: 97-125.

Sleap, M and Warburton, P. (1992). Physical activity levels of 5-11 year-old children in England as determined by continuous observation. *Research Quarterly for Exercise and Sport*, 63(3): 238-245.

Strong, W.B., Malina, R.M., Blimkie, C.J.R., Daniels, S.R., Dishman, R.K., Gutin, B., Hergenroeder, A.C., Must, A., Nixon, P.A., Pivarnik, J.M., Rowland, T., Trost, S. and Trudeau, F. (2005). Evidence based physical activity for school-age youth. *Journal of Pediatrics*, 146: 732-737.

Subramaniam, P.R. and Silverman, S. (2000). Validation of scores from an instrument assessing student attitude toward physical education. *Measurement in Physical Education and Exercise Science,* 4: 29-43.

Tomik, R. (2008). Students' membership in school sports clubs and their attitudes towards physical education and sport in various types of schools. *Human Movement*, 9(2): 142-149.

Trudeau, F., Laurencelle, L., Tremblay, J., Rajic, M. and Shephard, R.J. (1999). Daily primary school physical education: effects on physical activity during adult life. *Medicine and Science in Sports and Exercise*, 31: 338-342.

Twisk, J.W.R. (2001). Physical activity guidelines for children and adolescents. A critical review. *Sports Medicine*, 31(8): 617-627.

Wardle, J., Henning Brodersen, N., Cole, T.J., Jarvis, M.J. and Boniface, D.R. (2006). Development of adiposity in adolescence: five year longitudinal study of an ethnically and socioeconomically diverse sample of young people in Britain. *British Medical Journal*, 332: 1130-1135.

Williams, A. and Bedward, J. (1999). A more inclusive curriculum framework (QCA, 1999): making physical education relevant to adolescent girls. *British Journal of Physical Education*, Autumn: 6-10.

Zahner, L., Puder, J.J., Roth, R., Schmid, M., Guldimann, R., Phüse, U., Knöpfli, M., Braun-Fahrländer, C., Marti, B. and Kriemler, S. (2006). A school-based physical activity programme to improve health and fitness in children aged 6-13 years ("Kinder-Sportstudie KISS"): study design of a randomized controlled trial. *BioMed Central Public Health*, 6: 147-158.

In: Reviews in Pediatric Exercise Science
Editor: Michael Duncan, pp. 27-41
ISBN: 978-1-61470-978-7

Chapter III

Promoting Cardiovascular Health in the Primary School Curriculum

Moira N. McPherson, Kimberly Boardman, William J. Montelpare and Carlos E. Zerpa
Lakehead University, Canada.

Introduction

Cardiovascular disease is one of the leading causes of death worldwide (Institute of Medicine, 2010). Yet more important is the number of individuals affected by the progressive characteristics of the disease. Dai, Bancej, Bienek, Walsh, Stewart, and Wielgosz (2009) reported that about four percent of the total population of Canada is living with heart disease and one out of every three adult deaths in Canada can be attributed to some form of cardiovascular disease. Conditions such as obesity, hypertension, and diabetes, are known contributing factors to cardiovascular disease, and as such increase the prevalence of cardiovascular disease, globally.

The impact of cardiovascular disease on death rate and loss of quality of life years remaining is so profound that Donatelle (2009) suggested if all forms of cardiovascular disease were eliminated, the life expectancy in the United States could increase by seven years. In 2008 it was estimated that the economic burden of cardiovascular disease in the United States was more than 448.5 billion dollars (Rosamond et al., 2008). This estimated cost is attributed to several factors, such as, the cost of physician and nursing services, in-hospital care charges, as well as nursing home services, medications and various home health care needs. In addition to the direct medical costs of cardiovascular disease related illnesses, the financial burdens within a society are also impacted by the loss of productivity due to illness, absenteeism-replacement workers, health insurance increases, family hardship, and decreased quality of life years remaining.

One condition that reduces cardiovascular health is atherosclerosis. Atherosclerosis involves the thickening of the walls of the arteries and loss of elasticity as a result of atheroma plaque accumulation. Over time, a reduction in blood flow could result in a myocardial infarction, also known as a heart attack. In addition to the build-up of plaque, the potential accumulation of blood can result in the artery becoming weak and rupturing. There is an increased recognition that the atherosclerotic process can start in children as early as six months of age (Harrell, McMurray, Gansky, Bangdiwala, and Bradley, 1999).

A direct effect of atherosclerotic plaque development is the reduction of oxygenated blood supply to the myocardium. The resulting ischemic condition may cause a variety of degrees of chest pain also known as angina pectoris. Congestive heart failure occurs when the heart muscle is overworked or damaged and does not have the capacity to continue to circulate blood normally throughout the body. If the heart is weakened there will be a reduction in the driving pressure required to push blood throughout the arterial system. A decrease in arterial driving pressure will eventually reduce the pressure that moves the blood returning through the veins, and thereby lead to congestion in the body tissues. As a result, the heart muscle can hypertrophy, or become larger, and therefore decrease its efficiency. The decreased efficiency of the myocardium can limit blood flow throughout the body, and as a result, blood can accumulate in the lower extremities or the lungs (Kavey, Daniels, Lauer, Atkins, Hayman, and Taubert, 2003).

It is crucial that children be introduced to the controllable risk factors for cardiovascular disease and the potential health implications of poor heart health behaviours, at an early age. For example, congestive heart failure is a result of previous harm done to the heart muscle, yet the condition can be avoided if care is taken at a young age. Since children who are overweight often carry the risk factors of cardiovascular disease into adulthood, an increased number of adults are at risk of dying from cardiovascular disease or incurring co-morbidities such as adult onset diabetes, hypertension or chronic obstructive pulmonary disease (Veugelers and Fitzgerald, 2005; Sin, Anthonisen, Soriano, and Agusti, 2006, Fuster and Kelly, 2010).

Cardiovascular disease risk factors can be categorized into factors that can be controlled and factors that cannot be controlled. Among the factors that we cannot control are: heredity, age, sex and race. The factors that can be controlled include tobacco avoidance (smoking), frequency, intensity and duration of quality daily physical activity, stress, and the dietary consumption of saturated fats and cholesterol. These factors are controlled by behaviour choices that if attended to in the pre-pubescent years can change the risk for cardiovascular disease as well as many other health related problems.

The health consequences of a poor lifestyle, leading to progressive cardiovascular disease, are a heavy burden to the health care system and as such primary prevention through health education and illness awareness for primary school aged children is critical (Kavey, et al., 2003). Children may have the ability to improve their health status by consciously maintaining a healthy diet while adopting a lifestyle that includes daily physical activity and avoiding exposure to tobacco products (Donatelle, 2009).

Cardiovascular disease risk factors can be reduced through a variety of intervention strategies. School health interventions that focus on cardiovascular health provide a great opportunity to enhance the future health and well-being of children because they involve children during critical periods of growth and maturation (Veugelers and Fitzgerald, 2005).

The objective of this chapter is to discuss research that has examined the effectiveness of cardiovascular health intervention programs that have incorporated knowledge from the study of physical education and exercise science, and have been delivered in the primary school classroom. A second objective is to describe strategies for success in overcoming challenges to changing health behaviours.

Primary School Interventions Designed to Promote Cardiovascular Health

The study of exercise science has influenced the promotion of physical activity and of health and nutrition awareness and has targeted changes in adolescents' attitudes and behaviours toward sedentary lifestyle and poor-nutrition choices. The main tenets of school-based cardiovascular disease risk factor interventions include awareness to change unhealthy eating, tobacco avoidance, and involvement in regular physical activity.

Work by Arbeit, Johnson, Mott, Harsha, et al., (Arbeit, et al., 1992) is an example of an attempt to integrate a wider school and family/community approach to address cardiovascular disease prevention. In their work, Arbeit et al. combined the physical education curriculum with cardiovascular disease knowledge development through science classes, a healthy-choice nutrition lunch program, physical fitness testing, and a cardiovascular risk factor screening program, to determine if a comprehensive approach to health promotion could increase the frequency of positive targeted health outcomes in a group of intervention versus control schools.

While Arbeit, et al. (1992) did not find support for the contention that increased knowledge about healthy lifestyle behaviours would lead directly to behavioural change, the researchers were able to show, as we have now come to expect, that participants were more likely to demonstrate positive trends toward cardiovascular disease prevention when adopting a behavioural change that included greater participation in physical activity pursuits, and attention to dietary intake of unhealthy nutrition choices. Yet as Arbeit and co-workers also stated, the intervention was considered successful because of the comprehensiveness and multi-modal delivery of the cardiovascular disease prevention program, an approach that may not be considered feasible in some school settings.

One program that was specifically designed to evaluate children's food choices, knowledge about food, and self-efficacy with regard to diet was the Child and Adolescent Trial for Cardiovascular Health (CATCH) program. Developed during the early 1990s this program was created as a multi-centre school based intervention to promote healthy behaviours among elementary school students (Webber, Osganian, Luepker, Feldman, et al., 1995). The sample was based on 3714 students from 96 schools from four different regions within the United States. Although the main goal of CATCH was to reduce serum total cholesterol, secondary objectives were to reduce the consumption of saturated fats and salt, to increase the volume of daily physical activity, and to prevent the onset of cigarette smoking. The underlying rationale for this program was that making children aware of specific health concerns, and establishing positive lifestyle behaviours needs to be accomplished at a young age before behaviour patterns and lifestyle choices become entrenched.

As noted by the authors, the CATCH program demonstrated that a large-scale lifestyle change intervention program could maintain participant involvement and achieve objectives when there was sufficient will among the stakeholders (Webber et al., 1995). The success of CATCH was considered to be more than changing physical health outcomes within the sample cohorts, rather CATCH demonstrated a best practice solution for decision makers and school systems considering the adoption of a behaviour change program.

The Cardiovascular Health in Children Study (Harrell et al., 1999) used two different cardiovascular disease risk factor intervention strategies targeted at children in grades three and four who exhibited positive cardiovascular disease risk factors. Eighteen schools from the state of North Carolina participated in this public health education based program. In the first intervention, students were provided information from the American Heart Association school site kits, twice a week over an eight-week period. Students worked through materials that focused on 'heart healthy foods', the harmful effects of smoking, and the importance of participating in regular physical activity. In addition to the classroom-based presentations, students participated in a physical activity class three times each week.

For the second intervention, students were assigned to the risk-based group if they showed one or more cardiovascular disease risk factors. This second intervention strategy applied one of three separate approaches; i) a nutrition class, ii) a physical activity class, or iii) a "don't start smoking" class, which students attended based on their pre-existing risk factors (Harrell et al., 1999). The outcome of the intervention on these students was an improvement in self-reported physical activity scores and total healthy heart knowledge, with a concomitant decrease in the presence of earlier identified cardiovascular disease risk factors. Again supporting the contention that lifelong health behaviours are formed in the early years of life, and that elementary school provides a critical venue for intervention (Harrell et al., 1999).

Based on the earlier findings from the CATCH study, it was believed that a self-report classroom administered questionnaire was the best way to obtain valid measures of students' knowledge and attitudes toward healthy lifestyles. As a response to the alarming rates of childhood obesity the PATHWAYS Study was designed to change American Indian females' behaviour, knowledge and attitudes towards diet and physical activity (Stevens, Cornell, Story, French, Levin, Becenti, et al., 1999). Initial research from the PATHWAYS project relied heavily on previously conducted studies of nutrition health interventions in the development of an instrument that could be considered reliable and valid for subsequent applications.

The PATHWAYS Study was implemented in six American Indian cohorts at eight different schools. The questionnaire focused on four different areas: physical activity, diet, weight related attitudes, and cultural sensitivity. In total, the questionnaire consisted of 130 questions that were administered in three separate sections over a period of two to three days. Students completed each section of the survey in approximately 30 minutes.

After more than two years of psychometric evaluations, Stevens and co-workers reported that the PATHWAYS survey was reliable and valid, and although the plan was to continue development, the tool was deemed to be useable in subsequent research. As a result Caballero, Clay, Davis, Ethelbah, Holy Rock, and Lohman, et al. (2003) applied the PATHWAYS intervention strategy consisting of four components: classroom curriculum, food service, physical activity, and family involvement to a sample of 41 schools in seven American Indian communities within the USA. Each component had a specific structure that included a clearly articulated purpose and established measurement properties based on results from previous testing. For example, the classroom curriculum component used a schedule of delivering classroom lectures about healthy eating and increased physical activity to 3rd, 4th, and 5th grade students twice weekly for between 8 and 12 weeks. The food service intervention was a plan to work with school officials to change the lunchroom diet by reducing fat consumption while maintaining appropriate nutrient intake. The physical activity section was specifically directed to increasing energy expenditure in the school environment, and the family involvement approach was intended to assist families in creating a supportive environment for healthy behaviours.

The researchers (Caballero et al., 2003) concluded that although there was no significant decrease in percentage of body fat for persons in the intervention cohorts, overall the PATHWAYS program led to a significant reduction in dietary fat consumption both as a result of changes to the school menu as well as through changes to personal eating behaviours. Similarly, the authors found that providing a classroom curriculum that was culturally appropriate could lead to changes, both in health related knowledge, as well as in the adoption of healthy behaviours among children in this younger age cohort, a finding that supports the early introduction of knowledge development for lifelong positive healthy choices. Less of an impact was seen from changes to the implementation of physical activities during school time, through both explicit curriculum programming and intention to reduce sedentary behaviours. However, the researchers felt that the latter outcome was a result that required a sustained commitment over a long-term.

In 2003, the Children's Lifestyle and School-performance Study (CLASS) used a survey administered to grade 5 students in the province of Nova Scotia, Canada (Veugelers and Fitzgerald, 2005). This study targeted 242 of the 291 public schools in Nova Scotia and focused on nutrition, health and lifestyle behaviours. The selected survey was a modified version of the Harvard Youth/Adolescent Food Frequency Questionnaire. The CLASS survey included questions from the Harvard study pertaining to nutritional intake along with questions related to physical activity involvement.

In analyzing the precursors to obesity, the researchers concluded that the frequency of physical activity involvement was the only activity-related factor associated with being overweight. However, the researchers also concluded that parents, who achieved higher levels of education and had an income of over $60,000.00 per annum, were considered to have a lower risk of becoming overweight (Veugelers and Fitzgerald, 2005). The results of the CLASS study also suggested that integrated school programs which included: physical education, healthy lunches, health and nutrition education, training of staff, parental involvement, and concomitantly banning the sale of soft drinks, were successful in improving the students' dietary consumption of unhealthy foods and reducing overweight and obesity by some 59 and 72 percent, respectively (Veugelers and Fitzgerald, 2005).

The Physical Activity and Teenage Health (PATH) program is a school-based intervention that was instituted in three ethnically diverse New York City high schools (Bayne-Smith, Fardy, Azzollini, Magel and Schmitz, 2004). Four hundred and forty two adolescent females took part in a 12-week program that combined a regimen of vigorous physical activity and formal lectures on nutrition, exercise, stress, and smoking. The program was conducted five days per week over a 12-week duration. Heart health knowledge, health behaviours, and cardiovascular risk factors were assessed before and after the 12-week program using a questionnaire. Changes in physical fitness from the start to the end of the program were evaluated using a physical activity standardized measure. Lecture topics included: anatomy and physiology of the heart, cardiovascular risk factors and strategies for decreasing high-risk health behaviours (Bayne-Smith et al., 2004). In order to ensure consistency in delivery message and style, the Physical Education teachers responsible for program implementation participated in a training program prior to as well as during the intervention.

The student group was considered multi-culturally diverse with a high prevalence of cardiovascular disease risk factors, which if not dealt with early in life could have long-term health implications for many participants within the group (Bayne-Smith et al., 2004). Most important, the researchers were able to demonstrate that as a result of the health intervention in the selected cohort, there was a significant reduction in estimated percent of body fat, resting blood pressure, and heart health knowledge among study participants.

The Coronary Artery Risk Detection In Appalachian Communities (CARDIAC) program was developed as a cardiovascular disease screening intervention to address the rise in childhood obesity in primary schools in Western Virginia (Cottrell, Spangler-Murphy, Minor, Downes, Nicholson and Neal, 2005). In this cohort, the researchers found that in addition to a lack of general knowledge about healthy eating and ways that parents might provide more physical activity opportunities for children, there were also environmental factors identified that may have contributed to the higher rates of overweight or obese individuals in this geographic area. Constraints on grocery selection, poverty, and driving distance each contribute to a poor health trajectory for these individuals. Recognizing the need to change physical inactivity and diet, the approach targeted grade five students in the region, addressing not only the needs of the adolescents directly, but incorporating ways to increase parental knowledge about healthy diet and physical activity opportunities.

This study included an evaluation of the effectiveness of incorporating parents as part of the intervention. Students were given pedometers to track their daily step count and a journal to record their daily food intake. Parents also completed a questionnaire of perceptions of their child's health. Sadly, the results showed that 31% of the student participants were overweight or obese and that 65% of the parents of these children believed that their child received a sufficient amount of daily physical activity (Cottrell et al., 2005). The role of parents in controlling the health behaviours of children is central to long term health outcomes. Further, as Cottrell demonstrated, a parent's beliefs and behaviours are shaped by their level of knowledge and as such can directly influence the behaviours and health outcomes of their children.

Positive outcomes from previous research support the contention that developing knowledge about risk factors and health outcomes can lead to changes in attitudes and behaviours. School based health promotion programs and the application of health promoting school strategies (Rogers, Moon, Mullee, Speller, and Roderick, 1998; Macnab, Radziminski, Budden, Kasangaki, et al., 2010; Lynagh, Schofield, Sanson-Fisher, 1997) can have a positive impact on improving a student's level of knowledge about health related issues (Addison, Jenkins, White, and Young, 2006; Warren, Henry, Lightowler, Bradshaw and Perwaiz, 2008), and in some situations change behaviours that if ignored could lead to negative health consequences. For example, the *Eat Well and Keep Moving Program* developed by Warren, et al., (2008) exemplifies the incorporation of a program intended to decrease the consumption of foods high in saturated and total fat, increase fruit and vegetable intake, reduce television viewing time, and increase levels of physical activity with the traditional curriculum elements of math, science, language arts, and social science. This type of interdisciplinary approach provided opportunities for students to learn about health issues in a variety of non-traditional settings, including identifying links to community for free or low cost nutrition and physical activity programming for parents and students. Yet the challenge is not merely to implement programs of information about health risk factors, since Subramaniam and Silverman (2007) showed, students' attitude toward healthy lifestyle maintenance declines as they progress in grade level. Rather, the challenge is to create programs that can maintain positive attitudes as well as positive lifestyle behaviours for students and their families within their communities.

The Trial of Activity for Adolescent Girls (TAAG) program is an example of an approach designed specifically to accommodate links between schools and communities in order to increase the physical activity level of adolescent girls (Young, Steckler, Cohen, Pratt, Felton, Moe, et al., 2008). The TAAG program used a multi-dimensional intervention and included both health and physical education activities for schools as well as physical activity programs within the community. The outcomes of the TAAG program were evaluated through a formative research design using both oral and written reports that collected information from various stakeholders throughout the delivery of the TAAG intervention. The results indicated that the two critical factors required for successful implementation of healthy lifestyle programs that combine formal education with community based programming are the consistency of the programs that are delivered, along with the frequency of delivery and access to the programs.

Consistent with the argument that messages about cardiovascular disease prevention should be delivered to students at an early age (Swan and Gatzoulis, 2002), Arvidson (1990) developed the Children's Cardiovascular Health Promotion Attitude Scale (CVHPAS) for students between the ages of 8 and 12 years. The instrument is comprised of 22 multiple-choice questions using a four-point ordinal scale and focusing on four contributing factors to the development of cardiovascular disease: physical activity, nutrition, smoking, and stress. The instrument draws upon the concepts of modelled behaviour proposed by Bandura's Social-Learning Theory (1971), which states that modelling is not only used to produce imitative behaviours, but facilitates the internalizing of behaviours as the individual's own. Further applications of the survey to children between the ages of 8 and 12 showed that the CVHPAS has potential to provide health professionals and other researchers with valid and reliable measures of children's attitudes toward cardiovascular health.

More recent work by Toepperwein, Pruski, Blalock, Lemelle, and Lichtenstein (2008) provides strong support for the development of researcher-teacher partnerships in establishing a clear message about cardiovascular disease prevention through multi-modal delivery of early education. The work of Toepperwein, et al. (2008) is based on the understanding that atherosclerotic plaque and cardiovascular disease begins in early childhood and can be prevented through positive lifestyle changes that include a regimen of daily physical activity and an awareness to eating healthy. However, the greater challenge is in overcoming the illiteracy that exists among adults and children with respect to useful health information.

Toepperwein and co-workers indicated that the cardiovascular disease prevention message can be effectively delivered through the health curriculum within the formal structure of elementary school programs, and ultimately can be an effective modality to change lifestyle behaviours of children. The rationale for selecting students in grades 6 to 8 is based on the contention that this is a developmental period in the lives of children, where there is a potential to change health damaging attitudes, introduce health promoting choices, and take advantage of the emergence of independent thinking among children in this age cohort. Through an approach referred to as Teacher Enrichment Initiatives (TEI), researchers work with classroom teachers and school administrators to develop cardiovascular disease prevention curriculum/materials that can enhance the delivery of the prevention message and eventually create a behavioural change. TEI teachers are empowered to build on their strengths as facilitators of learning within the elementary age school student. Participating instructors work with curriculum designers and scientists to incorporate constructivist pedagogical principles in the development of lessons that challenge students to move out of their learning comfort zones. According to Toepperwein et al. (2008), each lesson includes specific learning objectives, relevant content materials and activities, as well as measurements of pre and post subject knowledge. Using this systematic approach enables teachers to follow a clear path of information presentation, while researchers can evaluate the effectiveness of the curriculum delivery.

As Toepperwein suggested, incorporating a process of evaluation into the TEI approach is essential to establishing the appropriateness of content-to-knowledge development in this age cohort, while determining the effectiveness of classroom instruction. Building a database of outcome assessments provides valuable evidence that the use of this curriculum delivery approach influences behavioural changes that have positive cardiovascular disease prevention outcomes. Most important however, is that while the evaluation measures can be used to modify content, delivery, and evaluation, they also help to shape the pedagogical development of the classroom teacher and in so doing are essential to the development of curriculum that improves health literacy.

In Canada, the Wizards of Motion program was designed by researchers at Lakehead University to introduce concepts of biomechanics and/or exercise physiology to elementary school students, while integrating healthy lifestyle messages (McPherson, Marsh, Montelpare, Van Barneveld and Zerpa, 2009). Using various curriculum delivery approaches, scientific experts in biomechanics, cardiovascular physiology, health, and education visited grade 5 and grade 7 classrooms with portable, self-contained laboratory experiences. The Wizards of Motion modules were intentionally designed to link closely with the Provincial Ministry of Education's science curriculum while enhancing classroom delivery and including an elementary school appropriate health message.

Boardman (2010) conducted an evaluation study of the Wizards of Motion Cardiovascular Module to determine the extent to which this specific module was effective in changing students' knowledge and attitudes related to cardiovascular disease and to adopting healthy lifestyle behaviours. An intervention was designed whereby scientific experts visited grade 5 elementary school classrooms and delivered a dynamic multimedia presentation that focused on basic cardiovascular physiology while highlighting factors that contribute to positive physical health. Students constructed a model of the cardiovascular system that demonstrated circulatory dynamics in response to changes in blood volume, capillary constriction, and pumping of the heart. The study used a two-group pre-post comparison design in which the intervention group ($n1= 39$ students) completed a knowledge test and an attitudes survey before and after receiving the intervention, while the control group ($n2= 31$ students) completed the same knowledge test and attitudes survey during the same time frame but did not receive the Wizards of Motion module.

The results showed that the Wizards of Motion module led to a statistically significant increase in post-test scores for both the knowledge test and the attitudes survey for the intervention group compared to the control group. The positive findings indicate that the intervention was effective in increasing the sample of students' level of knowledge about cardiovascular disease and changing their attitudes toward adopting healthy lifestyle behaviours. The success of increasing grade 5 student's knowledge and attitudes related to cardiovascular disease and adopting healthy lifestyle behaviours illustrates that a program such as the Wizards of Motion is a valuable education tool in order to assist in health promotion within elementary schools. The findings of the Wizards study support previous research, which has emphasized the importance of health education for young students.

Changing Health Behaviours

Cardiovascular disease risk factors are well known and can be reduced through a variety of intervention strategies. The health consequences of a poor lifestyle leading to progressive cardiovascular disease are a heavy burden to the health care system. The research that has been presented has shown clearly that primary prevention efforts must target young children (Kavey, et al., 2003). The global increase in the prevalence of cardiovascular disease rates support the argument that there is a need to educate the public about primary prevention. Yet, there are many challenges in this process. For example, Russell, Champika, Soysa, Wagoner and Dawson (2008) indicated that teaching cardiovascular disease prevention effectively is dependent on the level of knowledge about the specific condition in the community in which the prevention message is delivered. Likewise, there must be an intrinsic desire by the targeted individual to change their behaviours from those that have a negative health consequence to behaviours that lead to positive health outcomes.

Yet merely being told about a risk factor may not help to increase the knowledge of cardiovascular disease risk factors or enforce the cardiovascular disease prevention message effectively. Rather, providing accurate and meaningful evidence, like showing the relationship between a suggested risk factor and an outcome may better illustrate the magnitude of the risk factors within a specific cohort. For example, while there is a plethora of support for the evidence that an increase in percent body fat is a general risk factor for progressive cardiovascular disease, using location of fat – in particular the increase in abdominal fat, has become a more precise estimator of cardiovascular disease risk. Statistics, such as those reported by Schwandt, Bertsch, and Haas (2010) that the ratio of waist circumference to height of children in the UK rose from 5% to 17% in males and 1.5% to 11.7% in females in a twenty-year period from 1977 to 1997, provide a disquieting estimate of the increased risk of cardiovascular disease within this aging cohort.

In their studies, Schwandt and coworkers showed that using a simple, low cost measure like the ratio of waist circumference to height, the cardiovascular disease risk could be estimated with greater precision than when using a general estimate like the body mass index. This finding is important because it showed that through this simple measure researchers could calculate the estimator in population-based studies of large communities easily and thereby provide essential evidence to support the prevention message.

Similar evidence was shown by Maffeis, Banzato, and Talamini, et al. (2008) in a study using children from Italy to compare the estimates of metabolic and cardiovascular risk factors using i) waist circumference, ii) the ratio of waist circumference to height, and iii) body mass index. Similar to the Schwandt study, the research supports that there was tremendous value in estimating localized abdominal fat rather than merely describing BMI as a risk factor of cardiovascular disease. These findings are easily incorporated into the cardiovascular disease prevention message for children, because they are straightforward to acquire, and following collection, can generate useful discussion in explaining the importance of fat accumulation as a risk factor for cardiovascular disease.

Although there is widespread support for the delivery of the cardiovascular disease prevention message to children in the younger age groups (Fleming, Green, Martin, and Wicks, 2000), the behavioural changes that are sought through the education programs are difficult to initiate and maintain among pre-adolescent aged individuals. This is especially true if the school and/or home environments do not support the changes in lifestyle needed to reduce the risk factors.

The elementary school curriculum is widely recognized as the primary pathway through which to deliver health education messages (Bartlett, 1981; Nutbeam, 1992; Guinan, McGuckin, Ali, 2002; Collins, Kearns, Mitchell, 2006; Macnab, Radziminski, Budden, Kasangaki, et al., 2010). Schools need to develop and adopt heart healthy policies in order to promote an environment that encourages healthy eating and being physically active every day. Since adolescents spend approximately six hours each weekday in the classroom, teachers, administrators, and parents, need to be aware of the substantial positive effects heart healthy behaviour choices will have on the students' learning.

Two studies that build on the concept of using the elementary school to develop a child's knowledge about physical fitness and healthy eating behaviours were published by Shilts, Lamp, Horowitz, and Townsend (2009), and earlier by Burgeson, Wechsler, Brener, Young, and Spain (2001). In the Burgeson study, the researchers described the importance of promoting physical education for the health of young people, and the importance of developing school health policies and physical activity programs to enhance the level of fitness in youth. Burgeson and co-workers described the findings from the School Health Policies and Programs Study 2000, a US-based, nationwide review of state and regional requirements for physical education programming. Using a survey methodology, Burgeson collected data across the spectrum of elementary education, from the classroom level to the state level, and for all fifty states, to determine the extent to which schools delivered daily quality physical education and health, and to identify specific characteristics within the programs, such as student evaluations, guidelines and standards, exemptions for special needs, as well as staffing and professional preparation requirements. Their results indicated that more than 95% of elementary schools required that students take some form of physical education as part of the curriculum, and most elementary schools—more than 95%, provide regularly scheduled recess of some frequency and duration, daily.

However, daily recess was reserved for selected grades and not all grades received the same volume of recess nor did they receive the same frequency of recess during the day or week. Additionally, only some 66% of schools reported that students were able to access the schools athletic/recreational facilities outside of normal school hours.

Further, while elementary schools may have the potential to deliver the cardiovascular disease prevention message, in summarizing the actual delivery of daily quality physical and health education, Burgeson and colleagues reported that only eight percent of elementary schools in the United States provided daily quality physical education or its equivalent throughout the entire year.

In an attempt to demonstrate that nutrition awareness and physical education are essential components of the elementary school curriculum, Shilts, et al. (2009), investigated the effect of incorporating a program of healthy eating and regular physical activity skill development into the elementary school curriculum for children aged 11-14 years, to enhance academic performance. The researchers used a quasi-experimental crossover-controlled design for a sample of 95 grade six students, in which all participants were tested on specific standardized academic performance tests on three separate occasions (baseline, at 5 weeks and at 10 weeks).

The results showed that following the treatment period (week 5 to week 10) the children showed higher gains in academic achievements in comparison to the control period (baseline to week 5). Specifically, the intervention was associated with significantly higher performance scores on the standardized tests of listening and speaking, mathematical reasoning, and algebra and functions. According to Shilts these findings were to be expected given that previous research supports, in general, the contention that a student's health and academic achievements are linked, and that such indicators as school attendance, academic performance, and cognitive ability are correlated with nutritional status and measures of obesity. However, the results of Shilts and coworkers were the first to show that the combination of a nutrition education program with a program of physical activity skill and behaviour development had a directly positive influence on academic achievement, providing additional support for the inclusion of health education as a necessary part of the accepted elementary school curriculum.

Yet the conundrum, initially articulated by Bartlett (1981), that health education is, "*very effective in increasing knowledge, somewhat effective in improving attitudes, and, with a few notable exceptions, generally ineffective in changing health practices*", continues to challenge educators and public health officials. Behaviour change is a complex process and involves attention to both the level of knowledge and changes in attitude. Educating students about cardiovascular disease with the hopes of improving their level of knowledge does not necessarily mean that these students will change their health related behaviours. Health education interventions need to combine information that will lead to improvements in both knowledge and attitudes in order to acquire behavioural change. An individual must first have knowledge about healthy lifestyle behaviours in order to shape their attitude towards healthy lifestyle choices such as exercising. Students must be aware of why they should be adopting healthy lifestyle behaviours in order to justify their actions. The students' attitudes are formulated from numerous factors including their beliefs and past experiences. A student's attitude is central to the learning process and can contribute to the formation of intentions, which lead to actions (Miller et al., 1982; Torabi and Jeng, 2001).

Warren, et al., (2008) suggested that health education programs should strive to change behaviours so that there will be a measurable long-term influence on health. As Edelman and Mandle (2002) suggest, health education should result in behaviour change that is voluntary, but is a function of the integration of knowledge (past and present) with attitudes, personal skills, and environmental conditions.

A major problem faced by health educators in establishing a measurable behavioural change among students at the primary school level is that they may not be able to practice what they are taught. Quite simply, children between the ages of seven to fourteen do not have a great deal of decision-making since their parent or guardian is the authority (Rezendes, 2006). Children at this age are not responsible for purchasing food and making meals at home, although they have the ability to pester their parents/guardian into being more health conscious. Despite that students have been informed about the pitfalls of several lifestyle events to which they are exposed, because they do not have the ability to change their immediate circumstances they may choose to disengage from the material that they are presented or become frustrated in the learning process by the inability to act.

Empowerment for decision-making to change behaviour is only one of the challenges to a child adopting a lifestyle that will lead to long-term positive health outcomes. There are several other challenges, some of which include access to information, the development of prior knowledge, perception, and the environment, both physically and socially.

Conclusion

A fundamental premise of this chapter is that if we can change a child's level of knowledge about cardiovascular disease risk factors, then their understanding of lifestyle behaviours that lead to positive health outcomes will improve, as will their likelihood to make positive lifestyle choices. Lee, Tsang, Lee, and To (2003) suggested that by teaching health education across the curriculum, students are better prepared to make healthy choices because they develop a greater ability to read and comprehend health issues, as well as to understand the implications of healthy choices. Improving attitudes about making healthy choices will also have a long-term influence on an individual's health status. However, as Holt and Ricciardelli (2008) have indicated, the window of opportunity to shape positive health behaviours is narrow, and becomes smaller as children reach adolescence, develop into teenagers, and become young adults. Throughout this review, it was noted that the greatest opportunity to influence positive lifestyle decisions are in the pre-adolescent years.

While, the importance of health education and early intervention on increasing positive attitudes about cardiovascular disease prevention is evident, the strategy for development and implementation of a comprehensive elementary school based cardiovascular disease prevention curriculum that will lead to measureable changes in healthy behaviours requires continued efforts.

References

Addison, C., Jenkins, W., White, M., and Young, L. (2006). Implementation of a cardiovascular disease prevention program among school-aged children: A pilot study. *International Journal of Environmental Research and Public Health, 3* (3), 264-277.

Arbeit, M., Johnson, C., Mott, D., Harsha, D., Nicklas, T., Webber, L., et al. (1992). The Heart Smart Cardiovascular School Health Promotion: Behavior Correlates of Risk Factor Change. *Preventive Medicine, 21*, 1832.

Arvidson, C. (1990). Children's Cardiovascular Health Promotion Attitude Scale: An instrument development. *Doctoral disserataion (5202B)*, 745. (D. A. International, Compiler) Texas: Texas Women's University.

Bandura, A. *Behavior therapy from a social learning perspective.* London, England: International Congress of Psychology.

Bandura, A. (1971). *Psychological Modeling.* New York: Aldine-Atherton.

Bandura, A., and Walters, R. (1963). *Social learning and personality development.* NY: Holt, Rinehart and Winston.

Bartlett, E. (1981). The contribution of shcool health education to community health promotion: What can we reasonbly expect? *American Journal of Public Health, 71*, 1384-1391.

Bayne-Smith, M., Fardy, P., Azzollini, A., Magel, J., and Schmitz, K. (2004). Improvements in heart health behaviors and reduction in coronary artery disease risk factors in urban teenaged girls through a school-based intervention: The PATH program. *American Journal of Public Health, 94* (9), 1538-1543.

Boardman, K. (2010, June 1). Unpublished Masters Thesis. Lakehead University.

Burgeson, H. W., Brener, N. D., Young, J. C., and Spain, C. G. (2001). Physical Education and Activity: Results from the School Health Policies and Programs Study 2000. *Journal of School Health, 71* (7), 279-293.

Caballero, B., Clay, T., Davis, S., Ethelbah, B., Holy Rock, B., Lohman, T., et al. (2003). Pathways: a school-based, randomized controlled trial for the prevention of obesity in American Indian school children. *American Journal of Clinical Nutrition, 78*, 1030-1038.

Collins, D., Kearns, R., and Mitchell, H. (2006). An integral part of the children's education: Placing sun protection in Auckland primary schools. *Health and Place, 12*, 436-448.

Cottrell, L., Spangler-Murphy, E., Minor, V., Downes, A., Nicholson, P., and Neal, W. (2005). Kindergarten Cardiovascular Risk Surveillance Study: CARDIAC-Kinder. *American Journal of Health Behavior, 29* (6), 595-606.

Dai, S., Bancej, C., Bienek, A., Walsh, P., Stewart, P., and Wielgosz, A. (2009). Tracking Heart Disease and Stroke in Canada 2009.

Dontatelle, R. (2009). *Access to Health.* Toronto, Ontario: Pearson Education Canada Inc.

Edelman, C., and Mandle, C. (2002). *Health promotion: Throughout the lifespan.* Toronto, ON: Mosby.

Fleming, T., Green, J., J.C., M., and Wicks, M. (2000). Effectiveness of a cardiovascular health promotion education intervention on the attitudes of urban African American school-age children . *Journal of Community Health Nursing, 17* (1), 49-60.

Guinan, M., McGuckin, M., and Ali, Y. (2002). The effect of a comprehensive handwashing prgram on absenteeism in elementary schools. *American Journal of Infection Control, 30* (4), 217-220.

Harrell, J., McMurray, R., Gansky, S., Bangdiwala, S., and Bradley, C. (1999). A public health vs a risk based intervention to improve cardiovascular health in elementary school children: The Cardiovascular Health in Children Study. *American Journal of Public Health, 89* (10), 1529-1535.

Holt, K., and Ricciardelli, L. (2008). Weight concerns among elementary school children: A review of prevention programs. *Body Image, 5*, 233.

Institute of Medicine. (2010). *Promoting Cardiovascular Health in the Developing World: A Critical Challenge to Achieve Global Health.* (V. Fuster, and B. Kelly, Eds.) Washington, DC: National Academies Press.

Kavey, R., Daniels, S., Lauer, R., Atkins, D., Hayman, L., and Taubert, K. (2003). Heart Association guidelines for primary prevention of atherosclerotic cardiovascular disease beginning in childhood. *Circulation, 107*, 1562-1566.

Lee, A., Tsang, C., Lee, S., and To, C. (2003). A comprehensive "Healthy Schools Programme" to promote school health: the Hong Kong experience in joining the efforts of health and education sectors. *Journal of Epidemiology and Community Health, 57*, 174-177.

Lynagh, M., Schofield, M., and Sanson-Fisher, R. (1997). School health promotion programs over the past decade: A review of the smoking, alcohol and solar protection literature. *Health Promotion International, 12* (1), 43-60.

Maffeis, C., Banzato, C., and Talamini, G. (2008). Waist-to-height ratio, a useful index to identify high metabolic risk in overweight children. *Journal of Pediatrics*, 207-213.

Mcnab, A., Radziminski, N., Budden, H., Kasangaki, A., Zavuga, R., Gagnon, F., et al. (2010). Brighter Smiles Africa: Translation of a Canadian community-based health - promotion school program to Uganda. *Education for Health, 23* (2).

McPherson, M., Marsh, P., Montelpare, W., Van Barneveld, C., and Zerpa, C. (2009). An evaluation of a classroom science intervention designed to extend the bicycle helmet safety message. *American Journal of Health Education, 40* (2), 71-79.

Miller, P., Wilkoff, R., McMahon, M., Garrett, M., and Johnson, N. (1982). Development of a health attitude scale. *Nursing Research, 31* (3), 132-136.

Nutbeam, D. (1992). The health promoting school: closing the gap between theory and practice. *Health Promotion International, 7* (3), 151-153.

Rezendes, J. (2006). Bicycle Helmets: Overcoming barriers to use and increasing effectiveness. *Journal of Pediatric Nursing, 21* (1), 35-44.

Rogers, E., Moon, A., Mullee, M., Speller, V., and Roderick, P. (1998). Developing the Health Promoting School- A national survey of Healthy School Awards. *Public Health, 112*, 37-40.

Rosamond, W., Flegal, K., Furie, K., Go, A., Greenlund, K., Hasse, N., et al. (2008). Heart disease and stroke statistics. *Circulation, 117*, 25-146.

Russell, B., Soysa, C., Wagoner, M., and Dawson, L. (2008). Teaching prevention on sensitive topics: Key elements and pedagogical techniques. *Journal Primary Prevention, 29*, 413-433.

Schwandt, P., Bertsch, T., and Haas, G. (2010). Anthropometric screening for silent cardiovascular risk factors in adolescents: The PEP FAmily Heart Study. *Atherosclerosis, 211*, 667-671.

Shilts, M., Lamp, C., Horowitz, M., and Townsend, M. (2009). Pilot Study: EatFit impacts sixth graders' academic performance on achievement of mathematics and english education standards. *Journal of Nutrition Education and Behavior, 41*, 127-131.

Sin, D., Anthonisen, N., Soriano, J., and Agusti, A. (2006). Mortality in COPD: Role of comorbidities. *European Respiratory Journal, 28*, 1245-1257.

Stevens, J., Cornell, C., Story, M., French, S., Levin, S., Becenti, A., et al. (1999). Development of a questionnaire to assess knowledge attitudes and behaviors in American Indian children. *American Journal of Clinical Nutrition, 69* (4), 773-781.

Subramaniam, P., and Silverman, S. (2007). Middle school students' attitudes towards physical education. *Teaching and Teacher Education , 23*, 602-611.

Swan, L., and Gatzoulis, M. (2002). Early atherosclerosis...What does it mean? *European Heart Journal, 23* (17), 1317-1319.

Toepperwein, M., Pruski, L., Blalock, C., Lemelle, O., and Lichtenstein, M. (2008). Getting the word out: Teaching middle-school children about cardiovascular disease. *Journal of Clinical Lipidology, 2* (179-188).

Torabi, M., and Jeng, I. (2001). Health Attitude Scale construction: Importance of psychometric evidence. *American Journal of Health Behavior, 25* (3), 290-298.

Veugelers, P., and Fitzgerald, A. (2005). Effectiveness of school programs in preventing childhood obesity: A multilevel comparison. *American Journal of Public Health, 95* (3), 432-435.

Warren, J., Henry, C., Lightowler, H., Bradshaw, S., and Perwaiz, S. (2008). Evaluation of a pilot school programme aimed at the prevention of obesity in children. *Health Promotion International, 18* (4), 287-296.

Webber, L., Osganian, V., Luepker, R., Feldman, H., and al., e. (1995). Cardiovascular risk factors among third grade children in four regions of the United States: the CATCH Study. *American Journal of Epidemiology, 141*, 428-439.

Young, D., Steckler, A., Cohen, S., Pratt, C., Felton, G., Moe, S., et al. (2008). Process evaluation results from a school and community-linked intervention: the trail of activity for adolescent girls (TAAG). *Health Education Research, 23* (6), 976-986.

In: Reviews in Pediatric Exercise Science
Editor: Michael Duncan, pp. 43-65
ISBN: 978-1-61470-978-7

Chapter IV

Breakfast, Metabolism, Health and Cognitive Function in Young People

Keith Tolfrey, Julia K. Zakrzewski, Simon B. Cooper and Mary E. Nevill
Paediatric Exercise Science Research Group, Institute of Youth Sport, School of Sport, Exercise and Health Sciences, Loughborough University, Loughborough, UK.

Introduction

The often cited phrase 'breakfast is the most important meal of the day' may have been largely anecdotal and lacking empirical evidence originally, particularly where children and adolescents (young people) are concerned. However, this chapter will provide a critical overview of the literature that supports carers of young people who have gone great lengths to convince their charges of the virtues of breakfast; thus, demonstrating this practice has more substance than mere anecdote. The chapter is divided into two distinct halves; the first focusing on the link between breakfast consumption and young people's physical health – with a specific emphasis on breakfast composition, ready to eat cereals and breakfast glycaemic index (GI). The second half reviews how this first meal of the day might be a very important factor when examining cognitive function in young people – the focus is on the effects of breakfast consumption and composition on various components of cognitive function. Many of the studies in this section use chronological age to define maturation; whilst we recognise that this does not provide a valid indication of maturation, we have used the authors' definitions of children and adolescents if they failed to provide a recognised measure of maturation (e.g., secondary sexual characteristics, wrist-hand x-ray, peak height velocity). Sometimes we refer to adult-based studies when they provide the necessary foundation for other research that includes children and/or adolescents or to highlight areas that are particularly lacking in empirical findings from young people. Most of the terminology in the chapter should be familiar to the reader and should not require any specialised knowledge of the 'breakfast literature'; however, for clarity – breakfast skipping is defined as a habitual choice in free-living conditions (e.g., a child who chooses, for whatever reason, not to eat breakfast). In contrast, breakfast omission refers to an experimental manipulation that a study participant has consented to comply with when asked (e.g., it could include an adolescent who normally eats breakfast on a regular basis, but has completed some measurements after an overnight fast as part of an experimental study). Although the chapter cannot be considered an exhaustive, systematic review of the literature, we have made every effort to avoid any obvious bias in our presentation of the evidence and hope that it provides a platform for future research with young people in the specific areas that are critically reviewed below. Finally, despite numerous benefits relating to health and cognitive function, breakfast consumption has declined in young people and also declines from childhood to adolescents (Rampersaud, Pereira, Girard, Adams, and Metzl, 2005). Consequently, strategies to promote the regular consumption of a healthy breakfast in young people are warranted.

Breakfast and Health

Breakfast is commonly considered a key component of a healthy lifestyle. The relationship between breakfast consumption, including its composition, and various short and long term health outcomes has received increasing attention in recent years. Breakfast consumption may favourably affect nutrition, body composition and risk markers for chronic disease; all matters of considerable relevance given public health concerns of paediatric obesity and associated adverse health conditions, such as Type 2 diabetes (Cali and Caprio, 2008). Furthermore, the transition from adolescence to adulthood appears to be a high-risk period for weight gain (Gordon-Larsen, Adair, Nelson, and Popkin, 2004) and there is a temporal reduction in insulin sensitivity during the pubertal period (Goran and Gower, 2001).

This section reviews the literature that has examined health benefits of breakfast consumption in young people. The influence of breakfast composition is discussed later; specifically, the impact of ready-to-eat cereal consumption and breakfast glycaemic index. The evidence reviewed stems mainly from large observational studies, although experimental support is also available linking breakfast glycaemic index to health markers. Potential mechanisms mediating these relationships are discussed throughout and are summarised in Figure 1.

Breakfast Consumption

The nutritional benefits of regular breakfast consumption are well established (Rampersaud et al., 2005) and are particularly relevant for young people since inadequate nutrient intake during childhood may be associated with adverse health outcomes during childhood, adolescence and adulthood (Viteri and Gonzalez, 2002). Breakfast consumption has been associated with favourable diet quality and nutritional status in young people. More specifically, breakfast consumption is associated with higher micronutrient intakes and a greater likelihood of meeting recommended intakes for vitamins and minerals, including vitamins A and C, riboflavin, calcium, zinc, and iron (Nicklas, Bao, Webber, and Berenson,

1993; Nicklas, Reger, Myers, and O'Neil, 2000; Sjöberg, Hallberg, Höglund, and Hulthén, 2003).

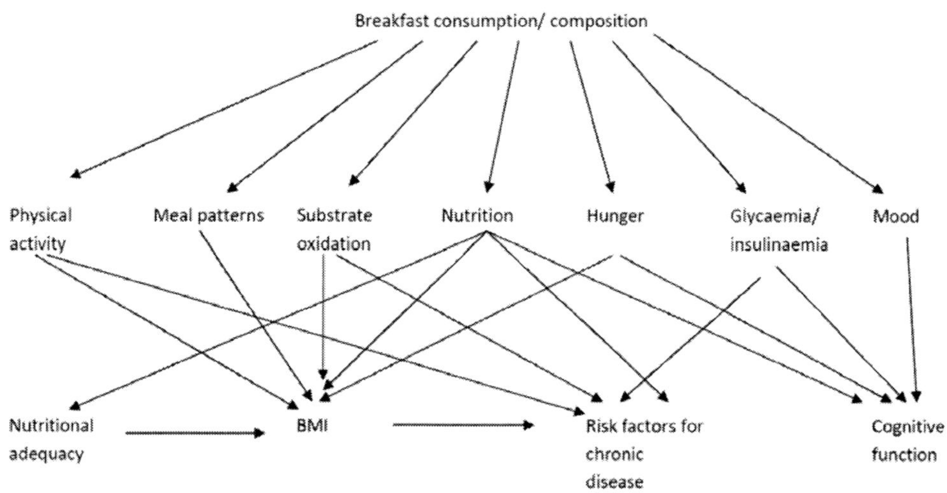

Figure 1. Potential mechanisms mediating relationships between breakfast consumption/composition and health and cognitive function.

The higher milk and calcium intake in breakfast consumers (Affentio et al., 2005; Barton et al., 2005) is critical for young people since bone calcium accretion is highest during adolescence (Weaver, 2000). Importantly, young people who skip breakfast do not seem to make up the nutrient deficits through other meals consumed during the day (Nicklas et al., 1993; Sjöberg et al., 2003). Breakfast consumption is also associated with higher daily total energy, carbohydrate, protein and dietary fibre intake and lower total and saturated fat intake (Nicklas et al., 1993; Affentio et al., 2005; Barton et al., 2005; Timlin, Pereira, Story, and Neumark-Sztainer, 2008), although the impact of breakfast consumption on sugar intake is unclear (Nicklas et al., 2000; Sjöberg et al., 2003).

Young people who consume breakfast habitually tend to have higher levels of physical activity and cardiorespiratory fitness (Kafatos et al., 2005; Sandercock, Voss, and Dye, 2010), a finding that may have particular relevance for girls since physical activity levels decline during adolescence (Armstrong and Welsman, 2006) and are lower compared with boys (Riddoch et al., 2007). Other health-compromising behaviours associated with breakfast skipping in adolescents include tobacco, alcohol and substance use, although it should be highlighted that it is not possible to infer causality between these relationships (Keski-Rahkonen, Kaprio, Rissanen, Virkkunen, and Rose, 2003; Timlin et al., 2008). Indeed, it seems plausible that adolescents who readily adopt a variety of unhealthy lifestyle choices may also skip breakfast.

Cross-sectional evidence has consistently shown that breakfast consumption is inversely associated with body mass index (BMI) and obesity in large diverse samples of young people (Affentio et al., 2005; Barton et al., 2005; Szajewska and Ruszcynski, 2010). Prospective studies indicate that habitual breakfast consumption is predictive of lower BMI (Affenito et al., 2005; Timlin et al., 2008) and its protective effect on weight gain increases in proportion to breakfast frequency (Timlin et al., 2008). Conversely, a reduction in BMI over time was associated with breakfast consumption in non-overweight, but breakfast skipping in overweight adolescents (Berkey, Rockett, Gillman, Field, and Colditz, 2003). Moreover, there is some uncertainty regarding whether such relationships are independent of confounding variables, such as physical activity, energy intake and parental education (Affenito et al., 2005; Barton et al. 2005; Timlin et al., 2008). Despite this, a recent systematic review concluded that breakfast consumption is associated with a reduced risk of overweight and obesity in young people (Szajewska and Ruszcynski, 2010). Although relationships between breakfast consumption and chronic disease risk factors are generally not well understood in young people, breakfast consumption has been associated with lower plasma cholesterol concentration (Resnicow, 1991) and adequate micronutrient intakes associated with breakfast consumption may reduce chronic disease risk (Willett, 1994).

Several behavioural and metabolic mechanisms may explain the relationship between breakfast consumption and health markers. Increased energy intake is unlikely to explain the higher BMI associated with breakfast skipping (Nicklas et al., 1993; Dubois, Girard, Potvin Kent, Farmer, and Tatone-Tokuda, 2009). However, skipping breakfast may promote eating patterns over the remainder of the day that favour gains in weight or body fat. Breakfast skipping can lead to overeating later in the day to compensate for the energy deficit at breakfast, particularly from the late evening snack (Schlundt, Hill, Sbrocco, Pope-Cordle, and Sharp, 1992; Dubois et al., 2009). Furthermore, overweight and obese young people skip breakfast more frequently, consume a lower proportion of energy at breakfast and consume a higher proportion of energy during dinner (Ortega et al., 1998; Maffeis et al., 2000). Interventions in adults have shown that consuming more energy earlier compared with later in the day may assist in weight loss (Keim, Van Loan, Horn, Barbieri, and Mayclin, 1997). As sedentary behaviour is more prevalent later in the day (Biddle, Gorely, Marshall, Murdey, and Cameron, 2004), it is likely that the energy consumed in the late afternoon or evening will be stored as glycogen and fat, rather than metabolised through physical activity. Breakfast skipping may also contribute to increased snacking, particularly high-fat snacks (Resnicow, 1991; Sjöberg et al., 2003). It therefore seems plausible that skipping breakfast leads to greater energy intake later in the day and snacking to compensate for the deficit, which predisposes obesity. Breakfast consumption may be a simple, yet effective, strategy to reduce energy intakes later in the day when young people may be less likely to expend the energy consumed.

It has also been suggested that breakfast consumption increases eating frequency and results in a more even distribution of energy intake throughout the day (Dubois et al., 2009). This may increase dietary induced thermogenesis and energy expenditure (Drummond, Crombie, and Kirk, 1996) and, consequently, contribute to healthy weight status. Indeed, meal frequency is inversely associated with obesity in young people (Toschke, Thorsteinsdottir, and Kries, 2009). The relationship between breakfast consumption and other health enhancing lifestyle factors, including increased physical activity and healthy food choices, is also likely to contribute to a lower BMI in breakfast consumers.

Collectively, these findings suggest that regular breakfast consumption is associated with a variety of nutritional and lifestyle-related health outcomes in large diverse samples of young people, which may prevent weight gain and nutrient deficiency. However, further research is required to establish possible links between breakfast consumption and risk factors for chronic disease. Future research should also consider methodological issues, such as the definition of breakfast consumption and skipping and the control of possible confounders (e.g., dietary factors, physical activity, socioeconomic status, parental obesity). Moreover, controlled, systematic experimental studies are required to infer causality and the mechanisms controlling these relationships require further investigation. However, randomised controlled trials involving the intentional manipulation of breakfast omission over a period of time may be challenging for ethical reasons.

Breakfast Composition

The relationship between breakfast and health benefits may not be due to consumption per se, but rather breakfast composition (Deshmukh-Taskar et al., 2010). However, compared with breakfast consumption, the effect of breakfast composition on health outcomes has rarely been examined systematically. Ready-to-eat cereals (RTEC) are commonly consumed for breakfast in westernised countries (Ruxton, O'Sullivan, Kirk, Belton, and Holmes, 1996; Albertson, Anderson, Crockett, and Goebel, 2003; Song et al., 2006). Studies assessing health benefits of RTEC consumption have typically compared RTEC consumers, other breakfast consumers (i.e., foods or beverages other than RTEC as the first meal) and breakfast skippers (Deshmukh-Taskar et al., 2010), whereas some simpler studies have not included other breakfast consumers for comparison (Gibson, 2003; Albertson et al., 2009).

Breakfasts containing cereal may be particularly beneficial for overall nutrient intake. Indeed, RTEC are typically low in fat, good sources of complex carbohydrates, fortified with vitamins and minerals and provide dietary fibre (Cotton, Subar, Friday, and Cook, 2004). Nutritional benefits of frequent RTEC consumption are similar to those of frequent breakfast consumption and include higher micronutrient, fibre, carbohydrate, protein and reduced fat and cholesterol intake (Ruxton et al., 1996; Gibson, 2003; Albertson et al., 2003; 2009), as well as improved biochemical indices of nutritional status, i.e., serum vitamin and mineral concentrations (Preziosi, Galan, Deheeger, Yacoub, Drewnowski, and Hercberg, 1999). Moreover, RTEC consumption is associated with greater nutritional benefits than other breakfasts in young people, including higher intakes of total carbohydrate, dietary fibre, and several micronutrients (Barton et al., 2005; Deshmukh-Taskar et al., 2010).

Similar to breakfast consumption, research in young people has associated frequent RTEC consumption with lower BMI and obesity risk (Albertson et al., 2003). In a study comparing RTEC consumption, other breakfast consumption and breakfast skipping, adolescent RTEC consumers had the lowest prevalence of obesity. Conversely, when children and adolescents were grouped together, obesity prevalence was lower in RTEC consumers compared with breakfast skippers, but not different between RTEC and other breakfast consumers (Deshmukh-Taskar et al., 2010). Similar studies are therefore needed to clarify the independent role of RTEC consumption in reducing obesity risk. Frequent RTEC consumption may also be protective against risk factors for chronic disease in young people, including reduced blood glucose (Kafatos et al., 2005) and low-density lipoprotein cholesterol (Gibson, 2003; Albertson et al., 2009) concentrations.

The positive relationship between breakfast consumption and RTEC consumption may partly explain the reported health benefits of RTEC consumption (Albertson et al., 2003). However, differences between RTEC and other breakfast consumers suggests the beneficial effect of breakfast consumption is enhanced with the inclusion of RTEC; thus, potential mechanisms relating RTEC consumption specifically with health markers warrant discussion. The nutrient fortification and low fat content of cereals may explain the relationship between RTEC consumption and nutrient intakes. In addition, lower fat intakes are associated with lower BMI in children (Maffeis et al., 2000) and may prevent weight gain in adults (Astrup, Grunwald, Melanson, Saris, and Hill, 2000). Increased calcium consumption, that often accompanies RTEC, is also related to lower BMI in children (Skinner, Bounds, Carruth, and Ziegler, 2003) and adult-based interventions indicate that increased calcium consumption may accelerate weight loss (Zemel, Thompson, Milstead, Morris, and Campbell, 2004).

Despite potential health-enhancing benefits of RTEC consumption, the nutritional content of these cereals varies considerably and there are concerns that the majority of RTEC marketed to children fail to meet national nutrition standards. These cereals are typically denser in energy, sugar and sodium, but sparser in fibre and protein compared with cereals that are not marketed specifically for children (Schwartz, Vartanian, Wharton, and Brownell, 2008). It has been suggested that the association between RTEC and health may be attributed to the consumption of whole-grain and not refined-grain cereals and there has been interest in the role of whole grains for diabetes in particular (Kochar et al., 2007; Kosti, Panagiotakos, and Zampelas, 2010). Conversely, it is possible that the health benefits of RTEC offset potential increases in added sugars. Moreover, the convenience and cost of RTEC as a breakfast food may facilitate the promotion of regular breakfast consumption in young people (Nicklas, McQuarrie, Fastnaught, and O'Neil, 2002).

Glycaemic Index (GI)

There has been considerable interest in potential health benefits of breakfasts containing whole grains and low glycaemic index (LGI) carbohydrates, as opposed to RTEC consumption. The concept of GI was introduced as a method of classifying different carbohydrate-rich foods according to their effect on postprandial glycaemia. It is defined as the incremental area under the two hour blood glucose curve following ingestion of 50 g available carbohydrate as a percentage of the corresponding area following an equivalent amount of carbohydrate from a standard reference product (glucose or white bread) (Jenkins et al., 1981). Values for GI range from 1 to 100 and carbohydrates can be classified as high (>70), moderate (56-69) or low (<55) GI. Foods classified as high GI (HGI) include refined grain products and potato, whereas LGI foods include whole grain products, legumes and fruits. A number of published tables now contain GI values for a variety of foods, including The International Tables of Glycaemic Index (Atkinson, Foster-Powell, and Brand-Miller, 2008). As the extent of postprandial glycaemia depends on both the GI and the amount of carbohydrate consumed, the glycaemic load (GL) was later proposed to provide an indication of the total glycaemic effect of the diet and is calculated as the product of the GI and total dietary carbohydrate divided by 100 (Brand-Miller et al., 2003).

Factors influencing GI include the type of monosaccharide (glucose, galactose, fructose, sucrose), amylose (unbranched) /amylopectin (branched) ratio and macronutrient and dietary fibre content. These food factors are affected by the method of preparation, processing, variety, origin, maturation and degree of ripeness. Although glycaemic and insulinaemic responses to consumed carbohydrate are typically well-related (Wolever and Bolognesi,

1996), the unexpectedly high insulinaemic index of milk (Ostman, Liljeberg Elmståhl and Björck, 2001) may be important when considering postprandial metabolism following breakfasts containing milk.

Dietary Glycaemic Index, Health and Disease in Young People

The rate of glucose entry into blood and duration of elevated blood glucose induce hormonal and metabolic changes that may affect health; mounting evidence suggests that the postprandial state contributes to the development of chronic disease (Heine et al., 2004). Reduced GI diets may have implications for reducing BMI, metabolic syndrome and cardiovascular risk factors, hyperglycaemia, fasted glucose and insulin and self-reported hunger in young people (Spieth et al., 2000; Fajcsak, Gabor, Kovacs, and Martos, 2008; Rovner, Nansel, and Gellar, 2009). Moreover, a reduced-GL diet may be more effective at improving BMI and insulin sensitivity compared with reduced-fat diet (Ebbeling, Leidig, Sinclair, Hangen, and Ludwig, 2003). Encouragingly, health benefits of lowering dietary GI may be achieved by lowering the GI of breakfast only (Pal, Lim, and Egger, 2008). However, conflicting evidence has shown dietary GI may not influence health markers in children (Cheng et al., 2009). Potential health-enhancing effects of reduced GI diets in young people are, therefore, encouraging but require greater research attention.

Acute Effect of Breakfast Glycaemic Index

Diets rich in LGI foods may reduce metabolic disease risk through both direct metabolic effects and reductions in body weight. Plausible mechanisms may arise from the contrasting metabolic responses to HGI and LGI foods, which have been investigated using randomised controlled trials in adults and to a lesser extent in young people.

Numerous studies in adults have shown that LGI compared with HGI mixed-breakfast meals reduce postprandial glycaemia and insulinaemia (Stevenson, Williams, Mash, Phillips, and Nute, 2006; Stevenson, Astbury, Simpson, Taylor, and Macdonald, 2009) and a few studies in adolescents provide similar findings (Ludwig et al., 1999; Ball et al., 2003), as displayed in Figure 2. In adults, LGI carbohydrate consumption may also attenuate glycaemic and insulinaemic responses to standard subsequent meals due to the 'second meal effect' (Liljeberg and Björck, 2000). Reduced blood glucose decreases the quantity of insulin required to clear glucose from the blood, which may up-regulate insulin receptors on cells and increase insulin sensitivity (Song, Sawamura, Ikeda, Igawa, and Yamori, 2000). Furthermore, the reduced postprandial glycaemic and insulinaemic response to LGI breakfasts has been proposed to affect satiety and substrate metabolism.

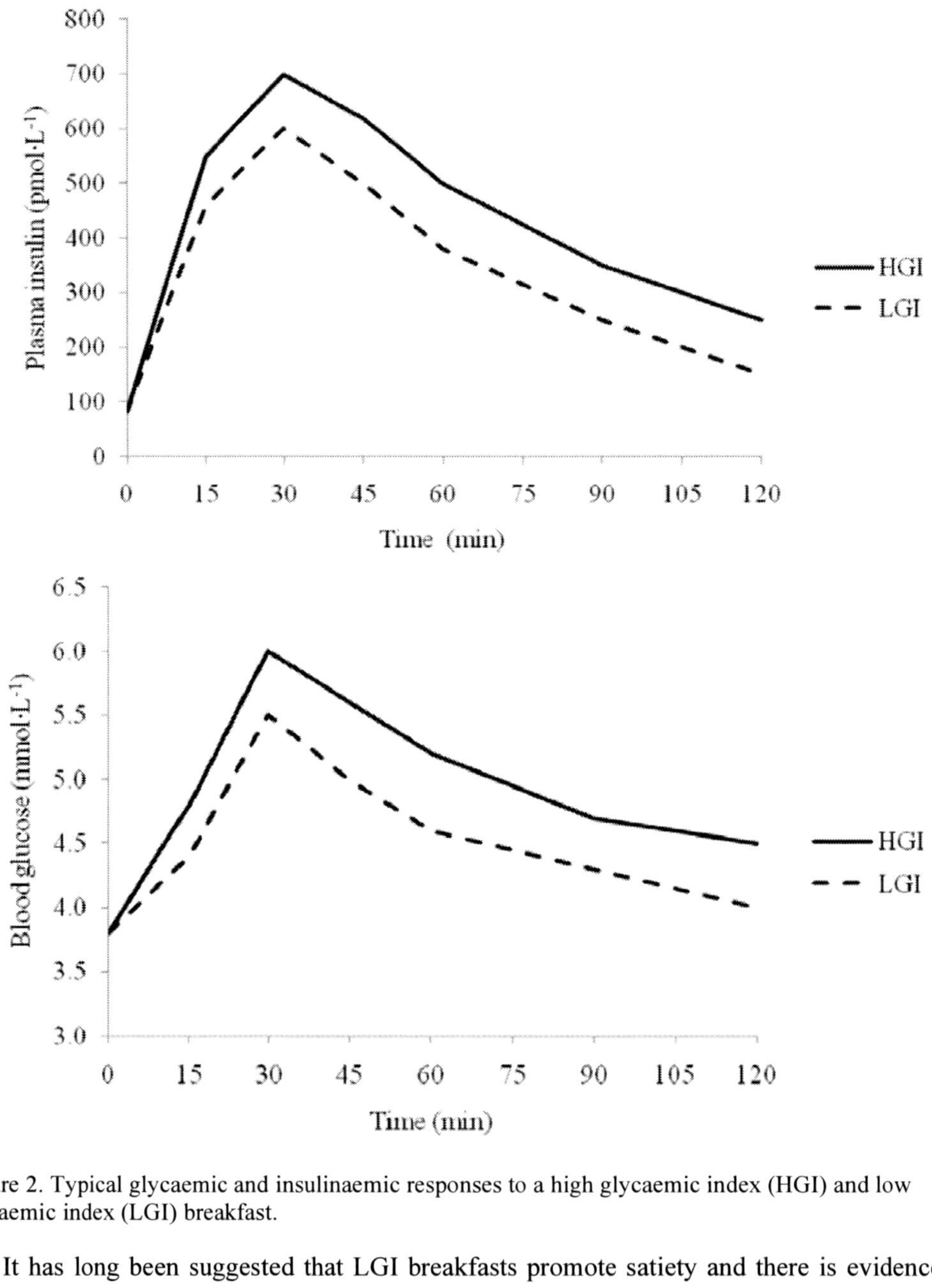

Figure 2. Typical glycaemic and insulinaemic responses to a high glycaemic index (HGI) and low glycaemic index (LGI) breakfast.

It has long been suggested that LGI breakfasts promote satiety and there is evidence to support this in young people (Ludwig et al., 1999; Ball et al., 2003; Warren et al., 2003). In a well-controlled study, Warren et al. (2003) reported lower lunchtime energy intake and hunger ratings after LGI, and LGI with added sugar, breakfasts compared with HGI and habitual breakfasts (which were also HGI) in children. Similar findings exist in obese adolescent boys, with voluntary energy intake and hunger ratings being greatest after a HGI, followed by a moderate GI and lowest after a LGI breakfast. Although the HGI and moderate GI breakfast were matched for key variables, the LGI breakfast contained less carbohydrate, more protein and more fat than the HGI breakfast, possibly confounding the GI comparison

(Ludwig et al., 1999). In contrast, another study reported similar energy intake and hunger ratings when comparing LGI meal replacement, a LGI whole-food meal and a moderately HGI meal replacement in overweight adolescents (Ball et al., 2003). Encouragingly, however, time to request additional food was prolonged following LGI breakfast consumption, indicating that overweight and obese adolescents are satisfied for a longer time period after LGI compared with HGI breakfast consumption (Ludwig et al., 1999; Ball et al., 2003). The lower energy intake and prolonged satiety following LGI breakfast consumption may partly explain the relationship between dietary GI and BMI. In turn, reduced BMI may contribute to other health benefits relating to LGI diets, including increased insulin sensitivity and reduced cardiovascular risk factors.

The lower glucose response following a LGI compared with HGI breakfast explained much of the lower voluntary food intake later in the day in obese adolescent boys (Ludwig et al., 1999); this suggested the blood glucose response might underpin the relationship between GI and satiety. The rapid absorption of glucose following HGI carbohydrate consumption stimulates insulin release, which promotes glucose uptake by the liver, skeletal muscle and adipose tissue, while suppressing both lipolysis in adipocytes and the release of glucose from the liver into the circulation. Subsequently, blood glucose concentration decreases rapidly. In contrast, the attenuated glucose response following LGI breakfast consumption stimulates more subtle hormonal responses and the prolonged and continued absorption of nutrients means that the fasted state is not reached until much later. The hunger response is, thus, prolonged following LGI carbohydrate consumption, which would promote longer term satiety.

Low rates of fat oxidation may be involved in the aetiology of obesity and accumulation of lipid within skeletal muscle can lead to abnormalities in insulin signalling and contribute to insulin resistance (Rogge, 2009). Maximising fat oxidation may therefore have important health implications for obesity and Type 2 diabetes. Although the health benefits of breakfast consumption are well established, fat oxidation is maximised in the fasted state because elevated insulin concentrations following carbohydrate consumption decrease lipolysis and fat oxidation (Wu, Nicholas, Williams, Took, and Hardy, 2003). The consumption of a LGI breakfast attenuates the insulin response and may, therefore, be a compromise between promoting both breakfast consumption and fat oxidation. In adults, increased fat oxidation during the immediate postprandial rest period has been reported following LGI compared with HGI breakfasts (Stevenson et al., 2009). However, numerous studies have not supported this finding (Díaz, Galgani, Aguirre, Atwater, and Burrows, 2005; Stevenson et al., 2006). Several studies have reported that LGI compared with HGI breakfast consumption results in higher fat oxidation during exercise performed 45 min to 3 h after breakfast (Sparks, Selig, and Febbraio, 1998; Wee, Williams, Tsintzas, and Boobis, 2005; Stevenson et al., 2006, 2009;). There is also evidence that the reduced fat oxidation following HGI breakfasts is largely due to the higher insulin response, which increases muscle glycogen stores and utilisation, resulting in higher carbohydrate and lower fat oxidation (Wee et al., 2005). However, another study demonstrated that a HGI breakfast resulted in higher exercise fat oxidation (Moore, Midgley, Thurlow, Thomas, and McNaughton, 2010). Furthermore, breakfast GI does not affect fat oxidation during rest or exercise when comparing a moderate GI and HGI breakfast (Backhouse, Williams, Stevenson, Nute, 2007) or when exercise is preceded by two LGI meals rather than breakfast alone (Stevenson, Williams, and Nute, 2005). Therefore, the manipulation of carbohydrate GI of a mixed breakfast meal on postprandial resting and exercise fat oxidation remains unclear. Moreover, similar studies in young people do not appear to be available. Discrepancies between studies may be due to differences in breakfast size and composition, exercise mode, intensity and duration, the time interval between breakfast and exercise and participant characteristics.

In conclusion, experimental studies have shown that LGI compared with HGI breakfast consumption results in reduced postprandial glycaemia and insulinaemia and, consequently, increased satiety and possibly fat oxidation. These findings may explain relationships between reduced dietary GI and improved health markers, such as BMI and cardiovascular risk factors. Substituting a HGI breakfast for a LGI breakfast may be particularly beneficial for overweight individuals through increased glycaemic control, fat oxidation and satiety. However, further research in young people is required to confirm findings from the adult-based literature.

Summary and Recommendations for Future Research

There is substantial evidence that breakfast consumption is associated with the health and well-being of young people, and the benefits seem to apply to a wide range of age, demographic, and socioeconomic groups. Observational studies support frequent breakfast consumption for improving nutrition and reducing obesity in young people. Health benefits of breakfast consumption may be enhanced with the inclusion of RTEC, particularly those containing LGI carbohydrates and whole-grain. Despite these health benefits, many young people often skip breakfast; thus strategies to promote breakfast consumption are warranted. However, it is noteworthy that breakfast is only one component of a healthy lifestyle and those involved in breakfast promotion should highlight this to the target audience. Future research should address relationships between breakfast and chronic disease and the impact of breakfast composition. Furthermore, experimental studies with stronger designs are required to test causality and possible mechanisms; however ethical barriers to invasive procedures with children and adolescents may impede progress in this area until non-invasive alternatives emerge.

Breakfast and Cognitive Function

Besides the health benefits of breakfast which have been discussed previously, the effects of breakfast consumption on cognitive function in young people have also been examined. In doing so, the focus has been largely on breakfast consumption compared to breakfast omission, whereas other studies have centred on the effects of breakfast composition (for example, breakfasts which differ in total energy content and G)). Studies in this area have assessed different elements of cognitive function, but have primarily focused on tests of memory and attention, two key components of cognitive function.

Studies investigating the effects of breakfast on cognitive function in young people have tended to examine children (up to 11 years old) (e.g. Pollitt, Leibel, and Greenfield, 1981; Mahoney, Taylor, Kanarek, and Samuel, 2005) and adolescents (12 to 16 years old) (e.g.

(Widenhorn-Müller, Hille, Klenk, and Weiland, 2008; Cooper, Bandelow, and Nevill, 2011) separately. Children (aged 3 – 11 years) have a larger brain weight relative to their body weight and a 50% greater metabolic rate per unit of brain weight compared to adults (Hoyland, Dye, and Lawton, 2009); thus, nutritional effects on cognitive function may be different in children, compared to both adolescents and adults. Furthermore, adolescents experience rapid growth and changes in metabolism during puberty, so the effects of breakfast on cognitive function are likely to be different to the effects in children and adults (Cromer, Tarnowski, Stein, Harton, and Thornoton, 1990; Kanarek, 1997). Therefore, examining these sub-categories of childhood separately is logical given that this is the approach taken in the literature. However, given that maturation is also likely to play a key role in determining the metabolic responses to different meals, the dichotomy between children (up to 11 years old) and adolescents (12 to 16 year olds) is made cautiously. This section will examine the evidence regarding the effect of breakfast consumption and composition on cognitive function in children and adolescents. Potential mediating mechanisms will also be examined.

Breakfast Consumption

Children

In a review of early studies in the area, Pollitt, Cueto, and Jacoby (1998) suggest that breakfast consumption has a positive effect on both visual attention and working memory in 9 to 11 year olds. However, breakfast consumption did not universally improve performance on all the tests of cognitive function used in these early studies, with performance on some tests actually improved following breakfast omission when compared to breakfast consumption (Pollitt et al., 1981). However, the authors concluded that overall the evidence suggests that breakfast omission affects memory and attention adversely in 9 to 11 year olds. Furthermore, the authors speculate that such effects could be mediated by metabolic changes in plasma glucose regulation in the brain (Pollitt et al., 1998).

More recently, breakfast consumption has been shown to enhance the accuracy of spatial memory in 6 to 11 year olds and the accuracy of working memory in 9 to 11 year olds (Mahoney et al., 2005). Conversely, there was no effect of breakfast consumption on attention in 6 to 11 year olds, suggesting beneficial effects of breakfast consumption on memory, but not attention, in young people. However, other studies have demonstrated a positive effect of breakfast consumption on attention in children, using a variety of measures. For example, using classroom observation, it has been reported that 9 year olds spent longer on task and displayed fewer lapses in attention following breakfast consumption compared to breakfast omission (Benton and Jarvis, 2007).

A test of attention commonly used in the literature is a form of continuous performance test (CPT). A CPT requires participants to identify a target sequence (e.g. 'X' followed by 'B') when monitoring a stream of letters and/or numbers. Following breakfast consumption, accuracy on a CPT in 9 to 12 year olds was enhanced (Conners and Blouin ,1982; Busch, Taylor, Kanarek, and Holcomb, 2002). Furthermore, Busch et al. (2002) also reported that breakfast consumption had no effect on response times on the CPT (i.e. the speed of attention), but given the improvement in accuracy, the results suggest that overall, breakfast consumption was beneficial for attention in children.

Adolescents

To date, four studies have examined the effects of breakfast consumption on cognitive function in adolescent populations (Cromer et al., 1990; Wesnes, Pincock, Richardson, Helm, and Hails, 2003; Widenhorn-Müller et al., 2008; Cooper et al., 2011). Although Cromer et al. (1990) reported that attention in 14 year olds was not affected by breakfast consumption, the cross-sectional study deign may have introduced some confounding factors, compared with a prospective design where cause and effect can be investigated. Indeed, using a prospective, cross-over design, Wesnes et al. (2003) found that breakfast consumption enhanced the accuracy of attention, but had no effect on working memory in 9 to 16 year olds. However, the results should be interpreted cautiously because the wide age range (spanning 9 to 16 year olds) suggests maturity dependant physiological differences between the participants could have influenced the study outcomes.

A similar problem is evident in the study of Widenhorn-Müller et al. (2008), where the participants ranged from 13 to 20 years old. The findings indicate that whilst breakfast consumption did not affect attention, participants did display a greater accuracy of visuospatial memory following breakfast consumption; however, breakfast consumption did not affect the accuracy of verbal memory.

In a recent study designed to overcome these short comings, the accuracy of attention and speed of working memory were improved in adolescents (11 to 14 years old) following consumption of a self-selected breakfast, compared to a breakfast omission control condition. In contrast, there were no effects of breakfast consumption on the speed of attention or accuracy of working memory (Cooper et al., 2011). However, given that the improvements in the speed of working memory and accuracy of attention were not combined with a decrease in performance on the other parameter (i.e. accuracy of working memory and speed of attention), these findings indicate that breakfast consumption enhanced cognitive function in an adolescent population.

Summary

Overall, the evidence reviewed here suggests that breakfast consumption, when compared to breakfast omission, is beneficial for cognitive function in both children and adolescents. However, it is important to note that some components of cognitive function have been unaffected by breakfast consumption, thus generalisations must be made cautiously. Comparisons between studies are difficult because of differences in research design, variations in the breakfasts provided, the different components and measures of cognitive function and the wide age range of the participants in some of the studies. However, evidence suggests that breakfast consumption enhances both memory and attention in children and adolescents, when compared to breakfast omission.

Breakfast Composition

In addition to the work examining breakfast consumption, the effects of breakfast composition on cognitive function have also been examined in various populations. In adults, the effect of breakfast macronutrient content (Fischer, Colombani, Lanhans, and Wenk, 2001), glycaemic load (Gilsenan, de Bruin, and Dye, 2009) and GI (Benton et al., 2003; Benton and Nabb, 2004; Nilsson, Radeborg, and Björk, 2009) have all been examined. However, this section is limited to literature specific to children and adolescents, thus it will only include the effects of breakfast GI and total energy content on cognitive function in children and adolescents.

Children

Studies examining the effects of breakfast composition on cognitive function in children have focused primarily on GI. One such study of 6 to 11 year olds showed an enhanced accuracy of secondary memory after a LGI when compared to a HGI breakfast, but there were no differences in the accuracy or speed of working memory between the HGI and LGI breakfasts (Ingwersen, Defeyter, Kennedy, Wesnes, and Scholey, 2007). In the same study, the LGI breakfast also reduced the decline in the accuracy of attention seen across the morning following a HGI breakfast. However, similar to the findings regarding the speed of memory, the speed of attention was not different between the breakfasts (Ingwersen et al., 2007). Again, it is not possible to generalise findings and conclude that a LGI breakfast was the most beneficial for cognitive function, because the effects were specific to selected components of cognitive function. Furthermore, the breakfasts provided were not matched for key variables such as total energy and macronutrient content, which may have confounded the results.

Using HGI and LGI breakfasts matched for total energy and carbohydrate content, Mahoney et al. (2005) found that a LGI breakfast led to greater accuracy of working memory in 6 to 8 year old girls and greater accuracy of spatial memory in 9 to 11 year old boys and girls. The LGI breakfast was also beneficial for the accuracy of auditory attention in 6 to 8 year old children, but there were no differences in visual attention or in the 9 to 11 year old children, when compared with the HGI breakfast. Collectively, these findings suggest that a LGI breakfast is most beneficial for children's cognitive function, but the precise effect may depend on both the component of cognitive function assessed and the age and sex of the children.

Manipulation of the total energy content of breakfast in children showed that a higher energy breakfast (700 kcal) improved both mood and cognitive function in 10 year old children, compared with a lower energy (172 kcal) breakfast (Wyon, Abrahamsson, Järtelius, and Fletcher, 1997; Benton and Jarvis, 2007). More recently, Benton and Jarvis (2007) found that 9 year old children who consumed a lower energy breakfast (on average 61 vs. 210 kcal) spent less time on task, thus displayed poorer attention. However, the adverse effects on cognitive function and mood of the lower energy breakfast were reversed by the consumption of a mid-morning snack (Benton and Jarvis, 2007), suggesting that breakfast may benefit children's cognitive function across the morning, but only if the breakfast is above a certain 'energy threshold'.

Adolescents

Complimenting findings in children, suggesting that a LGI breakfast is most beneficial for cognitive function, 9 to 16 year olds displayed smaller declines in memory and attention across the school morning after a LGI compared to HGI breakfast (Wesnes et al., 2003). Furthermore, performance on a word generation task improved after a LGI breakfast, compared to HGI breakfast, in 11 to 14 year olds (Micha, Nelson, and Rogers, 2008). In the same study, however, performance on the Stroop test (a classical test of attention and frontal lobe function) was enhanced following the HGI breakfast when compared to the LGI breakfast.

A further study to show a beneficial effect of a HGI breakfast on cognitive function measured verbal episodic memory in 14 to 17 year olds following HGI and LGI breakfasts (Smith and Foster, 2008). Although the authors suggested that the mechanism for the improved performance following the HGI breakfast could be higher blood glucose concentrations, which would be beneficial under the conditions of divided attention, non-significant between-condition differences in blood glucose concentrations failed to provide empirical support. Overall, the effects of breakfast GI on cognitive function in adolescents are equivocal, with some studies suggesting that selected components of cognitive function are enhanced by a LGI breakfast and other components enhanced by a HGI breakfast. Moreover, the reasons for the equivocal nature of the evidence are not clear, thus further research is required to extend knowledge in this area.

A more recent study with adolescents examined the effects of both the GI and GL of breakfast on cognitive function in 11-14 year olds (Micha, Nelson and Rogers, 2010). The findings suggest that following a breakfast which was LGI and HGL, participants performed better on a speed of information processing task, whereas immediate word recall (used to indicate memory) was enhanced following a HGI breakfast, regardless of the GL of breakfast (Micha et al., 2010). A limitation of this study was that participants consumed their usual breakfast (plus an optional snack) and were then allocated to groups according to the calculated GI and GL of the meal. Consequently, the study outcomes may have been confounded because the breakfasts were not matched for total energy or macronutrient content. Nonetheless, these results are interesting in that they combine the effects of GI and GL on cognitive function in adolescents, but the overall conclusions are still that some components of cognitive function are enhanced following a LGI breakfast, whereas others are improved after a HGI breakfast.

When examining the effects of breakfasts which differ in total energy content on cognitive function in 13-20 year olds, participants were asked to eat more than the first trial (habitual breakfast) for breakfast on their second trial (Michaud. Musse, Nicolas, and Mejean, 1991). During the second trial, energy intake was on average 63% higher and resulted in a greater accuracy of both working memory and attention when compared to habitual breakfast consumption. A caveat was that, despite the instructions to eat more on the second trial, 35% of participants consumed a higher energy intake on their first trial (habitual breakfast).

Furthermore, a potential learning effect cannot be discounted given the two breakfasts were not consumed in a counter-balanced order.

Summary

Studies that have examined the effects of breakfast composition on cognitive function in both children and adolescents have manipulated GI and total energy content. Generally, the evidence suggests a LGI breakfast is most beneficial for cognitive function in children. However, in adolescents, the evidence is more equivocal, where the effect of breakfast GI on cognitive function appears to be dependent on the component of cognitive function in question. A higher energy intake at breakfast is beneficial for cognitive function, but only two studies with children and one with adolescents have addressed this question to date.

Mechanisms

In addition to documenting the effects of breakfast consumption and composition on cognitive function in young people, some studies have attempted to provide potential mechanisms to explain the effects. An overview of the mechanisms by which breakfast consumption and composition could affect both health and cognitive function can be seen in Figure 1, with this section examining specifically those mechanisms relating to cognitive function. For example, it has been suggested that by alleviating hunger, breakfast consumption enhances mood and, subsequently, cognitive function in children (Pollitt, Gersovitz, and Gargiulo, 1978) and adolescents (Widenhorn Müller et al., 2008; Cooper et al., 2011). A further proposed mechanism is enhanced nutritional status associated with regular breakfast consumption, which may, in turn, improve cognitive function (Pollitt and Matthews, 1998). However, this chronic change in nutritional status is unlikely to explain the short-term, acute effects of breakfast consumption on cognitive function as reviewed above. It is possible, however, that in longer-term studies in children with poor baseline nutritional status, an improvement in nutritional status may contribute to enhanced cognitive function (Pollitt and Matthews, 1998).

More recently, it has been suggested that breakfast consumption modifies the metabolic responses to fasting and maintains a supply of nutrients to the central nervous system (Rampersaud, Pereira, Girard, Adams, and Metzl, 2005). Glucose has been identified frequently as a key nutritional mediator for cognitive function. This is unsurprising given that it is the only fuel that can be used by the brain directly. The leading role of glucose is well supported in adults, where glucose provision has been related to improved performance on the Stroop test (Dye, Lluch, and Blundell, 2000) and enhanced memory (Benton and Sargent, 1992).

In their review of early studies showing enhanced cognitive function following breakfast consumption in young people, Pollitt et al. (1998) suggest that such effects may be mediated by changes in glucose regulation. However, most studies in young people have not measured, or at least have not included serial measurements of blood glucose following their dietary interventions. Of the few studies that have measured blood glucose, some suggest it plays a leading role (Smith and Foster, 2008; Cooper et al., 2011), whereas others have shown glucose is not a key determinant of cognitive performance (Cromer et al., 1990; Michaud et al., 1991).

Interestingly, studies examining the effects of the GI of breakfast provide further insight into the potential mechanisms that may be at work. For example, Micha et al. (2008) found that whilst a HGI breakfast (and the associated higher blood glucose concentrations) is beneficial for performance on the Stroop test, a LGI breakfast (and the associated lower blood glucose concentrations) is beneficial for performance on a word generation task. This suggests that either blood glucose concentration (within the normal postprandial range, i.e. after high and LGI breakfasts) is not a key determinant of cognitive function and there are other mechanisms may be responsible, or that higher glucose concentrations are beneficial for some components of cognitive function, whereas they are detrimental for other components.

There is clear ambiguity in the literature regarding the effect of glucose on cognitive function in young people. Furthermore, no studies examining cognitive function in young people to date have measured insulin concentration following their dietary interventions. Given the central role of insulin in glucose regulation and the well documented effects of insulin on cognitive function (Laron, 2009 review), the simultaneous measurement of plasma insulin and glucose concentrations is recommended to further our understanding of diet-induced changes of cognitive function in young people.

Summary and Recommendations for Future Research

The evidence reviewed here suggests that breakfast consumption, when compared to breakfast omission, is beneficial for cognitive function in both children and adolescents. In addition, it appears that a LGI breakfast is the most beneficial for cognitive function in children, whereas findings in adolescents are equivocal, with some components of cognitive function enhanced after a HGI breakfast, whereas others are enhanced following a LGI breakfast. In addition, the limited evidence available suggests that breakfast must be above a certain 'energy threshold' to be beneficial for cognitive function. However, further work needs to be conducted to examine whether HGI and LGI breakfasts are beneficial for different components of cognitive function in adolescents and also to examine whether there is a 'threshold' total energy content of breakfast, above which breakfast becomes beneficial for cognitive function in young people. Importantly, future studies should extend current knowledge by: examining the possible independent influences of maturation and age, measure a range of cognitive functions using pre-validated, recognised measures, employ randomised, counter-balanced cross-over study designs, use breakfasts which are matched on all variables (e.g., energy and macronutrient content) other than the variable in question (e.g., GI) and finally, investigate potential mechanisms to explain any dietary induced effects on cognitive function.

Conclusions

Given the evidence reviewed here, it is clear that breakfast consumption and composition have key roles to play for both health and cognitive function in young people. Whilst the effects of breakfast consumption are well understood, the effects of breakfast composition are less clear and warrant further research. Furthermore, the mechanisms mediating the diet induced changes in health and cognitive function also require further research. Such benefits of regular breakfast consumption, coupled with the worrying decline in breakfast consumption amongst young people during recent years (Rampersaud et al., 2005), suggest that strategies designed to encourage young people to consume a healthy breakfast regularly are warranted.

References

Affenito, S.G., Thompson, D., Barton, B.A., Franko, D.L., Daniels, S.R., Obarzanek, E., Schreiber, G.B., and Striegel-Moore, R. (2005). Breakfast consumption in black and white adolescent girls correlates positively with calcium and fiber intake and negatively with body mass index. *Journal of the American Dietetic Association,* 105(6), 938-945.

Albertson, A.M., Affenito, S.G., Bauserman, R., Holschuh, N.M., Eldridge, A.L., and Barton, B.A. (2009). The relationship of ready-to-eat cereal consumption to nutrient intake, blood lipids, and body mass index of children as they age through adolescence. *Journal of the American Dietetic Association*, 109(9), 1557-1565.

Albertson, A.M., Anderson, G.H., Crockett, S.J., Goebel, M.T. (2003). Ready-to-eat cereal consumption: Its relationship with BMI and nutrient intake of children aged 4 to 12 years. *Journal of the American Dietetic Association*, 103(12), 1613-1619.

Armstrong, N., and Welsman, J.R. (1996). The physical activity patterns of European youth with reference to methods of assessment. *Sports Medicine*, 36(12), 1067-1086.

Astrup, A., Grunwald, G.K., Melanson, E.L., Saris, W.H., and Hill, J.O. (2000). The role of low-fat diets in body weight control: a meta-analysis of ad libitum dietary intervention studies. *International Journal of Obesity and Related Metabolic Disorders*, 24(12), 1545-1552.

Atkinson, F.S., Foster-Powell, K., and Brand-Miller, J.C. (2008). International tables of glycemic index and glycemic load values: 2008. *Diabetes Care*, 31(12), 2281-2283. doi:10.2337/dc08-1239.

Backhouse, S.H., Williams, C., Stevenson, E., and Nute, M. (2007). Effects of the glycemic index of breakfast on metabolic responses to brisk walking in females. *European Journal of Clinical Nutrition*, 1(5), 590-596.

Ball, S.D., Keller, K.R., Moyer-Mileur, L.J., Ding, Y.W., Donaldson, D., and Jackson, W.D. (2003). Prolongation of satiety after low versus moderately high glycemic index meals in obese adolescents. *Pediatrics*, 111(3), 488-494.

Barton, B.A., Eldridge, A.L., Thompson, D., Affenito, S.G., Striegel-Moore, R.H., Franko, D.L., Albertson, A.M., Crockett, and S.J. (2005). The relationship of breakfast and cereal consumption to nutrient intake and body mass index: the National Heart, Lung, and

Blood Institute Growth and Health Study. *Journal of the American Dietetic Association*, 105(9), 1383-1389.

Benton, D., and Jarvis, M. (2007). The role of breakfast and a mid-morning snack on the ability of children to concentrate at school. *Physiology and Behavior*, 90, 382-385. doi:10.1016/j.physbeh.2006.09.029.

Benton, D., and Nabb, S. (2004). Breakfasts that release glucose at different speeds interact with previous alcohol intake to influence cognition and mood before and after lunch. *Behavioral Neuroscience*, 118, 936-943. doi:10.1037/0735-7044.1185.936.

Benton, D., and Sargent, J. (1992). Breakfast, blood glucose and memory. *Biological Psychology*, 33, 207-210.

Benton, D., Ruffin, M., Lassel, T., Nabb, S., Messaoudi, M., Vinoy, S., Desor, D., and Lang, V. (2003). The delivery rate of dietary carbohydrates affects cognitive performance in both rats and humans. *Psychopharmacology*, 166, 86-90. doi:10.1001/s00213-002-1334-5.

Berkey, C.S., Rockett, H.R., Gillman, M.W., Field, A.E., and Colditz, G.A. (2003). Longitudinal study of skipping breakfast and weight change in adolescents. *International Journal of Obesity and Related Metabolic Disorders*, 27(10), 1258-1266.

Biddle, S.J., Gorely, T., Marshall, S.J., Murdey, I., and Cameron, N. (2004). Physical activity and sedentary behaviours in youth: issues and controversies. *Journal of the Royal Society of Health*. 124(1): 29-33.

Brand-Miller, J.C., Thomas, M., Swan, V., Ahmad, Z.I., Petocz, P., and Colagiuri, S. (2003). Physiological validation of the concept of glycemic load in lean young adults. *Journal of Nutrition,* 133(9), 2728-2732.

Busch, C.R., Taylor, H.A., Kanarek, R.B., and Holcomb, P.J. (2002). The effects of a confectionery snack on attention in young boys. *Physiology and Behavior*, 77, 333-340.

Cali, A.M., and Caprio, S. (2008). Obesity in children and adolescents. *Journal of Clinical Endocrinology and Metabolism*, 93(11):S31-S36.

Cheng, G., Karaolis-Danckert, N., Libuda, L., Bolzenius, K., Remer, T., and Buyken, A.E. (2009). Relation of dietary glycemic index, glycemic load, and fiber and whole-grain intakes during puberty to the concurrent development of percent body fat and body mass index. *American Journal of Epidemiology*, 169(6), 667-677.

Conners, K.C., and Blouin, A.G. (1982). Nutritional effects of behaviour of children. *Journal of Psychiatric Research*, 17, 193-201.

Cooper, S.B., Bandelow, S., and Nevill, M.E. (2011). Breakfast consumption and cognitive function in adolescent schoolchildren. *Physiology and Behavior*, in press. doi:10.1016/jphysbeh.2011.03.018.

Cotton, P.A., Subar, A.F., Friday, J.E., and Cook, A. (2004). Dietary sources of nutrients among US adults, 1994 to 1996. *Journal of the American Dietetic Association*, 104(6), 921-930.

Cromer, B.A., Tarnowski, K.J., Stein, A.M., Harton, P., and Thornton, D.J. (1990). The school breakfast program and cognition in adolescents. *Developmental and Behavioral Pediatrics*, 11, 295-300.

Deshmukh-Taskar, P.R., Nicklas, T.A., O'Neil, C.E., Keast, D.R., Radcliffe, J.D., and Cho S. (2010). The relationship of breakfast skipping and type of breakfast consumption with nutrient intake and weight status in children and adolescents: the National Health and

Nutrition Examination Survey 1999-2006. *Journal of the American Dietetic Association*, 110(6):869-878.

Díaz, E.O., Galgani, J.E., Aguirre, C.A., Atwater, I.J., and Burrows, R. (2005). Effect of glycemic index on whole-body substrate oxidation in obese women. *International Journal of Obesity*, 29(1), 108-114.

Drummond, S., Crombie, N., and Kirk, T. (1996). A critique of the effects of snacking on body weight status. *European Journal of Clinical Nutrition,* 50(12), 779-783.

Dubois, L., Girard, M., Potvin Kent, M., Farmer, A., and Tatone-Tokuda, F. (2009). Breakfast skipping is associated with differences in meal patterns, macronutrient intakes and overweight among pre-school children. *Public Health Nutrition*, 12(1), 19-28.

Dye, L., Lluch, A., and Blundell, J.E. (2000). Macronutrients and mental performance. *Nutrition*, 16, 1021-1034.

Ebbeling, C.B., Leidig, M.M., Sinclair, K.B., Hangen, J.P., and Ludwig, D.S. (2003). A reduced-glycemic load diet in the treatment of adolescent obesity. *Archives of Pediatrics and Adolescent Medicine*, 57(8), 773-779.

Fajcsak, Z., Gabor, A., Kovacs, V., and Martos, E. (2008). The effects of 6-week low glycemic load diet based on low glycemic index foods in overweight/obese children--pilot study. *Journal of the American College of Nutrition*, 27(1), 12-21.

Fischer, K., Colombani, P.C., Langhans, W., and Wenk, C. (2001). Cognitive performance and its relationship with postprandial metabolic changes after ingestion of different macronutrients in the morning. *British Journal of Nutrition*, 85, 393-405. doi:10.1079/BJN2000269.

Gibson, S. (2003). Micronutrient intakes, micronutrient status and lipid profiles among young people consuming different amounts of breakfast cereals: further analysis of data from the National Diet and Nutrition Survey of Young People aged 4 to 18 years. *Public Health Nutrition*, 6(8), 815-820.

Gilsenan, M.B., de Bruin, E.A., and Dye, L. (2009). The influence of carbohydrate on cognitive performance: a critical evaluation from the perspective of glycaemic load. *British Journal of Nutrition*, 101, 941-949. doi:10.1017/S0007114508199019.

Goran, M.I., and Gower, B.A. (2001). Longitudinal study on pubertal insulin resistance. *Diabetes*, 50(11), 2444-2450.

Gordon-Larsen, P., Adair, L.S., Nelson, M.C., and Popkin, B.M. (2004). Five-year obesity incidence in the transition period between adolescence and adulthood: the National Longitudinal Study of Adolescent Health. *American Journal of Clinical Nutrition*, 80(3):569-575.

Heine, R.J., Balkau, B., Ceriello, A., Del Prato, S., Horton, E.S., and Taskinen, M.R. (2004). What does postprandial hyperglycaemia mean? *Diabetic Medicine*, 21(3), 208-213.

Hoyland, A., Dye, L., and Lawton, C.L. (2009). A systematic review of the effect of breakfast on the cognitive performance of children and adolescents. *Nutrition Research Reviews*, 22, 220-243. doi:10.1017/S0954422409990175.

Ingwersen, J., Defeyter, M.A., Kennedy, D.O., Wesnes, K.A., and Scholey, A.B. (2007). A low glycaemic index breakfast cereal preferentially prevents children's cognitive performance from declining throughout the morning. *Appetite*, 49, 240-244. doi:10.1016/j.appet.2006.06.009.

Jenkins, D.J., Wolever, T.M., Taylor, R.H., Barker, H., Fielden, H., and Baldwin, J.M. (1981). Bowling AC, Newman HC, Jenkins AL, Goff DV. Glycemic index of foods: a physiological basis for carbohydrate exchange. *American Journal of Clinical Nutrition*, 34(3), 362-366.

Kafatos, A., Linardakis, M., Bertsias, G., Mammas, I., Fletcher, R., and Bervanaki, F. (2005). Consumption of ready-to-eat cereals in relation to health and diet indicators among school adolescents in Crete, Greece. *Annals of Nutrition and Metabolism*, 49(3), 165-172.

Kanarek, R. (1997). Psychological effects of snacks and altered meal frequency. *British Journal of Nutrition*, 77, S105-S120

Keim, N.L., Van Loan, M.D., Horn, W.F., Barbieri, T.F., and Mayclin, P.L. (1997). Weight loss is greater with consumption of large morning meals and fat-free mass is preserved with large evening meals in women on a controlled weight reduction regimen. *Journal of Nutrition*, 127(1), 75-82.

Keski-Rahkonen, A., Kaprio, J., Rissanen, A., Virkkunen, M., and Rose, R.J. (2003). Breakfast skipping and health-compromising behaviors in adolescents and adults. *European Journal of Clinical Nutrition*, 57(7), 842-853.

Kochar, J., Djoussé, L., and Gaziano, J.M. (2007). Breakfast cereals and risk of type 2 diabetes in the Physicians' Health Study I. *Obesity*, 15(12), 3039-3044.

Kosti, R.I., Panagiotakos, D.B., and Zampelas, A. (2010). Ready-to-eat cereals and the burden of obesity in the context of their nutritional contribution: are all ready-to-eat cereals equally healthy? A systematic review. *Nutrition Research Reviews*, 23(2), 314-322.

Laron, Z. (2009). Insulin and the brain. *Archives of Physiology and Biochemistry,* 115 (2), 112-116. doi:10.1080/13813450902949012

Liljeberg, H., and Björck, I. (2000). Effects of a low-glycaemic index spaghetti meal on glucose tolerance and lipaemia at a subsequent meal in healthy subjects. *European Journal of Clinical Nutrition*, 54(1), 24-28.

Ludwig, D.S., Majzoub, J.A., Al-Zahrani, A., Dallal, G.E., Blanco, I., Roberts, S.B. (1999). High glycemic index foods, overeating, and obesity. *Pediatrics*, 103(3), E26.

Maffeis, C., Provera, S., Filippi, L., Sidoti, G., Schena, S., Pinelli, L., and Tatò, L. (2000). Distribution of food intake as a risk factor for childhood obesity. *International Journal of Obesity and Related Metabolic Disorders*, 24(1), 75-80.

Mahoney, C.R., Taylor, H.A., Kanarek, R.B., and Samuel, P. (2005). Effect of breakfast composition on cognitive processed in elementary school children. *Physiology and Behavior,* 85, 635-645. doi:10.1016/j.physbeh.2005.06.023

Micha, R., Rogers, P.J., and Nelson, M. (2008). Glycaemic potency of breakfast predicts cognitive function in adolescent schoolchildren. *Proceedings of the Nutrition Society*, 67, E364. doi:10.1017/S0029665108000384

Micha, R., Rogers, P.J., and Nelson, M. (2010). The glycaemic potency of breakfast and cognitive function in school children. *European Journal of Clinical Nutrition*, 64, 948-957.

Michaud, C., Musse, N., Nicolas, J.P., and Mejean, L. (1991). Effects of breakfast-size on short-term memory, concentration, mood and blood glucose. *Journal of Adolescent Health*, 12, 52-57.

Moore, L.J., Midgley, A.W., Thurlow, S., Thomas, G., and Mc Naughton, L.R. (2010). Effect of the glycaemic index of a pre-exercise meal on metabolism and cycling time trial performance. *Journal of Science and Medicine in Sport*, 13(1), 182-188.

Nicklas, T.A., Bao, W., Webber, L.S., and Berenson, G.S. (1993). Breakfast consumption affects adequacy of total daily intake in children. *Journal of the American Dietetic Association*, 93(8), 886-891.

Nicklas, T.A., McQuarrie, A., Fastnaught, C., and O'Neil, C.E. (2002). Efficiency of breakfast consumption patterns of ninth graders: nutrient-to-cost comparisons. *Journal of the American Dietetic Association,* 102(2), 226-33.

Nicklas, T.A., Reger, C., Myers, L., and O'Neil, C. (2000). Breakfast consumption with and without vitamin-mineral supplement use favorably impacts daily nutrient intake of ninth-grade students. *Journal of Adolescent Health*, 27(5), 314-21.

Nilsson, A., Radeborg, K., and Björck, I. (2009). Effects of differences in postprandial glycaemia on cognitive functions in healthy middle-aged students. *European Journal of Clinical Nutrition*, 63, 113-120.

Ortega, R.M., Requejo, A.M., López-Sobaler, A.M., Quintas, M.E., Andrés, P., Redondo, M.R., Navia, B., López-Bonilla, M.D., and Rivas, T. (1998). Difference in the breakfast habits of overweight/obese and normal weight schoolchildren. *International Journal for Vitamin and Nutrition Research,* 68(2), 125-132.

Ostman, E.M., Liljeberg Elmståhl, H.G. and Björck, I.M. (2001). Inconsistency between glycemic and insulinemic responses to regular and fermented milk products. *American Journal of Clinical Nutrition*, 74(1), 96–100.

Pal, S., Lim, S., and Egger, G. (2008). The effect of a low glycaemic index breakfast on blood glucose, insulin, lipid profiles, blood pressure, body weight, body composition and satiety in obese and overweight individuals: a pilot study. *Journal of the American College of Nutrition*, 27(3), 387-393.

Pollitt, E., and Mathews, R. (1998). Breakfast and cognition: an integrative summary. *American Journal of Clinical Nutrition*, 67, 804S-813S.

Pollitt, E., Cueto, S., and Jacoby, E.R. (1998). Fasting and cognition in well- and undernourished schoolchildren: a review of three experimental studies. *American Journal of Clinical Nutrition*, 67, 779S-784S.

Pollitt, E., Gersovitz, M., and Gargiulo, M. (1978). Educational benefits of the United States school feeding program: a critical review of the literature. *American Journal of Public Health*, 68, 477-481.

Pollitt, E., Leibel, R.L., and Greenfield, D. (1981). Brief fasting, stress, and cognition in children. American *Journal of Clinical Nutrition*, 34, 1526-1533.

Preziosi, P., Galan, P., Deheeger, M., Yacoub, N., Drewnowski, A., and Hercberg, S. (1999). Breakfast type, daily nutrient intakes and vitamin and mineral status of French children, adolescents, and adults. *Journal of the American College of Nutrition*, 18(2):171-178.

Rampersaud, G.C., Pereira, M.A., Girard, B.L., Adams, J., and Metzl, J.D. (2005). Breakfast habits, nutritional status, body weight, and academic performance in children and adolescents. *Journal of the American Dietetic Association,* 105, 743-760.

Resnicow, K. (1991) The relationship between breakfast habits and plasma cholesterol levels in schoolchildren. *Journal of School Health*, 61(2), 81-85.

Riddoch, C.J., Mattocks, C., Deere, K., Saunders, J., Kirkby, J., Tilling, K., Leary, S.D., Blair, S.N., and Ness, A.R. (2007). Objective measurement of levels and patterns of physical activity. *Archives of Disease in Childhood.* 92(11), 963-969.

Rogge, M.M. (2009). The role of impaired mitochondrial lipid oxidation in obesity. *Biological Research for Nursing,* 10(4), 356-373.

Rovner, A.J., Nansel, T.R., and Gellar, L. (2009). The effect of a low-glycemic diet vs a standard diet on blood glucose levels and macronutrient intake in children with type 1 diabetes. *Journal of the American Dietetic Association*, 109(2), 303-307.

Ruxton, C.H., O'Sullivan, K.R., Kirk, T.R., Belton, N.R., and Holmes, M.A. (1996). The contribution of breakfast to the diets of a sample of 136 primary-schoolchildren in Edinburgh. *British Journal of Nutrition*, 75(3), 419-431.

Sandercock, G.R., Voss, C., and Dye, L. (2010). Associations between habitual school-day breakfast consumption, body mass index, physical activity and cardiorespiratory fitness in English schoolchildren. *European Journal of Clinical Nutrition*, 64(10), 1086-1092.

Schlundt, D.G., Hill, J.O., Sbrocco, T., Pope-Cordle, J., and Sharp, T. (1992). The role of breakfast in the treatment of obesity: a randomized clinical trial. *American Journal of Clinical Nutrition*, 55(3):645-651.

Schwartz, M.B., Vartanian, L.R., Wharton, C.M., and Brownell, K.D. (2008). Examining the nutritional quality of breakfast cereals marketed to children. *Journal of the American Dietetic Association*, 108(4), 702-705.

Sjöberg, A., Hallberg, L., Höglund, D., and Hulthén, L. (2003). Meal pattern, food choice, nutrient intake and lifestyle factors in The Göteborg Adolescence Study. *European Journal of Clinical Nutrition,* 57(12), 1569-1578.

Skinner, J.D., Bounds, W., Carruth, B.R., and Ziegler, P. (2003). Longitudinal calcium intake is negatively related to children's body fat indexes. *Journal of the American Dietetic Association*, 103(12), 1626-1631.

Smith, M.A., and Foster, J.K. (2008). The impact of a high versus a low glycaemic index breakfast cereal meal on verbal episodic memory in healthy adolescents. *Nutritional Neuroscience*, 11, 219-227. doi:10.1179/147683008X344110.

Song, W.O., Chun, O.K., Kerver, J., Cho, S., Chung, C.E., and Chung, S.J. (2006). Ready-to-eat breakfast cereal consumption enhances milk and calcium intake in the US population. *Journal of the American Dietetic Association*, 106(11), 1783-1789.

Song, Y.J., Sawamura, M., Ikeda, K., Igawa, S., and Yamori, Y. (2000). Soluble dietary fibre improves insulin sensitivity by increasing muscle GLUT-4 content in stroke-prone spontaneously hypertensive rats. *Clinical and Experimental Pharmacology and Physiology,* 27(1-2), 41-45.

Sparks, M.J., Selig, S.S., Febbraio, M.A. (1998). Pre-exercise carbohydrate ingestion: effect of the glycemic index on endurance exercise performance. *Medicine and Science in Sports and Exercise*, 30(6), 844-849.

Spieth, L.E., Harnish, J.D., Lenders, C.M., Raezer, L.B., Pereira, M.A., Hangen, S.J., and Ludwig, D.S. (2000). A low-glycemic index diet in the treatment of pediatric obesity. *Archives of Pediatrics and Adolescent Medicine*, 154(9), 947-951.

Stevenson, E., Williams, C., and Nute, M. (2005). The influence of the glycaemic index of breakfast and lunch on substrate utilisation during the postprandial periods and subsequent exercise. *British Journal of Nutrition,* 93(6), 885-893.

Stevenson, E.J., Astbury, N.M., Simpson, E.J., Taylor, M.A., and Macdonald, I.A. (2009). Fat oxidation during exercise and satiety during recovery are increased following a low-glycemic index breakfast in sedentary women. *Journal of Nutrition*, 139(5), 890-897.

Stevenson, E.J., Williams, C., Mash, L.E., Phillips, B., and Nute, M.L. (2006). Influence of high-carbohydrate mixed meals with different glycemic indexes on substrate utilization during subsequent exercise in women. *American Journal of Clinical Nutrition*, 84(2), 354-360.

Szajewska, H., and Ruszczynski, M. (2010). Systematic review demonstrating that breakfast consumption influences body weight outcomes in children and adolescents in Europe. *Critical Reviews in Food Science and Nutrition,* 50(2), 113-119.

Timlin, M.T., Pereira, M.A., Story, M., and Neumark-Sztainer, D. (2008). Breakfast eating and weight change in a 5-year prospective analysis of adolescents: Project EAT (Eating Among Teens). *Pediatrics*, 121(3), e638-645. doi:10.1542/peds.2007-1035.

Toschke, A.M., Thorsteinsdottir, K.H., and Kries, R.V. (2009). Meal frequency, breakfast consumption and childhood obesity. *International Journal of Pediatric Obesity*, 4(4), 242-248. doi:10.3109/17477160902763341.

Viteri, F.E., and González, H. (2002). Adverse outcomes of poor micronutrient status in childhood and adolescence. Nutrition Reviews, 60(5), S77-S83. doi:10.1301/00296640260130795.

Warren, J.M., Henry, C.J., and Simonite, V. (2003). Low glycemic index breakfasts and reduced food intake in preadolescent children. *Pediatrics*, 112(5), e414.

Weaver, C.M. (2000). The growing years and prevention of osteoporosis in later life. *Proceedings of the Nutrition Society*, 59(2), 303-306. doi:10.1017/S0029665100000331.

Wee, S.L., Williams, C., Tsintzas, K., and Boobis, L. (2005). Ingestion of a high-glycemic index meal increases muscle glycogen storage at rest but augments its utilization during subsequent exercise. *Journal of Applied Physiology*, 99(2), 707-714.

Wesnes, K.A., Pincock, C., Richardson, D., Helm, G., and Hails, S. (2003). Breakfast reduces the declines in attention and memory over the morning in schoolchildren. *Appetite*, 41, 329-331. doi:10.1016/j.appet.2003.08.009.

Widenhorn-Müller, K., Hille, K., Klenk, J., and Weiland, U. (2008). Influence of having breakfast on cognitive performance and mood in 13- to 20-year-old high school students: results of a crossover trial. *Pediatrics*, 122, 279-284. doi:10.1542/peds.2007-0944.

Willett, W. (1994). Micronutrients and cancer risk. *American Journal of Clinical Nutrition,* 59, S1162-S1165.

Wolever, T.M., and Bolognesi, C. (1996). Source and amount of carbohydrate affect postprandial glucose and insulin in normal subjects. *Journal of Nutrition*, 126(11),2798–2806.

Wu, C.L., Nicholas, C., Williams, C., Took, A., and Hardy, L. (2003). The influence of high-carbohydrate meals with different glycaemic indices on substrate utilisation during subsequent exercise. *British Journal of Nutrition*, 90(6), 1049-1056.

Wyon, D.P., Abrahamsson, L., Järtelius, M., and Fletcher, R.J. (1997). An experimental study of the effects of energy intake at breakfast on the test performance of 10-year-old children in school. *International Journal of Food Sciences and Nutrition,* 48, 5-12.

Zemel, M.B., Thompson, W., Milstead, A., Morris, K., and Campbell, P. (2004). Calcium and dairy acceleration of weight and fat loss during energy restriction in obese adults. *Obesity Research*, 12(4), 582-590. doi:10.1038/oby.2004.67.

In: Reviews in Pediatric Exercise Science
Editor: Michael Duncan, pp. 67-86
ISBN: 978-1-61470-978-7

Chapter V

Environmental Correlates of Physical Activity in Children and Adolescents

Stacey Hargreaves, Michael J. Duncan and Samantha Birch
Coventry University, UK.

Introduction

Physical activity when taken regularly is a health enhancing behaviour and reduces the risk for many chronic diseases. In children, future health benefits are also obtained by engaging in physical activity, such as a strong heart, healthy joints, strong bones and good mental health. Despite this, many children are not reaching their recommended levels of physical activity and overweight and obesity levels are increasing in children (Ferreira et al, 2006). Physical activity is the most important recommendation for a healthy lifestyle throughout the lifespan and if children are taught healthy habits in their early years may positively influence their health in adulthood (Strong et al, 2005). As the physical activity behaviours learnt in childhood is likely to continue into adulthood (Kjonniksen et al, 2008), it is important to address the deficit of physical activity to improve current and future health benefits (Craig and Mindell, 2008).

As levels of overweight have risen and physical activity declined worldwide, investigators have attempted to find the reasons for the increase in obesity in children and adolescents, and also the decrease in physical activity (van Sluijs et al, 2008; Giles-Corti, 2009; Schofield et al, 2009, Jones et al, 2010). They have found no single theory that explains all of the factors that contribute with genetic factors, socio-cultural variables and environmental factors all thought to contribute. As a change to the gene pool is unlikely to have taken place across the time span in which overweight and obesity has risen, it is likely that socio-cultural and environmental variables play a key part in level of overweight and obesity in children (Giles-Corti, 2009; Schofield et al, 2009, Jones et al, 2010). As a result, research is now needed to understand the interaction between environmental factors and physical activity and obesity in children and young people (Booth et al, 2005). The purpose of this review is to provide an overview of current research assessing the environmental correlates of physical activity in children and adolescents (Booth et al, 2005).

Environmental Correlates of Physical Activity

The changing nature of how children engage with their physical environment is one factor in the dramatic increase in children being overweight (Hillier, 2008). It has been suggested that children are spending more time within their homes and engaging in less physical activity outdoors. Consequently, many Children are no longer reaching their daily recommended level of physical activity and overweight and obesity levels are increasing (Ferreira et al, 2006). These recommended levels, that children and adolescents should engage in 60 minutes or more of physical activity each day (Centre for Disease Control and Prevention, 2010), are important because children who are physically active are less likely to become overweight, have better cardiovascular fitness and have improved health compared with less active children (Cooper et al, 2010b).

The Built Environment

The effects the environment can have on health can be in many forms, from emotional, physiological, and social to spiritual and intellectual wellbeing (Lake, 2006). One particular environmental influence which research is now showing to be a key environmental influence on physical activity is the built environment (Public Health Collaborating Centre, 2007) as the environment can influence health is through its physical design (the built environment), the socio-cultural rules that govern the environments and the socio-economic status of the environment (Feldman and Steptoe, 2004).

In any attempt to understand childhood obesity and physical inactivity, the 'built environment' must be considered. The built environment consists of neighbourhoods, roads, buildings, food sources and recreational facilities in which people live, work, are educated, eat and play (Sallis and Glanz, 2006) and describes everything that children encounter when they step outside their door in their immediate neighbourhood area. It is often based on the conception that children spend a large extent of their time near their homes (Hillier, 2008). There is strong evidence to show that modifying the built environment can increase children's physical activity, reduce their access to unhealthy foods and increase their access to healthy foods (Sallis and Glanz, 2006; Rahman et al, 2011).

However, the terms 'environment' and 'the built environment' do not always contain the same meaning. Cohen et al, (2006) distinguished four factors that can affect health. These were; the availability of healthful products (such as fruit and vegetables), and harmful products, such as (cigarettes and alcohol), physical structures in the environment, social structures and how the media influences the environment. Whereas, the term "the built environment" is mostly used by researchers to describe the many factors within the environment that can influence health.

The Impact of the Built Environment

Hillier (2008) defined the following being impacted by the built environment; physical activity, food access, crime and safety, outdoor advertising and racial and income disparities.

Physical Activity

There are numerous studies that describe how the built environment influences physical activity. Sallis and Glanz, (2006), Heath et al, (2006) and Handy et al, (2002) describe the influence on physical activity as the following:

1. Areas with mixed land use, greater residential and commercial densities, grid street networks, and sidewalks are associated with more walking, biking and transportation usage.
2. Children with access to parks, recreation facilities and programs are more physically active than those children without access.

Food Access

The food environment can also have an impact on health; this can have an influence on the individuals depending on what food resources they have. This could range from having fast food outlets locally in the area to the distance of the nearest fresh fruit and vegetable shops (Lake, 2006). It has also been found that people who have better access to supermarkets and limited access to convenience stores have improved and healthier diets and reduced levels of obesity (Rahman et al, 2011).

The research on the correlations of food access with physical activity is substantially growing. This has shown that food access such as fast-food restaurants, supermarkets and convenience stores vary in different neighbourhoods (Hillier, 2008). Zenk et al, (2005) and Horowitz et al, (2004) found that neighbourhoods with ethnic minorities and low income have a smaller number of supermarkets and less access to fresh and healthy foods such as fresh fruit and vegetables. It has also been indicated that those neighbourhoods with less access to fresh food have higher access to fast food restaurants and alcohol outlets (Morland et al, 2002). In contrast to this, Birch and Fisher, (1998) suggest that food access is more strongly linked to eating behaviour rather than being correlated with physical activity.

Frank et al, (2009) also considered how food outlets can affect physical activity and the variations across gender and race. They found there were a positive correlation of increased Body Mass Index (BMI) with females who ate fast food and a lower level of BMI for females with grocery store visitation and physical activity. They concluded that where people go for food differs significantly across gender and ethnicity. Many other studies have also found that the availability of healthful foods will predict healthier diets within the environment (Rose and Richards, 2004, Laraia et al, 2004).

Crime and Safety

The aptitude of how the environment can encourage active living and how individuals feel in the environment also can be closely related to health. The perceptions of how safe they feel in their environment could also have an effect on how much physical activity is participated in the environment (Lake, 2006). There has been less evidence in terms of BMI measurements that crime and safety in the environment has an effect on physical activity levels in children. However, the perceived perceptions of the parents in the neighbourhood in regards to safety can affect the level of activity children will engage in. For those parents who worry about road safety and crime in their neighbourhood are less likely to let their children outside unsupervised and will keep them indoors and more sedentary (Lumeng et al, 2006). In another study on the perceived perceptions of the environment, it was also found that adolescent girls are less interested in participating in community-based opportunities are more prone to engage in physical activity around the home. The study also concluded that those participants who did want to stay indoors were not engaging in significant physical activity to benefit their health and interventions need to focus on how to encourage children and adolescents out into the community (Dunton et al, 2003).

A study by Cox et al (2010) looked at the perspectives from children, teachers and parents regarding physical activity. They found that parents do want to encourage their children to be active but they found that some parents encourage their children to travel via cars and buses rather than biking or walking due to worry about the dangers that could happen to their child. However, Faulkner et al (2009) found that children who walk to school had much higher physical activity levels than those children who do not walk to school. They found that active school commuters tend to be overall more physically active than passive commuters. It has also been found that children who walk to school have a 50% increase of physical activity during the hour before and after school than children who travel by car (Cooper et al, 2005; Cooper et al, 2003; Sirard et al, 2005; Saksvig et al, 2007).

Neighbourhoods that are run down and have broken windows (known as the broken window syndrome) (Eggers and O'Leary, 1995) can often encourage crime and have increased safety risks. Lopez and Hynes, (2006) has suggested that in areas that have the "broken window syndrome", there is an increased chance that there would be less walking, less recreation opportunities and less physical activity engagement in these environments. When neighbourhoods are short of safe places to play and have factors such as neighbourhood crime, heavy trafficked streets and graffiti, children are prevented from being active outdoors and instead have increased indoor sedentary behaviour (Rahman et al, 2011). Time indoors promotes an increase in screen time such as watching TV and playing video games which is directly associated with child and adult obesity (Dietz and Gortmaker, 2001).

Outdoor Advertising

Outdoor advertising has also been found to be correlated with physical activity. Studies, although sparse, have found that there are more advertisements for alcohol and tobacco in areas with low income populations and racial minorities (Hackbarth et al, 2001; Kwate and Lee, 2007). One study found that the adverts influence the youth in their neighbourhoods and increase underage drinking in adolescents (Pasch et al, 2007), which could cause future health problems or even alcohol dependency (Van der Vorst et al, 2010). However, the extant data pertaining to the effects (either direct or in tandem with other variables) of advertising on physical activity and weight status is not expansive and future work is needed which investigates this issue in order for any conclusive statement to be made regarding the impact of outdoor advertising on physical activity and obesity in children and young people.

Racial and Income Disparities

Differences in race and income characterize physical activity, food access, eating, crime and outdoor advertising, and also overweight among children and adults (Day, 2006). It has been suggested that residential segregation can cause differences in the environment (Kawachi and Berkman, 2003). The differences in the environments can affect the way the people live their lives. They have fewer supermarkets which mean less healthy options but they are also exposed to an increased number of convenience stores and fast-food food outlets. It is also suggested that there was fewer opportunities for recreation and less access to physical activity settings (Powell et al, 2004). The study also found that communities with higher proportions of minority races such as American African and the race category 'other' are associated with fewer physical activity settings. There has also been an association that ethnic minorities and low income children watch more television than their white peers (Kumanyika and Grier, 2006). A study by (Tirodkar and Jain, 2003) found that there are more food commercials in shows that target black audiences and that within these food commercials, they are more likely to advertise unhealthy foods such as chocolate, sweets and fizzy drinks (Henderson and Kelly, 2005).

Studies Examining the Correlations of the Built Environment and Physical Activity in Children and Adolescents

There are many suggested environmental influences that can have an effect on children's physical activity and the structure of the environment can influence decisions such as where children will eat, what transport methods will be used, whether they will walk to their destinations and where they will socialise (Edwards and Tsouros, 2006). One other potential influence is the amount of time the child spends outdoors. Time outdoors has been found to be a correlate of children's physical activity in many studies (Cooper et al, 2010b, Loucaides et al, 2004; Public Health Collaborating Centre, 2007).

Ferreira et al, (2006) and Sallis et al, (2000) found that physical activity was associated with time outdoors. Baranowski et al, (1993) and Cleland et al, (2008) also found that there was an increased measurement of physical activity when children were outdoors. Correlations with time outdoors also indicated a low prevalence of overweight (Cleland et al, 2008) with higher independent mobility (Wen et al, 2009). Cleland et al, (2008) has also suggested that one method to prevent overweight and obesity is to encourage children to play outdoors. However, even though time outdoors is a beneficial factor to a child's health, Wen et al, (2008) reported that a significant proportion of children spend less than half an hour a day outdoors after school but have excessive screen time by watching TV, videos or playing computer games. The study by Wen et al (2008) also suggested that different environments play different roles in promoting independent mobility. Those environments that promote independent mobility have increased physical activity levels which can reduce the risk of obesity. Clearly, time spent outdoors is important in shaping opportunity for physical activity but it is also important when examining children's time spent outdoors to consider why they may not be going outside. Chan and Ryan, (2009) assessed the effects of weather conditions on physical activity and found that the weather has been identified as a perceived barrier to participate in physical activity. When the weather is poor such as cold temperatures or raining, people are more likely to use other transport methods rather than walking and cycling. However, it was found that there is an increase in physical activity in men when it is snowing. This is due to needing to chop woods for fires and also by using alternative methods to walking such as skating, snow-shoeing and cross-country skiing.

Work by Vries et al, (2010) examined the built environment correlates of the behaviour of children's walking and cycling. This study, which involved completing a seven day physical activity diary, found that the correlates of the children's walking and cycling behaviour differed by purpose by transportation, recreation and school, and also by the mode of commuting such as walking, cycling and combined. It was found that there was more physical activity taken place in neighbourhoods that had a higher number of pedestrian crossings and higher number of parking spaces. Similar to this, the safety of the environment is not the only problem. It is also believed that parents influence their children's behaviours and this affects the amount of physical activity that they participate in. Hennessy et al, (2010) found that for children whose parents gave higher levels of reinforcement or monitoring were associated with higher levels of physical activity than those children whose parents were uninvolved with their activities. Parental monitoring also resulted in a higher level of MVPA (Moderate to Vigorous Exercise).

Research is also beginning to find connections between the environment and sedentary behaviours. Children may spend more time being inactive indoors if they have no safe places to play. Problems such as heavy traffic can also reduce children from walking which then mean that children stay indoors and remain sedentary (Sallis and Glanz, 2006). This may mean that commuting to places then involves the use of the car which can the cause physical inactivity and overweight in children and adults. Time spent travelling in a car is associated with overweight adults so this could have the same affect on their offspring (Frank et al, 2004).

It has also been suggested that urban or rural settings may influence physical fitness in children (Findholt et al, 2010). Tsimeas et al, (2005) compared the fitness of children from both urban and rural areas and, although there were significant differences in activities between urban and rural children, the place of residence did not have a clear impact on physical fitness. Tsimeas et al, (2005) also reported that urban children had more body fat than rural children. Despite this, research has yet to fully elucidate the effect of living in urban or rural settings on physical activity in children in adolescents.

Communities

Neighbourhoods with lower-socioeconomic status have an increased risk of obesity as these communities frequently have restricted access to; food stores that have affordable and healthy options and recreational facilities (Rahman et al, 2011). Communities that live in poorer neighbourhoods have three times fewer supermarkets when compared to communities from wealthy neighbourhoods but have more convenience stores and fast food restaurants (Morland et al, 2002). This promotes un-healthful food choice and can cause unhealthy eating and poor nutrition (Hinkle and Wu, 2003). Physical activity can be promoted in neighbourhoods that have access to healthful eating and access to community gardens (Mikkelsen et al, 2007; Glanz and Yaroch, 2004).

Communities that have poor street connectivity, low density development patterns and a lack of safe walking destinations can impact health behaviours which can in the long term contribute to obesity and chronic illness (McCann and Ewing, 2003). Lopez, (2004) found that sprawling communities have a higher rate of adult obesity. Urban sprawl is defined as areas where homes are absent or far from amenities in the community and often have high speed roadways as the only route to reach destinations and driving is the method of transport used to reach destinations (Rahman et al, 2011). The more time driving could mean less time engaging in physical activity.

Parents as Role Models and Parental Support

Most studies have failed to find a relationship with parents as role models and physical activity. However, studies have found that in childhood, fathers appear to be seen as important role models as compared to mothers, especially in childhood (Davison et al, 2003; Fogelholm et al, 1999). It is also suggested that father's physical activity may be associated with their child's physical activity of either gender where mother's physical activity tends to be associated with the girls physical activity. However, a parent's physical activity has been found to be unrelated to their child's future physical activity levels (Ferreira et al, 2006; Strong et al, 2005). It is also hypothesized that encouragement and support from parents influences the behaviour of their offspring. Studies have demonstrated that activity programmes in the home where parents are trained to monitor their children's fitness had a significant increase in the physical activity in sedentary children (Trost and Loprinzi, 2008). Although in many studies of children where self reported PA is recorded, parental PA levels were most often assessed by parents them and adolescents were assessed by themselves and by parents. It is possible that the parental reports were perceived and the opinion of the parent and not a true indicator of how much physical activity have taken place (Ferreira, 2006).

Sedentary Time and TV Viewing

Sedentary time can be defined as when people are not active and can also be associated with increased adiposity in children (Steele et al, 2009). As sedentary time does not provide what activity the person has engaged in (Jago et al, 2010), the specific behaviours can be related to health outcomes (Biddle, 2007).

Television viewing is a commonly studied example of sedentary behaviour where increased television viewing has been related to a higher body mass in youth (Jago et al, 2005; Viner and Cole, 2005; Vandewater et al, 2004). Many children and adolescents exceed TV viewing recommendations but don't exceed or meet physical activity guidelines (Jago et al, 2005; Riddoch et al, 2004; Riddoch et al, 2007; Deverill et al, 2002). It is also important to consider the parents role as they are likely to be a significant influence on how much television is being viewed and how much physical activity they take (Gustafson et al, 2006; Davison et al, 2003; Jago et al, 2009; Thompson et al, 2009). Spending time watching television and playing video games can take away opportunities to engage in physical activity and can also impact eating habits as children who watch television are more likely to snack of junk food (Taveras et al, 2006; Harris et al, 2009).

Age is also an important consideration as physical activity levels of children decrease as they get older especially as they reach adolescence (Kimm et al, 2002; Caspersen et al, 2000). The age found to be where changes in physical activity occur is around 10-11 years old when the child is about to leave primary school and commence secondary school (Caspersen et al, 2000; Nader et al, 2008). Therefore, it is important to understand the factors that influence TV viewing and physical activity at this transitional age as a preventative of the development of cardiovascular and associated diseases (Jago et al, 2010).

How Schools Can Influence Physical Activity in Children

There are many opportunities where young people can engage in physical activity sessions in school. These include activities such as break times, PE classes, physical activity programmes, extracurricular sports, leisure time and use of playing fields and playgrounds (Ferreira et al, 2006). Schools also have trained employees who can deliver physical activity programmes and policies that promote and support physical activity and healthy lifestyles (Ferreira et al, 2006). Studies have found that school-based programmes that are well designed and well implemented can improve physical activity levels of young people (Timperio et al, 2004; Matson-Koffman, 2005; Stone et al, 1998). One study also found that PE lessons that are based outside generate more time in vigorous activities and had higher total energy expenditure than PE lesson that are taught indoors (Mckenzie et al, 1995). Another study found that correlates of higher engagement of physical activity in children were the size of the school, the availability of balls in the playground and the length of break times (Lindquist et al, 1999). However, Mckenzie et al, (2000) found that although there are physical activity facilities available within school, they are only used by few students during their leisure time at school (during lunch breaks and before and after school). Sallis et al, (2001) further explored these findings and found that the decision to use the facilities by the young people was based on the size and state of the facility and the existence of supervised and organised activities. Other researchers have found that schools are not providing enough time for physical activities (Simons-Morton et al, 1993; Simons-Morton et al, 1994; as mentioned by Ferreira et al, 2006).

Global Positioning Systems as a Tool to Study the Effect of the Environment on Physical Activity

There are an increasing number of studies conducted to examine how the environment correlates with physical activity. With the use of a global monitoring system, a study is able to identify the environment where the participants are engaged in activity (Cooper et al, 2010a; Cooper et al, 2010b; Duncan et al, 2009a; Duncan et al, 2009b; Fjortoft, 2004; Fjortoft et al, 2009; Maddison, 2009; Maddison, 2010; Quigg et al, 2010; Schutz and Chambaz, 1997; Troped et al, 2010; Wheeler et al, 2010). The Global Positioning System (GPS) is a new and potentially valuable tool to measure physical activity. It can also help to improve our understanding of physical activity by providing location information (Maddison et al, 2009).

Schutz and Chumbaz, (1997) first suggested that GPS could be used to measure human location. They suggested that the advantages of using a GPS was that they are small in size, non invasive non obtrusive free living measurements, they have a continuous measurement with data that can be accessed online, free access to the GPS satellites in any part of the world, the GPS is a reasonable cost, data can be stored and retrieved when required, the technique can be used to validate measurements of velocity of walking and running (Schutz and Chumbaz, (1997); as mentioned by Maddison et al, 2009).

Global positioning systems have also been used in sports to locate position, analyse speed and the overview of sporting performance, with sports including cross country skiing (Larsson and Henriksson-Larsen, 2005), football (Pino et al, 2007), golf (Peterson et al, 2005), orienteering (Larsson, 2003) and Australian football (Edgecomb and Norton, 2006). Such systems are used to research how individuals interact with the physical environment (Cooper et al, 2010b). The GPS is a valuable tool for field data collection as location data can be obtained using satellites which can be used in parallel with geographical Information Systems (GIS). GIS depends on pre-generated map layers of features such as streets and building. GIS is used in research on the associations between childhood obesity and the environment (Hillier, 2008). GIS allows spatial analysis which links physical activity with features such as green spaces (Quigg et al, 2010; as mentioned by Maas et al, 2008), playgrounds, parks and facilities (Cohen et al, 2008). Though the GIS can find these associations, they are unable to record the actual use of these findings, where a GPS combined with the GIS can resolve these difficulties (Maddison, 2010).

In practical terms, portable GPS monitors can be attached to the wrist of the participant, and can then be used to record geographical positions from satellites every fifth, second (Fjortoft et al, 2009). When GPS is combined with accelerometer data, associations between independent movement and physical activity can be defined (Mackett et al, 2007), how the child has travelled to school (Cooper et al, 2010b) and the location of bouts of moderate intensity physical activity (Jones et al, 2009). GPS monitors have also been used to map the travel routes to schools (Duncan et al, 2007). A study named the PEACH (Personal and Environmental Associations with Children's Health) project by Cooper et al, (2010b) investigated the positive association between time outdoors and physical activity in children. To examine this association, Global Positioning Systems (GPS) and accelerometers were worn by 1010 British primary school children after school for four weekdays. The results shown that the GPS measured time outdoors was a significant predictor of children's physical activity and that physical activity outdoors was increased in the summer months. It also found that more time in Greenspace is related to more time spent in moderate-to-vigorous physical activity (MVPA). In another similar study, Wheeler et al, (2010) examined time spent outdoors in greenspace and the effect that has on physical activity. Greenspace is defined as "Open, undeveloped land with natural vegetation" (Centre for Disease Control and Prevention, 2010). The results concluded that time is greenspace shown an increase in MVPA (Moderate to Vigorous Physical Activity) but the majority of outdoor activity volume occurs outside of greenspaces. The study suggests that green and non-green urban environments both play an important role in physical activity in children. In a similar study investigating MVPA and how the built environment can affect it, Troped et al, (2010) found that by using a GPS, they was able to show that the built environment around homes are positively related to physical activity and can influence how much physical activity is taken.

Another recent study by Maddison et al (2010) also examined GPS assessed physical activity in adolescents (n= 79). They found that on average, participants performed 74 minutes of moderate exercise activity per day and 7.5 minutes of vigorous activity per day. They also found that on weekends, physical activity patterns took place outside the home environment. Time spent in the school environment was also highlighted as the time where most inactivity took place; this could be due to lack of facilities within the school and also due the majority of the day sitting down in lessons.

Global Positioning Systems have also been used to track movement patterns in schoolyards. Fjortoft et al, (2009) investigated how 6-year old children used their school yards at break times and how the yard influenced physical activity. Two different schoolyards were used, with one in city and the other in a rural area. The results found that physical activity (mean heart rate) was similar in both schoolyards, however, the city schoolyard encouraged running and football and more physical activity in boys than the girls where the rural schoolyard was more attractive to girls than boys. In a similar study, Duncan et al (2009b) used a combined GPS and heart rate monitor to measure physical activity in primary school children. For this study, the levels of physical activity were measured during the school lunch break. The results suggested that children were relatively active during their lunch period and spent the majority of their time in motion. They also found that children who move at higher speeds expand more energy than those at slower speeds.

GPS has been further used to identify how much physical activity takes place in playgrounds and parks (Quigg et al, 2010). The study examined children aged between 5 to years old and found that only 1.9% of their recorded physical activity was taken place in parks and that there was a low percentage of children using parks and playgrounds. Although this percentage was low, they did find that there was an increased percentage with obese children, with this group recording 2.9% of physical activity in parks and playgrounds. Playgrounds have however been recognised in public health research as an area of play that can increase the physical activity levels of children (Floyd et al, 2008; Schoeppe and Braubach, 2007; Sallis and Glanz, 2006; Timperio et al, 2004). Veitch et al, (2006) agrees with this but found in their qualitative study that children can only access public places such as parks through parental time and inclination to take them there or if they have their own independent mobility. This could suggest why the study by Quigg et al, (2010) found that there was a higher proportion of physical activity taking place in parks on weekends rather than weekdays.

Research has also found that active commuting in the form of walking to school can benefit children (Cooper et al, 2010a). The study used an accelerometer combined with a GPS and was able to identify the level and location of children walking to school. The results found that children who walked to school had increased MVPA and overall higher total physical activity than those who travelled to school by car. They found that walking to school could be beneficial to health. Using GPS and Heart rate monitoring is a valuable method to investigate both the spatial location and the energy expenditure associated with children's physical activity (Duncan. al, 2009b). Duncan, et al, (2009b) agrees that GPS, especially if combined with heart rate monitors, GIS or accelerometer offers great potential in objectively measuring and studying the relationship of numerous environmental attributes to human behaviour in terms of physical activity. With GPS research, the advantage is that the satellite is able to map out where activity has taken place thus giving a clear idea of how the environment affects the individual. However, a limitation to those studies are that whilst indoor, there is limited signal received and cannot indicate how indoor environments can affect physical activity.

Potential Limitations with the GPS

One reported limitation with the GPS was participant compliance with wearing the GPS (Cooper et al, 2010a). Cooper et al reported that this was difficult to assess as the GPS data is only recorded if the device is switched on and has satellite signals. A second limitation highlighted by many studies (Cooper et al, 2010a; Quigg et al, 2010; Maddison and Mhurchu, 2009; Wheeler et al, 2010; Duncan et al , 2009a; Cooper et al, 2010b) was the limited battery life of the GPS which meant the participants had to switch the GPS on and off. It is also mentioned that the GPS is only effective in outdoor areas that are not covered by trees or other structures (Duncan et al, 2009b), however they do suggest that with the combination of a heart rate monitor, the GPS can continue measuring energy expenditure, intensity, duration and frequency indoors and outdoors. Other issues have been on the method to interpret and analyse the data as there are large amounts of activity data that are produced from the GPS (Maddsion et al, 2010 and this important to understand as it shows how the individuals move within their environment. Another issue reported by Wheeler et al, (2010) found that the initialisation period of the GPS could mean that activity is being missed or misclassified as indoors when they individual is outdoors. They also found that there is sometimes misclassification of data points when around different urban structures such as tall buildings and difficulty to interpret data when the individual is in a car or public transport. However, they still found that the GPS was a valuable tool to physical activity and the environment.

Conclusion

Regular physical activity is a health enhancing behaviour for children and adolescents. Although there is a significant amount of data to support this, many children and adolescents are still not reaching their daily recommended levels of physical activity. There are various factors suggested of why physical activity is decreasing and a more frequently suggested factor is the how the environment affects physical activity.

When examining environmental correlates of physical activity, there are limitations present. Much literature has parents, children and adolescents reporting perceived perceptions of the environment by the use of questionnaires. Even though many studies do also objectively measure physical activity, how the environment is perceived will be different for each individual. The use of the GPS monitors for this type of study will give more detailed data about the environment. Though the monitors do have their own limitations, the use of the satellite to provide maps of where physical activity takes place will provide more accurate information and the environment can be examined and contrasted in great detail.

As overweight and obesity levels are increasing and physical activity levels are decreasing (Van Sluijs et al, 2008; Giles-Corti, 2009; Schofield et al, 2009, it is apparent that the environment does have an impact on physical activity. In order to reduce overweight and obesity in children, interventions are needed to not only understand how the environment influences physical activity but strategies to increase physical activity in children and adolescents. More research is also needed to examine racial and ethnic variation and to compare data against other countries.

References

Baranowski, T., Thompson, W., DuRant, R., Baranowski, J. and Puhl, J. (1993) 'Observations on physical activity in physical locations: age, gender, ethnicity, and month effects'. *Research Quarterly for Exercise and Sport*, 64 (2), 127-133.

Biddle, S. (2007) 'Sedentary behaviour'. *American Journal of Preventive Medicine* 33 (6), 502-504.

Biles-Corti, B., Kelty, S., Zubrick, S. and Villanueva, K. (2009) 'Encouraging walking for transport and physical activity in children and adolescents; How important is the built environment?' *Sports Medicine* 39 (12), 995-1009.

Birch, L. and Fisher, J. (1998) 'Development of eating behaviours among children and adolescents'. *Pediatrics*, 101, 539-549.

Booth, K., Pinkston, M., Walker, S. and Poston, C. (2005) 'Obesity and the built environment'. *Journal of the American Dietetic Association*, 105, S110-S117.

Caspersen, C., Pereira, M. and Curran, K. (2000) 'Changes in physical activity patterns in the United States, by sex and cross-sectional age'. *Medicine and Science in Sports and Exercise* 32 (9), 1601-1609.

Centre for Disease Control and Prevention (2010) 'Healthy Places Terminology'. [Online] Available from <http://www.cdc.gov/healthyplaces/terminology.htm> [26th November 2010].

Centre for Disease Control and Prevention (2010) 'Physical Activity for Everyone' [online] Available from <http://www.cdc.gov/physicalactivity/everyone/guidelines/children.html> [26th November 2010].

Chan, C. and Ryan, D. (2009) 'Assessing the effects of weather conditions on physical activity participation using objective measures'. *International Journal of Environmental Research and Public Health*, 6, 2639-2654.

Cleland, V. Crawford, D., Baur, LA., Hume, C., Timperio, A. and Salmon, J. (2008) 'A prospective examination of children's time spent outdoors, objectively measured physical activity and overweight'. *International Journal of Obesity*, 32, 1685-1693.

Cohen, D., Ashwood, S., Scott, M., Overton, A., Evenson, K., Voorhees, C., Bedimo-Rung, A. and McKenzie, T. (2006) 'Proximity to School and Physical Activity among Middle School Girls: The Trial of Activity for Adolescent Girls Study'. *Paediatrics.* 118(5), e1381–e1389.

Cohen, D., Ashwood, S., Scott, M., Overton, A., Evenson, K., Staten, L., Porter, D., McKenzie, T. and Catellier, D. (2008) 'Public Parks and Physical Activity Among Adolescent Girls' *Paediatrics,* 118 (5), e1381- e1389.

Cooper, A., Andersen, L. Wedderkopp, N., Page, A., Froberg, K. (2005) 'Physical activity levels of children who walk, cycle, or are driven to school'. *American Journal of Preventive Medicine* 29 (3), 179-184.

Cooper, A., Page, A., Foster, L. and Qahwaki, D. (2003) 'Commuting to school: are children who walk more physically active?' *American Journal of Preventive Medicine* 25 (4), 273-276.

Cooper, A., Page, A., Wheeler, B., Griew, P., Davis, L. Hillsdon, M. and Jago, R. (2010a) 'Mapping the walk to school using accelerometry combined with a global positioning system'. *American Journal of Preventive Medicine* 38 (2), 178-183.

Cooper, A., Page, A., Wheeler, B., Hillsdon, M., Griew, P. and Jago, R. (2010b) 'Patterns of GPS measured time outdoors after school and objective physical activity in English children: the PEACH project'. *International Journal of Behavioural Nutrition and Physical Activity* 7 (31), 1-9.

Cox, M., Schofield, G and Kolt, G. (2010) 'Responsibility for children's physical activity: Parental, child, and teacher perspectives'. *Journal of Science and Medicine in Sport,* 13, 46-52.

Craig, R. and Mindell, J. (2008) 'Health Survey for England 2006, Volume 2: Obesity and other risk factors in children'. *The Information Centre.* Leeds.

Davison, K., Cutting, T. and Birch, L. (2003) 'Parents' activity-related parenting practices predict girls' physical activity'. *Medicine and Science in Sports and Exercise* 35 (9), 1589-1595.

Davison, K., Werder, J. and Lawson, C. (2008) 'Children's' active commuting to school: current knowledge and future directions'. *Preventing Chronic Disease* 5 (3), 1-11.

Day, K. (2006) 'Active living and social justice: Planning for physical activity in low-income, black, and Latino communities'. *Journal of the American Planning Association* 72 (1), 88-99.

Dietz, W. and Gortmaker, S. (2001) 'Preventing obesity in children and adolescents'. *Annual Review of Public Health* 22, 337-353.

Deveriill, C., Doyle, M., Erens, B., Falaschetti, E, Hedges, B., Malbut, K, Primatesta, P., Stamatakis, E. and Wardle, H. (2002) 'The Health of Children and Young People'. *Health Survey for England 2002.* Edited by: Sprotson, K., Primatesta, P. London: Stationary Office.

Duncan, M., Mummery, W. and Dascombe, B. (2007) 'Utility of global positioning system to measure active transport in urban areas'. *Medicine and Science in Sports and Exercise,* 39, 1851-1857.

Duncan, J., Badland, H. and Mummery, K. (2009a) 'Applying GPS to enhance understanding of transport related physical activity'. *Journal of Science and Medicine in Sport* 12, 549-556.

Duncan, J., Badland, H. and Schofield, G. (2009b) 'Combining GPS with heart rate monitoring to measure physical activity in children: A feasibility study'. *Journal of Science and Medicine in Sport* 12, 583-585.

Dunton, G., Jamner, M. and Cooper, D. (2003) 'Assessing the perceived environment among minimally active adolescent girls: Validity and relations to physical activity outcomes'. *The American Journal of Health Promotion* [online] Available from <http://www.activelivingresearch.org/alr/files/AJHP_10_Dunton.pdf> [28th October 2010].

Edgecomb, S. and Norton, K. (2006) 'Comparison of global positioning and computer bases tracking systems for measuring player movement distance during Australian Football'. *Journal of Science in Sport and Medicine* 9, 25-32.

Edwards, P and Tsouros, A. (2006) 'Promoting physical activity and active living in urban Environments: the role of local governments'. *World Health Organisation* [online] Available from http://www.euro.who.int/__data/assets/pdf_file/0009/98424/E89498.pdf.

Eggers, W. and O'Leary, J. (1995) 'Broken Windows Syndrome'. *Policy Review* [online] 74. Available from <http://www.sjvgreens.org/broken.shtml> [28th November 2010].

Faulkner, G., Buliung, R., Flora, P and Fusco, C. (2009) 'Active school transport, physical activity levels and body weight of children and youth: A systematic review'. *Preventive Medicine*, 48, 3-8.

Feldman PJ, Steptoe A. (2004) 'How neighbourhoods and physical functioning are related: the roles of neighbourhood socioeconomic status, perceived neighbourhood strain, and individual health risk factors'. *Annals of Behavioural Medicine: a Publication of the Society of Behavioural Medicine* 27(2):91–9.

Ferreira, I, Horst, K., Wendel-Vos, W., Kremers, S., Lenthe, F. and Brug, J. (2006) 'Environmental correlates of physical activity in youth- a review and update. *Obesity reviews* 8, 129-154.

Findholt, N., Michael, Y., Davis, M. and Brogoitti, V. (2010) 'Environmental influences on children's physical activity and diets in rural Oregon: Results of a youth photovoice project'. *Online Journal of Rural Nursing and Health Care* 10 (2), 11-18.

Fjortoft, I. (2004) 'Landscape as playscape: the effects of natural environment on children's play and motor development'. *Children, Youth and Environments.* 14 (2), 21-44.

Fjortoft, I., Kristoffererersen, B. and Sageie, J. (2009) 'Children in schoolyards: Tracking movement patterns and physical activity in schoolyards using global positioning system and heart rate monitoring'. *Landscape and Urban Planning* 210-217.

Floyd, M., Crespo, C., Sallis, J., (2008) 'Active living research in diverse and disadvantaged communities stimulating dialogue and policy solutions'. *American Journal of Preventive Medicine* 34, 271-274.

Fogelholm, M., Nuutinen, O., Pasenen, M., Myohanen, E. and Saatela, T. (1999) 'Parent-child relationship of physical activity patterns and obesity'. *International Journal of Obesity and Related Metabolic Disorders*, 23, 1262-1268.

Frank, L., Andresen, M. and Schmid, T. (2004) 'Obesity relationships with community design, physical activity, and time spent in cars'. *American Journal of Preventive Medicine,* 27 (2), 87-96.

Frank, L., Kerr, J., Saelens, B., Sallis, J., Glanz, K. and Chapman, J. (2009) 'Food outlet visits, physical activity and body weight: variations by gender and race-ethnicity'. *British Journal of Sports Medicine* , 43, 124-131.

Glanz, K. and Yaroch, A. (2004) 'Strategies for increasing fruit and vegetable intake in grocery stores and communities: policy, pricing and environmental change'. *Preventive Medicine* 39, S75-S80.

Gustafson, S. and Rhodes, R. (2006) 'Parental correlates of physical activity in children and early adolescents'. *Sports Medicine* 36 (1), 79-97.

Hackbarth, D., Snopp-Wyatt, D., Katz, D., Williams, J., Silvestri, B. and Pfleger, M. (2001) 'Collaborative research and action to control the geographic placement of outdoor advertising of alcohol and tobacco products in Chicago'. *Public Health Reports,* 116, 558-67.

Handy, S., Boarnet, G., Ewing, R, Killingsworth, R. (2002) 'How the built environment affects physical activity: Views from urban planning'. *American Journal of Preventive Medicine* 23, (2S), 64-73.

Harris, J., Bargh, J. and Brownell, K. (2009) 'Priming effects of television food advertising on eating behaviour'. *Health Psychology* 28, 404-413.

Heath, G., Hebert, K. and Lancaster, K. (2006) 'The effectiveness of urban design and land use and transport policies and practices to increase physical activity': A systematic review. *Journal of Physical Activity and Health,* 3 (Suppl. 1): S55-S76.

Henderson, V. and Kelly, B. (2005) 'Food advertising in the age of obesity: Content analysis of food advertising on general market and African American television'. *Journal of Nutrition Education and Behaviour,* 37 (4), 191–96.

Hennessy, E., Hughes, S., Goldberg, J., Hyatt, R. and Economos, C. (2010) 'Parent-child interactions and objectively measured child physical activity: a cross-sectional study'. *International Journal of Behavioural Nutrition and Physical Activity*, 7, 1-14.

Hillier, A. (2008) 'Childhood overweight and the built environment: Making technology part of the solution rather than part of the problem'. *The ANNALS of the American Academy of Political and Social Science*, 615, 56-82.

Hinkle, A. and Wu, E. (2003) 'California adolescent nutrition and fitness program and California Pan Ethnic Health Network. Addressing the obesity epidemic-public policies for healthy eating and physical activity environments. [Communities of colour issue briefing paper] [Online] <Available from http://www.canfit.org/pdf/CANFit-CPEHNbrief.pdf.> [03rd March 2011].

Horowitz, C., Colson, K., Hebert, P. and Lancaster, K. (2004) 'Barriers to buying healthy foods for people with diabetes: Evidence of environmental disparities'. *American Journal of Public Health,* 94, (9), 1549-54.

Jago, R., Anderson, C., Baranowski, T. and Watson, K. (2005) 'Adolescent patterns of physical activity: Differences by gender, day and time of day'. *American Journal of Preventive Medicine* 28(5), 447-452.

Jago. R., Baranowski, T., Baranowski, J., Thompson, D. and Greaves, K. (2005) 'BMI from 3-6y of age is predicted by TV viewing and physical activity, not diet'. *International Journal of Obesity Related Metabolic Disorders* 29 (6), 557-564.

Jago, R., Thompson, J., Page, A., Brockman, R., Cartwright, K., Page, A. and Fox, K. (2009) 'Licence to be active: parental concerns and 10-11 year old children's ability to be independently physically active'. *Journal of Public Health* 31 (4), 472-477.

Jago, R., Fox, K., Page, A. and Thompson, J. (2010) 'Parent and child physical activity and sedentary time: Do active parents foster active children?' *BMC Public Health,* 10 (194), 1-9.

Jones, A., Coombes, E., Griffin, S. and van Slujis, E. (2009) 'Environmental supportiveness for physical activity in English schoolchildren: a study using Global Positioning Systems'. *International Journal of Behavioural Nutrition and Phys Activity,* 6, 42.

Jones, A., van Sluijs, E., Ness, A., Haynes, R. and Riddoch, C. (2010) 'Physical activity in children: Does how we define neighbourhood matter?' *Health and Place* 16, 236-241.

Kagagambe, E. (2002) 'Comparison of dietary intakes of micro- and macronutrients in rural, suburban and urban populations in Costa Rica'. *Public Health and Nutrition* [online] 5, 835-842.

Kawachi I. and L. F. Berkman. (2003) 'Introduction. In *Neighbourhoods and health*, edition 1', 1-17. New York: Oxford University Press.

Kimm, S., Glynn, N., Kriska, A., Barton, B., Kronsberg, S., Daniels, S., Crawford, P., Sabry, Z. and Liu, K. (2002) 'Decline in physical activity in black girls and white girls in adolescence'. *The New England Journal of Medicine* 347 (10), 709-715.

Kjonniksen, L., Torsheim, T. and Wold, B. (2008) 'Tracking of leisure-time physical activity during adolescence and young adulthood: a 10-year longitudinal study'. *International Journal of Behavioural Nutrition and Physical Activity* 5, 69.

Kumanyika, S., and S. Grier. (2006) 'Targeting interventions for ethnic minority and low-income populations'. *The Future of Children,* 16 (1), 187-207.

Kwate, N. and Lee, T (2007) 'Ghettoizing outdoor advertising: Disadvantage and panel density in black neighbourhoods'. *Journal of Urban Health,* 84 (1), 21-31.

Laraia, B., Siega-Riz, A., Kaufman, J. and Jones, S. (2004) 'Proximity of supermarkets is positively associated with diet quality index for pregnancy'. *Preventive Medicine,* 39 (5), 869-875.

Lake, A. (2006) 'Obesogenic environments: exploring the built and food environments. *The Journal of The Royal Society for the Promotion of Health,* 126 (6), 262-267.

Larsson, P. (2003) 'Global positioning System and Sports Specific Testing'. *Sports Medicine* 33 (15), 1093-1101.

Larsson, P. and Henriksson-Larsen, K. (2005) 'Combined metabolic gas analyzer and dGPS analysis of performance in cross-country skiing'. *Journal of Sports Sciences* 23 (8), 861-870.

Lindquist, C., Reynolds, K. and Goran, M. (1999) sociocultural determinants of physical activity among children. *Preventive Medicine* 29, 305-312.

Lopez, R. (2004) 'Urban sprawl and risk of being overweight or obese'. *American Journal of public health* 94, 1574-1579.

Lopez, R. and Hynes, P. (2006) 'Obesity, physical activity, and the urban environment: public health research needs'. *Environmental Health,* 5 (25), 1-10.

Loucaides, C., Chedzoy S and Bennett, N. (2004) 'Differences in physical activity levels between urban and rural school children in Cyprus'. Health *Education Research: Theory and Practice* 19 (2), 138-147.

Lumeng, J., Appugliese, D., Cabral, H., Bradley, R. and Zuckerman, B. (2006) 'Neighbourhood safety and overweight status in children'. *Archives of Pediatric and Adolescent Medicine* 160 (1), 25-31.

Maas, J., Verheij, R., Spreeuwenberg, P., Groenewegen, P. (2008) 'Physical activity as a possible mechanism behind the relationship between green space and health: A multilevel analysis'. *BMC Public Health* [online] Available from <http://www.biomedcentral.com /content/pdf/1471-2458-8-206.pdf> [20th January 2011].

Mackett, R., Brown, B., Gong, Y., Kitazawa, K., and Paskins, J. (2007) 'Children's Independent Movement in the Local Environment'. *Built Environment*, 33(4), 454-468.

Maddison, R. and Mhurchu, C. (2009) 'Global positioning system: a new opportunity in physical activity measurement'. *International Journal of Behavioural Nutrition and Physical Activity* 78 (6) 1-8.

Maddison, R., Jiang, Y., Hoorn, S., Exeter, D., Mhurchu, C. and Dorey, E. (2010) 'Describing patterns of physical activity in adolescents using global positioning systems and accelerometer'. *Paediatric Exercise Science*, 22, 392-407.

Matson-Koffman, D., Brownstein, J., Neiner, J. and Greaney, M. (2005) 'A site specific literature review of policy and environmental interventions that promote physical activity and nutrition for cardiovascular health: what works?' *American Journal of Health Promotion* 19, 167-193.

McCann. B. and Ewing, R. (2003) Smart Growth America Surface Transportation Policy Project. '*Measuring the health effects of sprawl: A national analysis of physical activity, obesity and chronic disease'* [online] Available from http://www.smartgrowthamerica.org/report/healthsprawl8.03.pdf. [03rd March 2011].

McKenzie, T., Marshall, S., Sallis, J. and Conway, T. (2000) 'Leisure-time physical activity in school environments: an observational study using SOPLAY'. *Preventive Medicine* 30, 70-77.

Mikkelsen, L. and Chehimi, S. (2007) 'The links between the neighbourhood food environment and childhood nutrition'. Princeton, NJ: Robert Wood Johnson Foundation.

Morland, K., Wing, S., Roux, A. and Poole, C. (2002) 'Neighbourhood characteristics associated with the location of food stores and food service places'. *American Journal of Preventive Medicine,* 22 (1), 23-29.

Nader, P., Bradley, R., Houts, R., McRitchie, S. and O'Brien, M. (2008) 'Moderate-to-vigorous physical activity from ages 9-15 years'. *Journal of the American Medical Association* 36 (1), 79-97.

Pasch, K. Komro, K., Perry, C, Hearst, M and Farbakhsh. K. (2007) 'Outdoor alcohol advertising near schools: What does it advertise and how is it related to intentions and use of alcohol among young adolescents?' *Journal of Studies on Alcohol and Drugs,* 68 (4), 587-96.

Peterson, M., Froman, N. and Grollman, M. (2005) 'Impact of DGPS post processing techniques and course mapping and on evaluation of outdoor athletic performance in walking golf'. *Proceedings of the 18th International Technical Meeting of the Satellite Division of The Institute of Navigation.*

Pino, J., Martinez-Santos, R., Moreno, M. and Padilla, C. (2007) 'Automatic analysis of football games using GPS on real time'. *Journal of Sports Science and Medicine* 6-11.

Powell, L., Slater, S. and Chaloupka, F. (2004) 'The relationship between community physical activity settings and race, ethnicity, and socioeconomic status'. *Evidence-Based Preventive Medicine* [online] 1 (2), 135-44. Available from <http://www.impacteen.org/journal_pub/pub_PDFs/EBPM-1-2-Powell%20et%20al1. pdf>[10th November 2010].

Public Health Collaborating Centre- Physical Activity (2007) 'Review 2- Correlates of physical activity in children: A review of quantitative systematic reviews'. *Promoting physical activity for children* [online], 1-51. Available from <http://www.children-on-the-move.ch/dateien/dokumentation/NICE_PromotingPhysicalActivityChildrenReview2QuantitativeCorrelates.pdf> [01st November 2010].

Quigg, R., Gray, A., Reeder, A., Holt, A. and Waters, D. (2010) 'Using accelerometers and GPS units to identify the proportion of daily physical activity located in parks and playgrounds in New Zealand children'. *Preventive Medicine,* 50, 235-240.

Rahman, T., Cushing, R., Cushing, B. and Jackson, R. (2011) 'Contributions of built environment to childhood obesity'. *Mount Sinai Journal of Medicine* 78, 49-57.

Rose, D. and Richards, R. (2004) 'Food store access and household fruit and vegetable use among participants in the US Food Stamp Program'. *Public Health Nutrition* [online] 7 (8), 1081-88.

Riddoch, C., Anderson, L., Wedderkopp, N., Harro, M., Klasson-Heggebo, L., Sardinha, L., Cooper, A. and Ekelund, U. (2004) 'Physical activity levels and patterns of 9-and 15-yr-old European children'. *Medicine and Science in Sports and Exercise* 36 (1), 86-92.

Riddoch, C., Mattocks, C., Deere, K., Saunders, J., Kirkby, J., Tilling, K., Leary, S., Blair, S. and Ness, A. (2007) 'Objective measurement of levels and patterns of physical activity'. *Archives of Disease in Childhood* 92 (11), 963-969.

Saksvig, B. Catellier, D. and Pfeiffer, K. (2007) 'Travel by walking before and after school and physical activity among adolescent girls'. *Archives of Paediatrics and Adolescent medicine* 161 (2), 153-158.

Sallis, J., Conway, T., Prochaska, J., McKenzie, T., Mashall, S. and Brown, M. (2001) The association of school environments with youth physical activity. *American Journal of Public Health* 91, 618-620.

Sallis, J., Prochaska, J. and Wendell, T. (2000) 'A review of correlates of physical activity of children and adolescents'. *Medicine and Science in Sports and Exercise* [online] 963-975.

Sallis, J. and Glanz, K. (2006) 'The role of the built environments in physical activity, eating and obesity'. *The Future of Children* [Online] 16 (1), 89-108.

Schoeppe, S. and Braubach, M. (2007) 'Tackling obesity by creating healthy residential environments'. *World Health Organisation* 1-96.

Schutz, Y. and Chambaz, A. (1997) 'Could a satellite-based navigation system (GPS) be used to assess the physical activity of individuals on earth'. *European Journal of Clinical Nutrition* 51 (5),

Simons-Morton, B., Taylor, W., Snider, S. and Huang, I. (1993) 'The physical activity of fifth grade students during physical education classes'. *American Journal of Public Health* 83, 262-264.

Simons-Morton, B., Taylor, W., Snider, S.and Huang, I. Fulton, J. (1994) 'Observed levels of elementary and middle school children's physical activity during physical education classes'. *Preventive Medicine* 23, 437-441.

Sirard, J., Riner, W., McIver, K. and Pate, R. (2005) 'Physical activity and active commuting to elementary school'. *Medicine and Science in Sports and Exercise* 37 (12), 2062-2067.

Steele, R., van Sluijs, E., Cassidy, A., Griffin, S. and Ekelund, U. (2009) 'Targeting sedentary time or moderate-and vigorous-intensity activity: independent relations with adiposity in a population-based sample of 10-y-old British children'. *American Journal of Clinical Nutrition* 90 (5), 1185-1192.

Stone, E., McKenzie, T., Welk, G. and Booth, M. (1998) 'Effects of physical activity intervention in youth. Review and syntheses. *American Journal of Preventive Medicine* 15, 298-315.

Strong, W., Malina, R., Cameron, J., Daniels, S., Dishman, R., Gutin, B., Hergenroeder, A., Must, A., Nixon, P., Pivarnik, J., Rowland, T., Trost, S. and Trudeau, F. (2005)

'Evidence based physical activity for school-age youth'. *Journal of Paediatrics* [online] 146, 732-737.

Taveras, E., Sandora, T. and Shih, M. (2006) 'The association of television and video viewing with fast food intake by preschool-age children'. *Obesity (Silver Spring)* 14, 2034-2041.

Thompson, J., Jago, R., Brockman, R., Cartwright, K., Page, A. and Fox, K. (2009) 'Physically active families-de-bunking the myth?' A qualitative study of family participation in physical activity. *Child: Care, Health and Development* 36 (2), 265-274.

Timperio, A., Crawford, D., Telford, A. and Salmon, J. (2004) 'Perceptions about the local neighbourhood and walking and cycling among children'. *Preventive Medicine* 48, 316-320.

Timperio, A., Salmon, J. and Ball, K. (2004) 'Evidence-based strategies to promote physical activity among children, adolescents and young adults: review and update'. J*ournal of Sports Science in Medicine* 7, 20-29.

Tirodkar, M. and Jain, A. (2003) 'Food messages on African American television shows' *American Journal of Public Health* 93 [online] (3), 439-41.

Troped, P., Wilson, J. and Matthews, C., Cromley, E., Melly, S. (2010) 'The Built Environment and Location-Based Physical Activity'. *American Journal of Preventive Medicine* [Online] 38 (4), 429-438.

Trost, S and Loprinzi, P (2008) 'Exercise- Promoting healthy lifestyles in children and adolescents'. *Journal of Clinical Lipidology* [online] 2, 162-168.

Van der Vorst, H., Engels, R. and Burk, W. (2010) 'Do parents and best friends influence the normative increase in adolescents' alcohol use at home and outside the home?(Report)'. *Journal of Studies on Alcohol and Drugs* 71 (1) 105-114.

Vandewater, E., Shim, M. and Caplovitz, A. (2004) 'Linking obesity and activity level with children's television and video game use'. *Journal of Adolescence* 27(1), 71-85.

Van Sluijs, E., Page, A., Ommundsen, Y. and Griffin, S. (2008) 'Behavioural and social correlates of sedentary time in young people'. *British Journal of Sports Medicine* [online] 44, 747-755.

Van Sluijs, E., Skidmore, P., Mwanza, K., Jones, A., Callaghan, A., Ekelund, U., Harrison, F., Harvey, I., Panter, J., Wareham, N., Cassidy, S. (2008) 'Physcial activity and dietary behaviour in a population-based sample of British 10-year old children: the SPEEDY study (Sport, Physical Activity and Eating Behaviour: Environmental Determinants in Young People)'. *BMC Public Health* 8, 388.

Viner, R. and Cole, T. (2005) 'Television viewing in early childhood predicts adult body mass index'. *Journal of Paediatrics* 147 (4), 429-435.

Vries, S., Hopman-Rock, M., Bakker, I., Hirasing, R. and Mechelen, W. (2010) 'Built environment correlates of walking and cycling in Dutch urban children: results from the SPACE study'. *International Journal of Environmental Research and Public Health* [online] 7, 2309-2324.

Wen, L., Kite, J., Merom, D. and Rissel, C. (2009) 'Time spent playing outdoors after school and its relationship with independent mobility: a cross-sectional survey of children aged 10–12 years in Sydney, Australia'. *International Journal of Behavioural Nutrition and Physical Activity* [online] 6 (15), 1-8.

Wheeler, B., Cooper, A., Page, A. and Jago, R. (2010) 'Greenspace and children's physical activity: A GPS/GIS analysis of the PEACH project'. *Preventive Medicine* 51, 148-152.

Zenk, S., Schulz, A., Israel, B., James, S., Boa, S. and Wilson, M. (2005) 'Neighbourhood racial composition, neighbourhood poverty, and the spatial accessibility of supermarkets in metropolitan Detroit'. *American Journal of Public Health* 95 [online] (4), 660-67.

In: Reviews in Pediatric Exercise Science
Editor: Michael Duncan, pp. 87-96
ISBN: 978-1-61470-978-7

Chapter VI

Body Image Perception and its Relationship with Nutritional Status in Childhood and Adolescence

Edio Luiz Petroski, Andreia Pelegrini and Diego Augusto Santos Silva
Universidade Federal de Santa Catarina, Brasil.

Introduction

Along the years, bodily beauty ideals have undergone some changes, given the concern with physical appearance increasingly evident in contemporary society, which leads people to worry excessively about it.

Body image perception can be defined as the individual's accuracy of judging his own body size, shape and weight in relation to its proportion, while body image dissatisfaction is defined as the negative assessment of one's own body, being usually diagnosed through patterns of body silhouettes and questionnaires, which focus concerns about weight, shape and body fat (Smolak, 2001).

In recent years, thinness has been promoted as a standard of female beauty and images shown by the media, considered ideal, have become progressively thinner. Body shape changes end up by leading to significant increased body image dissatisfaction among women.

Thus, the proportion of people who are dissatisfied with their physical appearance has increased in recent decades, with smaller proportions in western countries.

In relation to nutritional status, although subjects with normal body weight can be dissatisfied with their body image, overweight students are the most susceptible. In recent years, the obesity prevalence increased significantly in developed and developing countries, which worsens the body image dissatisfaction among children and adolescents.

In this sense, body image dissatisfaction has aroused great interest among researchers, mainly due to the close relationship between this and eating disorders (anorexia and bulimia). Adolescent girls dissatisfied with their body image often adopt abnormal eating behaviors and inadequate weight control practices, such as the use of diuretics, laxatives, self-induced vomiting, and exhausting physical activity. Thus, body image dissatisfaction in adolescence has been identified as the most important risk factor for developing eating disorders such as anorexia and bulimia (Alves, Vasconcelos, Calvo, and Neves, 2008).

Eating disorders (anorexia nervosa and bulimia nervosa) are characterized by a morbid fear of gaining weight, obsessive concern with food, persistent desire for becoming thin and body image distortion, causing biological and psychological damage and increased morbidity and mortality.

Thus, this chapter aims to present the topic body image perception and its relationship with nutritional status and eating disorders in childhood and adolescence.

Instruments for Body Image and Eating Disorder Assessment

Body image assessment, which refers to how much the person is satisfied with his body, is probably the most common aspect of body image. The most commonly used methods to assess body image satisfaction are figures (body silhouettes) and questionnaires. Furthermore, the instruments used to assess eating disorders are also largely based on questionnaires. Body satisfaction measures can be obtained by a variety of psychometric instruments, which have been widely reviewed, describing the main components related and body image disorders among adolescents and adults (Thompson and Van Den Berg, 2002).

A method used to verify body image dissatisfaction was proposed and validated by Brown, Cash and Mikulka (1990) and adapted by Loland (1998). The satisfaction scale of the body parts proposed by Brown et al. (1990) consists of nine evaluation areas: face, hair, low back, mid back, high back, muscle tone, weight, height and general appearance. The scale ranges from 1, very dissatisfied to 5, very satisfied. The satisfaction scale of the body parts adapted by Loland (1998), in addition to areas covered by the scale of Brown et al. (1990), introduces six new areas, totaling 15 areas: face, hair, buttocks, hips, thighs, legs, stomach, waist, breast / chest, back / shoulders, arms, muscle tone, weight, height, all areas.

According to Loland (1998), several researchers have used the "Multidimensional Body Self Relation Questionnaire" - MBSRQ - proposed by Brown et al. (1990) to assess body image, which consists of 34 items. This instrument uses two subscales: seven items of the appearance evaluation to measure the total body image evaluation and nine items containing satisfaction scales of body areas to assess body image dissatisfaction-satisfaction with discrete body areas, such as face, weight, and muscle tone.

One of the most known scales of body figures (Figure Rating Scale) is that of Stunkard, Sorensen, and Schlusinger (1983). It consists of a series of schematic figures of human silhouettes that range from very thin (underweight) to very obese (overweight), developed from a sample composed of 125 men and 204 women. Participants are asked to select two figures: the first figure is the one they believe to be the most representative of their current body shape (body shape concerns) and the second figure is the one they consider ideal. The discrepancy between them is a measure of body shape dissatisfaction. Although with some criticism, it has been used in adolescents to determine the ideal body image perception. Even though the scale does not highlight muscle development, boys who have thin silhouettes perceive larger figures as of greater muscle development. Participants are asked to select two figures: the first figure is the one they believe is the most representative of their current or real body size, then, the second, a body figure that they consider ideal or that they would like to have.

Tiggeman and Wilson-Barrett (1998) created a version of body scales for children, who had to select two figures: the first one refers to the current body silhouette (the way the child sees himself) and the second one is related to the ideal body silhouette (the way the child would like to be). If the real and ideal body silhouette selected is the same, the child has no body image dissatisfaction. In case two different body silhouettes are selected, there is evidence of body image dissatisfaction, being represented by the discrepancy between the body figures. The questions that must be used for children are those of the Figure Rating Scale.

Another instrument that has been widely used to investigate body image dissatisfaction is the Body Shape Questionnaire - BSQ (Cooper, Taylor, Cooper and Fairburn, 1987). The BSQ is a Likert scale with 34 self-administered items constructed to measure in the last four weeks the concern with body shape and weight, especially the frequency in which individuals with and without eating disorders experience the sensation of "feeling fat". The BSQ provides a continuous and descriptive assessment of body image disturbances in clinical and non-clinical populations and can be used to evaluate the role of this disturbance in the development, maintenance and response to anorexia and bulimia nervosa treatment.

The questionnaire has 34 questions and each question has 6 possible answers: 1. "Never," 2. "Rarely", 3. "Sometimes," 4. "Often," 5. "Very often" and 6. "Always." Score below 80 is considered no dissatisfaction; between 80 and 110, mild dissatisfaction; between 111 and 140, moderate dissatisfaction; and greater than 140, severe dissatisfaction.

Among the instruments used to identify anorexia nervosa and bulimia nervosa, the Eating Attitudes Test, EAT-26, proposed by Garner, Olmsted, Bohr and Garfinkel (1982) stands out. Validation and internal consistency reliability of the test, represented by Cronbach's alpha 0.80, were considered satisfactory due to the fact that this value is close to 1.00. In this sense, the EAT-26 is an adequate instrument for application in adolescents, helping in the pre-diagnosis of possible cases of eating disorders.

The EAT-26 is a self-administered questionnaire with questions such as the Likert scale with six answer options ("Never", "Seldom", "A Few Times", "Sometimes", "Often" and "Always", whose score range from 0 (zero) to 3. Answers "Never", "Seldom", "A Few Times" scorer 0 (zero) points, and answers "Sometimes", "Often" and "Always" score 1, 2 and 3 points, respectively. In question 25, the score is considered the other way round, scoring 0 (zero) points alternatives "Sometimes", "Often" and "Always ", and 1, 2 and 3 points alternatives "A Few Times" "Seldom" and "Never", respectively. The final score of the questionnaire can range from 0 (zero) to 78 points. Subjects totaling 20 points in the questionnaire are classified as of risk food behavior.

Body Image Dissatisfaction and Nutritional Status

The modern western culture has emphasized the thinness, denigrated overweight and stigmatized obese people, so that obese people internalize these messages and feel bad about their physical appearance.

Obesity can lead to severe psychological consequences. In many instances, dissatisfaction with life, social responsibilities and distress about body image produced by obesity are beneficial, motivating people to want to lose weight.

Many overweight people can feel that the best way to improve body image is to reduce body weight. This seems to be true, as seen in studies evaluating body image distortion before and after a weight reduction program, where it was found that the body image perception was improved in those who lost weight (Sarwer, and Thompson, 2002). However, another perspective on the relationship between weight loss and body image does not necessarily improve body satisfaction, as other studies have shown that body image can be improved with different cognitive behavioral therapies. These studies show that body image perception can be improved when obese individuals are encouraged to change their lifestyle and accept their body better.

According to Ricciardelli and McCabe (2001), the increase in body mass index (BMI) is related to worsened body dissatisfaction in adolescent girls.

Children receive daily messages for the construction of an ideal body image and of a beauty standard of attractiveness. The messages are persistent and are present even in toys. In toys with male human figures of today, muscularity is more evident than in toys of 20 or 30 years ago, unreal proportionalities of a human being at any age. The so-called "Barbie" doll is an example of idealized thinness as female body shape. The internalization of these body ideals may also promote increased body dissatisfaction, since these culturally accepted ideals are difficult to reach or are unattainable for most boys and girls (Presnell, et al., 2004).

There is evidence that body image is formed even before adolescence, and that children assimilate it with their families, teachers, friends and media that fat is "bad" and thinness is "good", and they learn this lesson quite before adolescence. When the attitudes of preschool children from both sexes, aged 2-5 years are evaluated in relation to fat and normal individuals represented by puppets, it was found that early at this age group, there is evidence of prejudice against fat figures. Fat figures in general, received more negative ratings than normal figures, and among the fat, girls received more negative ratings than boys (Turnbull, Healslip and Mcleod, 2000).

In a population-based study conducted with Chinese children and adolescents (3 - 15 years), it was observed that approximately 60% were dissatisfied with their body image, being most prominent among obese children and adolescents, i.e., 37.5% of obese boys and 47.2% of obese girls were moderately dissatisfied. Moreover, body image dissatisfaction showed that 69.7% of obese boys and 69.6% of obese girls wanted to be thinner (Li, Hu, Ma, Wu, and Ma, 2005). In adolescents (12 to 17 years) from California, it was observed that approximately 24% of girls were dissatisfied with their bodies, compared with 22% of boys. Furthermore, it was found that high body mass index and low / regular health status are factors that contribute to body image dissatisfaction among Californian adolescents. Adolescents who reported poor health status were four times more likely to report body dissatisfaction when compared to adolescents who reported excellent health status. Likewise, adolescents with BMI equal to or above percentile 85 were three times more likely to report body dissatisfaction than those with BMI below percentile 85 (Wilkosz, Chen, Kennedy, and Rankin, 2011).

A study conducted in 24 countries and regions of Europe, Canada and the United States revealed that among adolescent boys, the highest body image dissatisfaction rates were observed in Italy (39.9%), United States (37.7%) and Greece (35.2%), while among adolescent girls, the highest body image dissatisfaction rates were found in Czech Republic (61.8%), Slovenia (56.8%) and Italy (55.2%). These Results show that body image dissatisfaction is more common among girls. In addition, age and overweight were positively associated with body dissatisfaction in all countries investigated (Al Sabbah, et al., 2009).

Studies conducted in different Brazilian regions show high body image dissatisfaction rates among children and adolescents. Pelegrini and Petroski (2009) analyzed the association between body image dissatisfaction and nutritional status in adolescents (14 to 18 years) and found that 65.5% of adolescents were dissatisfied with their body image, and while girls wanted to reduce their body size silhouette, boys wanted to increase their size. It was also found that overweight girls were more likely to have body dissatisfaction. Another study with adolescents aged 11 to 14 years found that 75.8% of adolescent girls were dissatisfied with their body shape, of which 61.5% had the desire to reduce their body weight (Scherer, Martins, Pelegrini, Matheus, and Petroski, 2010).

A recent study conducted with adolescents from 26 Brazilian state capitals and Federal District aimed to describe the correlation between body image and nutritional status and to verify the association between body image and nutritional status with behaviors related to body weight, showed that the concordance between nutritional status and body image was low (kappa index = 0.33). Almost half the overweight students rated themselves as with adequate weight and 27% as thin. A higher proportion of overweight adolescents were making use of extreme weight reduction practices, compared to those with healthy weight and underweight (Castro, et al., 2010).

Another aspect that influences body image dissatisfaction is sexual maturation, since there are reports in which among girls at menarche age, the majority wanted to reduce body weight. This demonstrates that body image undergoes changes during maturation (represented by the presence of menarche), since the body goes through many changes resulting from puberty, with increased adiposity (Scherer, et al., 2010). The increment of body fat in post-menarche adolescents leads most adolescents to show the desire to lose weight due to increased body image dissatisfaction. Another study to identify body shape satisfaction was conducted with 1070 high school students. The following question was formulated: Are you satisfied with your body weight? Participants responded wither 'Yes' or 'No'. For schoolgirls who answered "No", the reason for dissatisfaction was asked. It was observed that 48.2% of students were dissatisfied with their body weight. The reasons reported by students for their dissatisfaction were: 74.2% of students rated themselves as overweight and would like to lose weight, 20.2% rated themselves as underweight and would like to gain weight, and 5.6%, indicated other reasons of more aesthetic nature such as being taller, having thicker legs or larger breasts, among others. The authors also observed that students dissatisfied with their body weight and who wanted to lose weight were those who had matured earlier (Petroski, Velho, and De Bem, 1999).

The results of studies that investigated the relationship between ethnicity and body image are controversial. Researches conducted with Caucasian and Nipponese adolescents in Brazil have found that Caucasian adolescents showed greater body image dissatisfaction than Nipponese adolescents (Sampei, et al., 2009).

Another study (Pelegrini, Glaner, and Petroski, 2011) conducted with a sample composed of 641 adolescents (303 boys and 338 girls), 368 living in urban areas and 273 in rural areas aged 11 to 17 years, with the aim of verifying the reasons for the prevalence of body image dissatisfaction among adolescents, used the scale of nine body silhouettes proposed by

Stunkard, et al. (1983). The set of body silhouettes was shown to adolescents, who answered to two questions: What is the silhouette that best represents your current body appearance (real)? Which is the body silhouette that you would like to have (ideal)? When the variation between ideal and real silhouette was zero, the adolescents were classified as satisfied, and if not zero, dissatisfied. If the difference was positive (real - ideal), there was a desire to reduce weight and, when negative, there was a desire to increase weight. In case of dissatisfaction, adolescents answered one more question: What is the main reason for your dissatisfaction? The answers were categorized into the following reasons: aesthetics, health, improve daily life. The prevalence of body image dissatisfaction was 60.4%. Girls (65.7%) had greater body dissatisfaction than boys (54.5%), while boys wanted to increase the size of their body silhouette (26.4%), girls wanted to reduce it (52.4%). When dissatisfaction was analyzed in relation to "desire to increase" and "desire to reduce" the size of the body silhouette, it was observed that the main reasons given by adolescents who wished to increase the size of their body silhouette were: improvement in daily activities, family opinion and the desire to be physically strong (44.8%) and aesthetics (32.0%). On the other hand, the reasons reported by adolescents who wanted to reduce the size of their body silhouette were, in descending order: self-esteem (88.7%), health (86.4%) and aesthetics (64.9%).

Body dissatisfaction appears to be a reality in adolescence, and a study with schoolchildren from 13 to 17 years of age showed that, according to the BMI, underweight and overweight adolescents were, respectively, 3.1 and 8.5 times more likely to have body image dissatisfaction than their peers with normal weight. As for body adiposity, adolescents with high Σ2SF were 2.08 times more likely to have body dissatisfaction (ideal weight as reference) (Petroski, Pelegrini, and Glaner, 2009).

A longitudinal study with a five-year monitoring period conducted with American schoolchildren showed that body image satisfaction has declined significantly, except for older girls. Furthermore, a significant reduction, which is higher among older adolescents than among younger adolescents and among some ethnic groups of males, was observed and that the shift in body satisfaction depends on the BMI category (Eisenberg, Neumark-Sztainer, and Paxton, 2005).

According to researches, it was observed that body image dissatisfaction is a highly frequent phenomenon in adolescents from both sexes. In addition, the nutritional status significantly influences body dissatisfaction, especially among overweight or obese adolescents.

Body Image Dissatisfaction and Symptoms of Eating Disorders

Eating disorders generally have their onset in childhood and adolescence. Changes in eating behavior can be divided into two stages: 1) disorders that occur early in childhood and that represent changes in the child's relationship with food and 2) disorders that appear later and consist of eating disorders themselves, called anorexia nervosa and bulimia nervosa.

Anorexia nervosa is characterized by severe weight loss at the expense of strict self-imposed diets in the pursuit of thinness, body image distortion and amenorrhea. Low self-esteem and body image distortion are the main components that reinforce the search for a constant weight loss, leading to exhausting physical exercise, fasting and a more intensive use of laxatives or diuretics.

According to the results obtained by a literature review, Fleitlich, Larino, Cobelo and Cordás, (2000) showed that the most widely known risk factors for anorexia nervosa are age and sex. The most common age of onset is adolescence, and there is an increased prevalence among women. Furthermore, the authors found studies that showed that anorexia was expressed only in higher economic classes. However, more recent researches have identified a similar incidence also in lower social classes. The prevalence of eating disorders varies according to methodology and sample used.

In studies conducted with adolescents in Canada and UAE, the prevalence of anorexia and bulimia symptoms were respectively 14% and 23.4% (Eapen, et al., 2006). The literature also shows higher prevalence of symptoms of these eating disorders, as in the case of Jordanian adolescent girls (10 to 16 years) who had a prevalence of 40.5% (Mousa, Mashal, Al-Domi, and Jibril, 2010).

In Brazil, studies conducted in São Paulo and Rio Grande do Sul showed prevalence of symptoms of eating disorders by 21.1% and 27.6%, respectively (Dunker, and Philippi, 2003; Martins, Pelegrini, Matheus, and Petroski, 2010). Another study with adolescent girls aged 11 to 14 years found that 75.8% of them were dissatisfied with their body shape, of which 61.5% had the desire to reduce body weight. Regarding the relationship between BMI and symptoms of ED, most adolescent girls who wanted to reduce body weight showed symptoms of ED (Scherer, Martins, Pelegrini, Matheus, and Petroski, 2010).

Body dissatisfaction is related to eating disorders in adolescent girls (Thompson, and Smolak, 2001), and even in children (Gardner, Stark, Friedman, and Jackson, 2002). Studies have shown that body image dissatisfaction in adolescent boys is also associated with eating disorders (Keel, Fulkerson, and Leon, 1997; Leon, Fulkerson, Perry, and Early-Zald, 1995).

According to the studies reviewed, there is a high prevalence of body image dissatisfaction and symptoms of eating disorders, which are alarming, given the association between these phenomena, and symptoms of eating disorders can develop into clinical cases. In this context, the need for interventions in schools in order to prevent the development of this phenomenon in ever-younger ages should be highlighted.

Conclusion

The high prevalence of body image dissatisfaction is evident in childhood and adolescence. In addition, the presence of symptoms of eating disorders in ever-younger ages can be observed. It is recommended that school health professionals and provide opportunities to children and adolescents vulnerable to body dissatisfaction to accept their body shape and help in choosing healthy body shape.

References

Al-Sabbah, H., Vereecken, C.A., Elgar, F.J., Nansel, T., Aasvee, K., Abdeen, Z., et al. (2009). Body weight dissatisfaction and communication with parents among adolescents in 24 countries: international cross-sectional survey. *BMC Public Health, 9*:52.

Alves, E., Vasconcelos, F.A., Calvo, M.C., and Neves, J. (2009). Prevalência de sintomas de anorexia nervosa e insatisfação com a imagem corporal em adolescentes do sexo feminino do município de Florianópolis, Santa Catarina, Brasil. *Caderno de Saude Publica, 24*(3), 503-512.

Brown, T.A., Cash, T.F., and Mikulka, P.J. (1990). Attitudinal body-image assessment: factor analysis of the body-self relations questionnaire. *Journal of Personality Assessment, 55*, 135-144.

Campagna, V.N., and Souza, A.S. (2006). Corpo e imagem corporal no início da adolescência feminina. *Boletin de Psicologia, 56*(124), 9-35.

Cash, T.F. (2002). The management of body image problems. In: K.D. Brownell, and C. G. Fairburn (Eds.), *Eating disorders and obesity: A comprehensive handbook* (pp. 599-603). New York: Guilford Press.

Castro, I.R.R., Levy, R.B., Cardoso, L.O., Passos, M.D., Sardinha L.M.V., Tavares, L.F. et al., (2010). Imagem corporal, estado nutricional e comportamento com relação ao peso entre adolescentes brasileiros. *Ciência e saúde* coletiva, 15(suppl.2), 3099-3108.

Cooper, P,J., Taylor, M.J., Cooper, Z., and Fairburn, C.G. (1987). The development and validation of the body shape questionnaire. *International Journal of Eating Disorders, 6*(4), 485-494.

Dunker, K.L., and Philippi, S.T. (2003). Hábitos e comportamentos alimentares de adolescentes com sintomas de anorexia nervosa. *Revista de Nutrição, 16*(1), 51-60.

Eapen, V., Mabrouk, A.A., and Bin-Othman, S. (2006). Disordered eating attitudes and symptomatology among adolescent girls in the United Arab Emirates. *Eating Behaviors, 7*(1): 53-60.

Eisenberg, M.E., Neumark-Sztainer. D. and Paxton, S.J. (2006). Five-year change in body satisfaction among adolescents. Journal of Psychosomatic Research, 61: 521-527.

Fleitlich, B.W., Larino, M.A., Cobelo, A. and Cordás, T.A. (2000). Anorexia nervosa na adolescência. *Jornal de Pediatria, 76 (Supl.3): S323-S329.*

Gardner, R.M., Stark, K., Friedman, B.N., and Jackson, N.A. (2000). Predictors of eating disorder scores in children ages 6 through 14 - a longitudinal study. *Journal Psychosomatic Research, 49*(3), 199-205.

Garner, D.M., Olmsted, M.P., Bohr, Y., and Garfinkel, P.E. (1982). The eating attitudes test: psychometric features and clinical correlates. *Psychology Medicine, 12*(4), 871-878.

Keel, P.K., Fulkerson, J.A., and Leon, G.R. (1997). Disordered eating precursors in pre- and early adolescent girls and boys. *Journal of Youth and Adolescence, 26*(2),203-216.

Leon, G.R., Fulkerson, J.A., Perry, C.L., and Early-Zald, M.B. (1995). Prospective analysis of personality and behavioral vulnerabilities and gender influences in the later development of disordered eating. *Journal Abnormal Psychology, 104*(1), 140-149.

Li, Y., Hu, X., Ma, W., Wu, J., and Ma, G. (2005). Body image perceptions among Chinese children and adolescents. *Body Image, 2*(2), 91–103.

Lobera, I.J., Candau, J.R., Ríos, P.B., Berriatúa, C.M., Jaramillo, R.D., González, M.T. M. et al. (2009) Conducta alimentaria e imagen corporal em una muestra de adolescentes de Sevilla. *Nutrición Hospitalaria, 24*(5), 568-573.

Martins, C.R., Pelegrini, A., Matheus, S.C., and Petroski, E,L. (2010), Insatisfação com a imagem corporal e relação com estado nutricional, adiposidade corporal e sintomas de anorexia e bulimia em adolescentes. *Revista de Psiquiatria do Rio Grande do Sul, 32*(1), 19-23.

Mumford, D.B., Whitehouse, A.M., and Choudry, I.Y. (1992). Survey of eating disorders in English-medium schools in Lahore, Pakistan. *International Journal of Eating Disorders, 11*(2), 173-184.

Muth, J.L., and Cash, T.F. (1997). Body-image attitudes: what difference does gender make? *Journal of Applied Social Psychology, 27*, 1438-1452.

Pelegrini, A., and Petroski, E.L. (2010). The Association Between Body Dissatisfaction and Nutritional Status in Adolescents. *Human Movement, 11*(1), 51-57.

Pelegrini, A, Glaner, MF,and Petroski, EL. (2011) Reasons and prevalence of body image dissatisfaction in adolescents. *Ciência and Saúde Coletiva* (In press).

Petroski, E.L., Velho, N.M., and De Bem, M.F.L. (1999). Menarche age and satisfaction with body weight. *Revista Brasileira de Cineantropometria and Desempenho Humano, 1*(1), 30-36.

Petroski, E.L., Pelegrini, A. and Glaner, M.F. Body image dissatisfaction among rural and urban adolescents. *Motricidade,*, Dec. 2009, vol.5, no.4, p.13-25.

Presnell, K., Bearman., S.K., and Stice, E. (2004). Risk Factors for Body Dissatisfaction in Adolescent Boys and Girls: A Prospective Study. *International of Journal of Eating Disorder, 36*(4), 389–401.

Ricciardelli, L. A., and McCabe, M. (2001). Children's body image concerns and eating disturbance: a review of the literature. *Clinical Psychology Review*, 21, 325-344.

Rosen, J. C., Jones, A., Ramirez, E., and Waxman, S. (1996). Body shape questionnaire studies of validity and reliability. *International of Journal of Eating Disorders, 20*(3), 315-359.

Sampei, M.A., Sigulem, D.M., Novo, N.F., Juliano, Y., and Colugnati, F.A.B. (2009). Atitudes alimentares e imagem corporal em meninas adolescentes de ascendência nipônica e caucasiana em São Paulo (SP). *Jornal de Pediatria, 85*(2), 122-128.

Sarwer, D.B., and Thompson, J.K. (2002). Obesity and body image disturbance. In: T.A. Wadden, and A.J., Stunkard (Eds.), *Handbook of Obesity Treatment* (pp. 447-464). New York: Guilford Press.

Scherer, F.C., Martins, R.M., Pelegrini, A., Matheus, S.C., and Petroski, E.L. (2010). Body image among adolescents: association with sexual maturation and symptoms of eating disorders. *Jornal Brasileiro Psiquiatria, 59*(3), 198-202.

Smolak, L.M. (2001). Body image in children. In J.K. Thompson, and L. Smolak, editors. *Body image, eating disorders and obesity in youth: Assessment, prevention and treatment.* (pp. 41-66). Whashington, DC: American Psychological Association.

Stunkard, A.J., Sorensen, T., and Schulsinger, F. (1983) Use of the Danish Adoption Register for the study of obesity and thinness. In:, S.S., Kety, L.P., Rowland, R.L., Sidman, and S.W., Matthysse (Eds.), *The Genetics of Neurological and Psychiatric Disorders* (pp. 115-120). New York: Raven Press.

Thompson, J.K., and Van Den Berg, P. (2002). Measuremente body attitudes among adolescents and adults. In. T. F. Cash and T. Pruzinsky (Eds.) Body image – A handbook of theory, research, and clinical practice. (pp. 142-154). Guilford Press, New York.

Turnbull, J.D.,Healslip, S., and Mcleod, H.A. (2000). Pre-school children's attitude to fat normal male and female stimulus figures. *International Journal of Obesity, 24*(12), 1705-1706.

Wang, Z., Byrne, N.M., Kenardy, J.A., and Hills, A.P. (2005). Influences of ethnicity and socioeconomic status on the body dissatisfaction and eating behaviour of Australian children and adolescents. *Eating Behaviors, 6*(1), 23-33.

Wilkosz, M.E., Chen, J.L., Kenndey, C., and Rankin, S. (2011). Body dissatisfaction in California adolescents. *Journal of the American Academy of Nurse Practitioners, 23*(2),101-109.

Scherer FC, Martins RM, Pelegrini A,, Matheus SC, and Petroski EL, (2010). Body image among adolescents: association with sexual maturation and symptoms of eating disorders. *Jornal Brasileiro de Psiquiatria, 59*(3):198-202.

In: Reviews in Pediatric Exercise Science
Editor: Michael Duncan, pp. 97-113
ISBN: 978-1-61470-978-7

Chapter VII

The Efficacy of Exercise in Enhancing Children's Reading Ability

Esther Curley, Michael J. Duncan and Samantha Birch
Coventry University, UK.

Introduction

Evidence to support the positive health benefits of physical activity abounds. Research demonstrates a dose-response relationship, in that as physical activity levels increase so do the associated health gains (Janssen, and LeBlanc, 2010). Physical inactivity on the other hand increases a person's risk of suffering non-communicable diseases, such as cardiovascular disease, diabetes and cancer (World Health Organisation 2010). In view of these risks, children's physical activity levels give reason for concern, as only 32% of boys and 24% of girls in England were reported to have achieved recommended guidelines in 2008 (The NHS Information Centre, 2010). Unfortunately given the self-reported nature of this data, young people's inactivity levels may be somewhat higher than testified (Basterfield, *et al.,* 2008).

To date, the main objectives driving Government plans to increase physical activity levels, appear to have been focused around reducing individual health costs of inactivity and the economic burden to society and the National Health Service (Department of Health, 2009). It seems that academic gains are a less prominent motivating factor behind the promotion of physical activity, yet studies indicate that exercise can enhance the health of the brain and facilitate learning (Cotman, Berchtold, and Christie, 2007). The effects of physical activity on school children's academic performance however, remain unclear, due to studies drawing mixed results (Taras, 2005).

Educational attainment is the strongest predictor of adult life outcomes/chances (National Literacy Trust, NLT, 2005). For instance, individuals with low literacy skills are more likely to experience social exclusion, be unemployed by the time they reach 30 years of age (NLT, 2010) or find themselves turning to youth offending (Audit Commission, 2004). Data from longitudinal studies, such as the National Child Development Study (Centre for Longitudinal Studies, CLS, 2008), depict how education can mould young people's direction in life. For instance poor educational attainment has been found to be the strongest risk factor associated with young pregnancy; as well as playing a key role in disadvantage, low wages, and unemployment (CLS, 2008). Such data underscores the importance of promoting good literacy skills. Statistics show that one in six people in the UK experience poor literacy (NLT, 2010), and one in three children, aged between 6 and 16 years, are identified with special educational needs (SEN) (Department for Children, Schools, and Families, DCSF, 2010). The prospect of a child with SEN and reaching national expectations, five A-C grades at GCSE level (General Certificate of Secondary Education in the UK), is low if they come from a low income family (DCSF, 2010). Only 7.5% of children dealing with the combined challenge of SEN and disadvantage, managed to achieve national expectations in 2009 (DCSF, 2010).

A review conducted by the Office for Standards in Education, Children's Services and Skills (Ofsted, 2010), into the best teaching practices in England, found that systematic phonic teaching lay behind the success of 12 outstanding schools boasting high standards of reading. However, the view of effective reading tuition did not reference the contribution that physical activity may have upon a child's academic or literacy attainment. School administrators and parents may harbour fears that increased time allotted to physical activity may reduce more valuable time that could be spent in the classroom improving performance in core subject areas. This issue has been acknowledged by a number of studies, which have found that despite a failure to always observe significant academic improvement as a result of physical activity, academic performance was not compromised (Ahamed, *et al* 2007, Carlson *et al* 2008, and Trudeau, and Shephard, 2008).

Berg (2010) presents a review of empirical findings in an attempt to raise the profile of physical education (PE) in schools. His review includes a number of studies to support anatomical and physiological changes in the brain following bouts of exercise. For instance, animal studies have shown that the production of brain-derived neurotrophic factor (BDNF) increases in the hippocampus, as a result of several days of running. BDNF is a neurotrophic factor or protein, proposed to enhance the survival and growth of neurons in the brain, whilst the hippocampus plays a part in spatial memory (Kolb, and Whishaw 2011) and learning (Vayman, Ying, and Gomez-Pinilla, 2003). Berg (2010) is encouraged by animal studies which have found a link between increased BDNF in rats and their ability to solve mazes quicker, as such findings may benefit cognitive functioning and learning in humans. An investigation into the link between exercise-induced cognitive enhancement and BDNF action, discovered that by blocking BDNF in rats, former exercise-induced improvements in learning was eliminated (Vayman, Ying, and Gomez-Pinilla, 2004). Although a number studies have demonstrated that synaptic-plasticity changes in the brain are enhanced by exercise, and that BDNF is utilised in exercise to improve learning acquisition and memory retention (Berg, 2010, Vayman, Ying, and Gomez-Pinilla, 2004, and Vayman, Ying, and Gomez-Pinilla, 2003), further research is needed to clarify the type, frequency and amount of exercise needed in order for significant benefits to be experienced (Cotman, Berchtold, and Christie, 2007). In addition, a call has been made for animal studies to increase their relevance to humans, since human studies tend to analyse the completion of tasks co-ordinated by the forebrain, whilst animal studies usually assess hippocampus-dependent learning (Cotman, Berchtold, and Christie, 2007).

Exercise and Academic Achievement

Current literature appears unclear as to what types of physical activity benefit what areas of learning in school-aged children. Taras (2005) concludes from his review of 14 studies, that although physical activity may improve a pupil's concentration, to date, literature does not demonstrate a clear association between physical activity and enhanced academic performance. However, the article reasons that the current lack of evidence should not be viewed as means to justify restrictions to children's PE, rather a reason to conduct further exploration so that the relationship between physical activity and academic performance may be better understood. It is difficult to draw a firm conclusion based on a relatively small number of studies, particularly as Taras (2005) based a proportion of the review on abstract articles rather than complete records. In addition, at least a third of the studies included for review had relied on self-reported measures of physical activity levels, a method subject to risks of under or over reporting. Such discrepancies were demonstrated by Watkinson *et al's* (2010) study in which self-rated levels of physical activity were compared to measures provided by heart rate monitors. The study found that those who were classified as inactive were most likely to perceive themselves as active and thus overestimate levels of activity.

Trudeau, and Shephard's (2008) review of the effects of school PE on academic performance examined the results from 7 quasi-experimental and 10 cross-sectional studies. The quasi-experimental studies provided data corresponding to the effects of reduced school tuition (by up to 4 hours in certain cases) in order to accommodate extra time for PE. Although additional PE time did not lead to significant academic improvements, academic results for experimental and control groups were comparative, thus leading the review in question to conclude that learning efficiency was enhanced as a result of increased physical activity (Trudeau, and Shephard 2008).

The cross-sectional studies on the other hand, generally showed a positive association between physical activity and academic performance, with only 2 studies having reported an inverse association with academic attainment. However, a causal relationship cannot be construed from the cross-sectional data as physical activity levels may drop or rise depending on the time point figures were collected. It is encouraging that the positive relationship between physical activity and academic performance remained significant, despite confounding variables such as the socio-economic status (SES), a significant predictor of children's physical activity levels (Borraccino, *et al.,* 2009, Drenowatz, *et al.,* 2010, and Raudsepp, 2006) and academic achievement (Dollman, Boshoff, and Dodd 2006, and Walker, Petrill, and Plomin, 2005) having been controlled for in a number of these cross-sectional studies. Furthermore, the positive associations between physical activity and academic achievement were drawn from large samples of between 5810 and 11957 participants (apart from one study where n=921), increasing the likelihood that the results were derived from a representative samples. Nevertheless, the magnitude of the samples cannot guarantee that the target population were accurately represented in all cases, as the self-report nature of data collection utilised in the cross-sectional studies can be subject to non-response and therefore susceptible to a degree of selection bias. Although Nelson and Gordon-Larsen (2006) based their findings (e.g. those who were more active were more likely to achieve higher grades and less likely to partake in risky behaviours) on a large sample of US middle and high school population drawn from the National Longitudinal Study of Adolescent Health (n = 11957), the authors acknowledge that the exclusion of data from students who were severely disabled (n = 132), pregnant (n = 160) or Native American (n = 74), may have lead to a sample which was not strictly representative. Additional limitations include the variation in self-reported outcome measures and the resulting inability to make direct comparisons between studies. For instance Dwyer, *et al* (2001) measured academic achievement on a 5 point ability scale (e.g. 1 equalled poor scholastic performance and 5 equalled excellent) provided by the school principal, and Pate, *et al* (1996) measured academic attainment by means of a student's self-perception of academic performance. Besides the comparability issues associated with different outcome measures, one may also question the validity of the self-reported data. It is impossible to know what the ratings provided by the school principals in Dwyer, *et al's* (2001) study for example, are based upon, and one may question whether the principals provided scores which best reflected their school's performance. In addition Pate, *et al's* (1996) self-perceived ratings of academic success may have been over or under embellished, and so in all cases the provision of standardised scores would have lead to more meaningful data which would have facilitated interpretation and comparability.

Exercise and Cognitive Functioning

Research into the effects of physical activity on cognitive functioning has predominately focused on older adults (Kramer, *et al.,* 2005). A meta-analysis of studies investigating aerobic fitness training and its effects on cognitive functioning in adults over the age of 55 years, found that the greatest effect was seen in the tasks which involved executive control processes (e.g. working memory and task co-ordination) (Kramer, *et al.,* 2005). In addition, the same meta-analysis found that aerobic exercise combined with strength and flexibility training rather than aerobic training alone, had a greater impact on cognitive functioning. Attention is now pointing towards younger populations in order to assess the effects of physical activity on children's cognitive functioning as it unknown whether the findings drawn from adult studies can be generalised to a younger population (Tomporowski, 2003). Despite providing researchers with a research gap to fill, many researchers appear to have taken a rather defensive stance (e.g. Hillman, *et al.,* 2009; Taras, 2005) in an attempt to stop the global decline in time reserved for PE in schools (Hardman, and Marshall, 2000). It has been argued that as soon as the physical benefits of PE were accepted in the 1970s and its place within the school curriculum warranted, there was no longer any need to justify its cognitive benefits (Sibley, and Etnier, 2003). However, with world-wide surveys confirming beliefs that PE is undervalued and often shelved in an effort to improve performance in more 'academic' subjects (Hardman, and Marshall, 2000), coupled with the increasing challenges of childhood obesity and physical inactivity levels (WHO, 2011), the need to refocus on the important role that physical activity can play in children's lives has reappeared.

A review of 21 studies which had investigated the effects of acute exercise on children's/adolescent's behaviour and cognitive functioning, based the majority of its evaluation on studies which had focused on populations with clinical disorders (Tomporowski, 2003). Of the 4 studies that had examined the acute effects of exercise on children without clinical disorders, significant improvements in mathematics computation was observed in one study following 50 minutes vigorous physical activity rather than 20, 30 or 40 minutes (Gabbard, and Barton, 1979). In another, mathematics computation was enhanced significantly after 30 and 40 minutes of paced walking rather than 20 minutes, and enhanced performance was only observed when analysed at midday and in the afternoon, rather than in the morning (McNaughton, and Gabbard, 1993). A further study which entailed a sample of second, third and fourth grade children, found that 15 minutes of vigorous aerobic exercise only enhanced fourth-grade children's performance on the Woodcock Johnson Test of Concentration, yet 15 minutes of stretching exercises had no significant effects on either of the grades (Caterino, and Polak, 1999).

The remainder of Tomporowski's (2003) review concentrated on the effects of antecedent exercise on behaviour and cognitive functioning in children with attention-deficit disorders, autism or learning disorders, behavioural disorders and mental retardation. Disruptive behaviours were less frequent following exercise interventions which differed in duration and intensity. Exercise also facilitated cognitive functioning in adolescents with mild retardation, although the effects were greater for participants with the higher fitness levels (VO_{2max} greater than 45 ml/kg $\cdot$ min^{-1}). However, the benefits of exercise in some cases were short lived. For instance, the disruptive behaviours of autistic children were found to reduce after a high intensity 15 minute run, yet effects only lasted for a period of approximately 90 minutes. Similar results were observed in Trainable Mentally Retarded children; reduced rates of inappropriate behaviour were observed immediately after exercise, yet between 1 and 2 hours post exercise, a regression to increased rates of inappropriate behaviour were noted.

In summary, Tomporowski's (2003) review does provide some evidence that behaviour and cognitive functioning can improve as a result of acute exercise, however the bulk of the studies leant towards the study of subjects with clinical disorders making it difficult to generalise findings to populations without clinical disorders. Given the diverse types of individual characteristics, cognitive demands and exercise intensities under review, it is impossible to reach a strong conclusion regarding the effectiveness of acute exercise on children's cognitive performance. In addition, results were largely based on small samples of around 4 participants. A limitation of small studies is the risk that they can over-estimate the strength of an association and therefore such data should form the basis of larger confirmatory research (Hackshaw, 2008).

Research into the neuroelectric changes that may underlie cognitive functioning has been conducted via the recording of the P3 component of event-related potentials (ERPs) (Hillman, *et al.,* 2009). This is a non-invasive technique that maps the brains electrical activity in response to a specific sensory event (Kolb, and Whishaw, 2011). P3 is a positive brain-wave occurring around 300 milliseconds after presentation of a stimulus (Kolb, and Whishaw, 2011). Unlike the more apparent measures of cognitive performance, ERPs provide an opportunity to study covert aspects of cognitive processes that take place leading up to, and in response to, a stimulus (Hillman, *et al.,* 2009). Based on previous research, Hillman *et al's* (2009) study into the effects of acute moderately-intense aerobic exercise on cognitive control, hypothesised that following a single bout of exercise; children would present greater P3 amplitude (thought to indicate improved allocation of attentional resources) as well as shorter P3 latency (thought to indicate a quicker stimulus classification/cognitive processing speed) compared to baseline measures.

Twenty children with an average age of 9.6 years participated in the within-subject design study that required participants to attend a laboratory on two separate days. On the first visit, one half of the participants received a 20 minute seated resting session and the remainder received a 20 minute aerobic session on a motor-driven treadmill at around 60% of their maximum heart rate. Both groups then completed a modified flanker task whilst wearing an electrode cap. On removal of the electrode cap, standardised achievement tests (WRAT3) were administered to assess reading, spelling and mathematical ability, finally followed by a cardiorespiratory fitness assessment. On the second visit each group was required to swap conditions and repeat the former cognitive assessments. Data analysis showed significant improvements in the children's reading comprehension following an acute bout of aerobic exercise comparative to rest. However this was not the case for spelling or arithmetic. Improved response accuracy during incongruent flanker task trials were recorded post aerobic exercise, yet an acute bout of exercise did not enhance the pace of children's responses. A general exercise-induced increase in P3 amplitude was observed in the fronto-central, central, and parietal regions, though the greatest P3 amplitude was reached in the central-parietal region in response to incongruent trials post exercise. The utilisation of neuroimaging in earlier studies have also reported greater activation in the prefrontal and parietal regions of highly fit or aerobically trained adults, compared with adults of low fitness, when tasks demanding inhibitory control were administered (Colcombe, *et al.,* 2004). Hillman, *et al* (2009) believe that the aforementioned results and previous findings (Colcombe, *et al.,* 2004), suggest that the parietal region is open to exercise interventions, and that younger populations may too profit from benefits to the neural networks effecting cognitive control during inhibitory control. Although these results indicate that an acute bout of aerobic exercise may be an effective means of enhancing children's cognitive control of attention and academic performance, it is possible that other factors, such as motivation, may have influenced the subject's performance. The study appears to have recruited volunteers, reimbursed for their involvement, which as a result may have exposed the research to a source of bias. The sample's mean (SD) IQ, according to the Kaufman Brief Intelligence Test, was 120.7 (10.2), a classification of above average to upper extreme intelligence (Kamphaus, 2005). Such demographic data along with the recruitment method utilised, suggests that the study attracted children who possessed a strong motivation to succeed in their studies, whilst individuals with a greater need for an academic intervention were not represented.

Exercise and Reading Ability

Poor reading skills may hinder some individuals from achieving national academic expectations. Individuals diagnosed with dyslexia experience difficulties with language and literacy related skills such as phonological processing and rapid naming (British Dyslexia Association, n.d.). Although the cause(s) of developmental dyslexia is not clear, explanations include the magnocellular deficit hypothesis (Dyslexia Research Trust, n.d., and Stein, and Walsh, 1997), the phonological deficit hypothesis (Joly-Puttuz 2008), the cerebellar deficit hypothesis (Nicolson, Fawcett, and Dean, 2001), and neuro-developmental delays, which links the persistence of primary reflexes with specific learning difficulties (Goddard Blythe, 2006, Jordan-Black, 2005, and McPhillips, Hepper, and Mulhern, 2000). Over the last 10 years there has been increased interest in the efficacy of exercise in enhancing reading ability specifically. However, the extant data on this topic are equivocal due to the range of participant groups employed, differences in assessment of reading ability and variation in the frequency, intensity, time and type of exercise prescribed.

Reynolds, Nicolson and Hambly (2003) present the findings of an exercise-based intervention, described as Dyslexia Dyspraxia Attention Treatment (DDAT), aimed to remediate dyslexia-related disorders and children struggling with reading difficulties through the retraining of the cerebellum. The DDAT programme is described as a 'complex programme of integrated sensory stimulation incorporating visumotor and vestibular therapy.' The programme takes the cerebellar deficit hypothesis (Nicolson, Fawcett and Dean 2001) one step further by theorising that the retraining of the cerebellum will result in the remedy of cerebellar impairments (proposed as the cause of dyslexia) and as a result normal learning will follow. Cerebellar and vestibular function was tested as part of the Dyslexia Screening Test by measuring the number of beads that could be threaded in 30 seconds (measure of manual dexterity), as well as the degree of forward/backward sway after being gently pushed in the back (measure of postural stability). In addition to the DST, measures of cerebellar/vestibular functioning were also tested via Dynamic Posturography and Electronystagmography. Dynamic Posturography equipment assessed the participant's ability to suppress disruptive visual information, their skill at recovering from unexpected movement of supporting surface or walls, and their motor reaction when faced with irregular floor surfaces. Electronystagmography assessed eye movement by recording the participant's visual tracking ability, and saccade accuracy and latency when presented with a moving target.

The DDAT treatment involves the use of a balance board, throwing and catching, as well an array of stretching and co-ordination exercises. However, the study does not disclose the entire sequence of exercises for commercial reasons. The Dyslexia Screening Test (DST) identified 35 children considered to be at risk of reading difficulties and then randomly divided them into the treatment (10 male, 8 female, mean age 9.4 years, mean DST 0.74 vs. 0.72) or control group (9 male, 8 female, mean age 9.4 years, mean DST 0.72) matched according to gender, age and DST score. The treatment group completed the 10 minute DDAT programme at home, twice daily for 6 months, while the control group received normal school support as they continued with their normal daily routine. The study reported significant improvements in the intervention group's reading (number of words read in one minute), nonsense passage reading (mixing real words with pseudo words), semantic fluency (the number of animals participants could name in a minute), rapid naming (time taken to name pictures of objects), phonemic segmentation, postural stability and bead threading dexterity. The results of the standardised school tests showed that the intervention group achieved a 19 month gain in reading age, significant improvements in comprehension and writing, yet significant improvements were not observed for mathematics. In terms of the control group, significant improvements were observed for nonsense passage reading and phonemic segmentation. The results of the standardised school tests were not presented for the control group, as at the end of the 6 month period they undertook the DDAT programme, which meant that the aforementioned school tests would have included 3 months treatment. Reynolds, Nicolson, and Hambly (2003) concluded that the DDAT intervention was an effective means of improving cerebellar function, cognitive skills and literacy performance. At present the intervention, rebranded as the Dore Programme (www.dore.co.uk) is a commercial treatment available at around £2000 for individuals struggling with a range of learning difficulties.

The DDAT intervention has received much criticism for its methodological and statistical limitations (e.g., Snowling, and Hulme, 2003; McArthur, 2007). Snowling and Hulme (2003) put forward a catalogue of methodological flaws in an attempt to demonstrate why Reynolds, Nicolson, and Hambly (2003) are not justified in their claims. For instance, Snowling and Hulme (2003) suggested that statistical analysis should have been conducted on raw DST scores, rather than deciles, which are an ordinal scale of measurement. Averaging scores based on an ordinal scale of measurement was pronounced misleading, as differences may be amplified between scores close to the mean, whilst differences at the lower and upper end of the distribution are reduced (Snowling, and Hulme, 2003). By grouping different scores into deciles, valuable information may be hidden as a consequence (Snowling, and Hulme, 2003). Significant improvements in the DDAT group's reading scores were based on these scores (deciles), utilised in a total of 22 t-tests. Consequently the result was condemned invalid as conducting copious t-tests increases the likelihood of finding significant differences by chance (Snowling, and Hulme, 2003) and furthermore the assumptions for this particular statistical test were violated (Pallant, 2007). Alternatively, it was advised that a more suitable test would have been analysis of covariance, using raw scores, in order to control for differences in the two group's reading scores at baseline (Snowling, and Hulme, 2003). However the critique judged the study's lack of control group as its main limitation. It was suggested that parents of the control group could have spent an equivalent amount of time supporting their children with reading, which would have provided a comparative treatment (placebo) and a means of reducing the 'Hawthorne effect. To expand on Snowling, and Hulme's, (2003) review, further limitations are evident in the DDAT intervention (Reynolds, Nicolson, and Hambly 2003) as baseline measures show an imbalance between the control (mean delay of 4.4 months) and intervention (mean delay of 10.6 months) group's reading delay. As these scores ranged from 45 months delay to 22 months ahead, one may question why some of these subjects were classified as children with reading difficulties. The internal validity of the study was compromised by the fact that 7 participants from the intervention group, along with 5 from the control, all underwent small group support twice per week. It is therefore impossible to determine whether the academic improvements can be attributable to the exercise programme or additional support. Furthermore, as the programme was conducted at home without the supervision of trained personnel, adherence remains unknown as well.

Reynolds, and Nicolson (2007) conducted a further follow-up study in order to evaluate whether the gains associated with the DDAT programme had been maintained over the following 18 months, and to respond to criticisms of the original study (Reynolds, Nicolson, and Hambly 2003). By the time statistical analysis was conducted, the initial intervention group and original control group, now referred to as the delayed treatment group, had completed the exercise programme 6 to 12 months prior. As had been recommended (Snowling, and Hulme, 2003) analysis of covariance was conducted, using baseline data as the covariate, results from the final follow-up tests as the dependent variable, and group as the independent variable. In terms of the initial differences in performance scores, significant statistics were not reported. Given the lack of statistical effects and the small differential effect sizes observed, the researchers chose to pool the data for both groups prior to further analysis. Data analysis on the follow-up data reported that although the exercise-based intervention had discontinued, improvements in working memory, phonological skill, and semantic fluency had been maintained. Strangely, the standardised school tests reported an overall improvement of 32 months in reading age yet these achievements were not reflected in the DST scores. These differences may cause one to question the reliability and validity of the two assessments (Rack, *et al.,* 2007).

Despite claims that the DDAT programme offers long-lasting cognitive and literacy benefits (Reynolds, and Nicolson 2007), critics remain unconvinced (Rack, *et al.,* 2007, McArthur, 2007). Study reviews highlight the lack of an external reference point to due to the pooling of data (Rack, *et al.,* 2007). Attention is drawn again to the follow-up study's continued use of deciles, thought to deem the significant results 'meaningless' (Rack, *et al.,* 2007). It is suggested that literacy gains reported by Reynolds and Nicolson (2007), may have been due to test-retest effects, an effect which could have been avoided by using a randomised controlled trial (McArthur, 2007).

Support for the cerebellar explanation is mixed. Raberger and Wimmer (2003) assessed the relationship between balancing deficits, rapid naming and reading difficulties in four groups of children, including those solely with reading difficulties, a group with reading difficulties plus attention deficit hyperactivity disorder (ADHD), children with ADHD only, and a group of children without reading difficulties or ADHD. Cerebellar impairment has been explained by problems with phonemic segmentation and rapid naming speed, and balancing difficulties whilst performing a secondary task (Nicolson, Fawcett, and Dean 2001). However, Raberger and Wimmer (2003) failed to find a difference in balancing ability when the group of children with reading problems and the group of children without impairment were compared. Yet when ADHD was included in the analysis, poor balancing was found. The group with reading difficulties only and the group with reading difficulties plus ADHD displayed problems with poor rapid naming, although the group with ADHD alone did not. The study acknowledged limited support for the cerebellar deficit hypothesis in that problems with slower information processing speed were found to correspond with reading difficulties, yet poor balancing was not associated with reading difficulties alone.

Kibby, *et al* (2008) used quantitative magnetic imaging to examine whether any anatomical differences existed in the cerebellar of 20 children with dyslexia and 20 children without dyslexia, and the correlations with cognitive functioning. Findings gave partial support to the cerebellar deficit hypothesis of dyslexia (Nicolson, Fawcett, and Dean, 2001), in that several children with dyslexia exhibited atypical cerebellar morphologic structure. This was manifested by atypical cerebellar asymmetry, and in the rapid naming test, a smaller hemisphere volume correlated moderately with a higher error frequency. Although Nicolson, Fawcett, and Dean (2001) have reported that cerebellar dysfunction is particularly associated with a deficit in naming speed, Kibby *et al* (2008) found that the different asymmetry groups (i.e. with hemisphere symmetry, reversed asymmetry, or typical rightward asymmetry) were comparable in phonological processing skills which included naming speed, and that only 14 of the dyslexic sample experienced rapid naming difficulties. In addition, only 2 children diagnosed with dyslexia satisfied all of the main symptoms said to be indicative of a dysfunctional cerebellar. In view of the limited correlations, Kibby, *et al* (2008) proposed that there may be subtypes of dyslexia and therefore a single theory may not be appropriate for the heterogeneity equated with dyslexia, or else as Zeffiro, and Eden's (2001) suggested, the central problem is possibly sited elsewhere in the brain.

Zeffiro, and Eden (2001) draws attention to the symptoms of cerebellar disease as observed by the late work of Holmes, (1939): postural hypotonia, asthenia and muscle fatigue, problems managing the rate, range and force of voluntary movements, and finally disturbances of associated movements which may be manifest the passive swinging of lifeless arms as a result of shoulder movement. The suggestion that impairments to the cerebellar are at the source of dyslexia has prompted questions, firstly as to why classic signs of cerebellar disease are not overtly exhibited in persons with dyslexia, and secondly, why sufferers of cerebellar disease do not also display phonological or reading difficulties (Zeffiro, and Eden, 2001). Alternatively, signs normally attributed to cerebellar impairments may be due to inferior input from other regions of the brain, for instance, oculomotor difficulties could be a sign of cerebellar damage or changes to the processing of information from the extrastriate cortex (Zeffiro, and Eden, 2001).

Further non-tuition based interventions, designed to support individuals struggling with literacy and academic attainment, have been based on the theory that retention of primary reflexes are the underlying cause of a range of learning difficulties (Goddard Blythe, 2006; McPhillips, Hepper, and Mulhern, 2000). A randomised, individually matched, double-blind, placebo controlled study observed significant reductions in persistent reflexes in an experimental group following a 12 month home administered movement programme, along with significant gains of between 19.6 (Neale analysis of reading ability) and 15.3 (Wechsler, objective reading dimensions) months in reading age (McPhillips, Hepper, and Mulhern, 2000). However, it is worth noting that significant literacy improvements were also reported for the placebo group who were required to repeat non-specific movements each day, whilst control groups continued with their normal daily activities. All groups showed significant progress in writing speed, spelling age and spoonerisms. Significant gains in rapid naming speed along with significant reductions in ATNR persistence and saccadic frequency were isolated to the experimental group. Of the 70 known primary reflexes, the intervention required the daily 10 minute repetition of only four, namely the tonic labyrinthine reflex (TLR), the Moro reflex (MR), the symmetrical tonic neck reflex (STNR), and the ATNR. ATNR was proposed as a good indicator of total reflex persistence as well as an important function in visual development, however, empirical evidence to explain the remaining choice of reflexes was not offered. The placebo group were required to repeat a daily sequence of non-specific movement. The findings appear to have been derived from a well-designed study; participants were well matched and randomly assigned to different treatment groups which reduced the possibility of random error (Mitchell, and Jolley, 2010); a placebo-control group and non-treatment control group allowed for any effects in addition to any potential 'Hawthorne effects' to be evaluated, as well as maturation being controlled for (May-Benson, and Koomer, 2010); and a double-blinded design helped to reduce the threat of bias as the administrator/assessor and participant were unlikely to have manipulated the results in support of the hypothesis (Mitchell, and Jolley, 2010).

However, the study was not without limitations, and interpretation of the results should be done with care. The study recognised that it may have fallen victim to a certain degree of sampling bias as the study participants were associated with parents who had volunteered their participation, and so motivation may have partially influenced the results. Good 'at-home' parenting, which involves taking an interest in your child's educational progress, is reported to be a significant factor in how well a child progresses in school, carrying even more weight than the parent's level of education or socio-economic status (The National Literacy Trust, 2005). In addition, there was a higher ratio of boys to girls in the sample (16 females and 50 males met the inclusion criteria) and as statistics indicate that girls in England outperform boys in Key Stage 2 English (Department for Education, 2010), one could question whether the reading delays were partly down to gender. The small scale of the study also hinders confidence in the results, as there is a chance that the small sample sizes may have over-estimated the strength of association (Hackshaw, 2008). A questionnaire was circulated post intervention in order to monitor for potential confounding variables such as school attendance, illness, extra specialised support, and/or change in circumstances, yet there was no evidence of statistical adjustments reported, to indicate that such factors that may have contributed to the treatments effectiveness, had been controlled for. Tests such as analysis of covariance may not have been conducted, as small samples can produce unreliable statistical results when controlling for confounders (Hackshaw, 2008). A full description of the intervention is not disclosed and this lack of transparency could elicit reader mistrust: independent replication to aid an informed decision would be impossible. The researchers may harbour a fear that total exposure may draw interest away from their training course (www.primarymovement.org) which provides teachers with the complete sequence of movements at a charge.

Although these findings need to be considered tentatively, the aforementioned study (McPhillips, Hepper, and Mulhern, 2000) has shown that the retention of primary reflexes may be a risk factor in certain reading problems. However, as the primary author developed the programme and was involved in the research, there is a chance of reporting bias. It is therefore good to discover that the interventions effectiveness has been investigated by an alternative researcher on a larger scale (Jordan-Black, 2005).

A large comparative study (n = 683 children, aged 6-11 years) has been conducted over a period of 2 years in order to investigate the effects of the Primary Movement programme on reading performance, mathematical ability, spelling and ATNR levels (Jordan-Black 2005). Alongside the comparative study, a second quasi-experimental study tracked the progress of four parallel groups of children, comprising of an experimental and control group from Year 3 (n = 82) and an experimental and control group from Year 5 (n = 97). Control groups continued with normal daily activities. In contrast to prior home administration (McPhillips, Hepper and, Mulhern 2000), the decision was taken to administer the intervention to complete classes of children over a period of one academic year, as previous findings (McPhillips, and Sheehy, 2004), have indicated that mild levels of retained reflexes can be present in children with average and above reading levels. Baseline data for both studies (reading ability assessed by WORD, mathematics by Wechsler Objective Numerical Dimensions, Non-Reading Intelligence Tests for Year 3 and 5 as Year 7 were too old, and ATNR by means of the Schilder test) were collected at the end of the academic year in spring and summer 2002, then the longitudinal study and quasi-experimental treatment groups began the movement intervention the following school year. Reassessment was not carried out until the end of the following academic year in spring and summer 2004.

For the comparative study, multiple regression analysis reported verbal IQ to be the strongest predictor of reading, over and above ATNR levels, gender, month of birth and free school meals, which was consistent with previous research (McPhillips, and Sheehy, 2004) Verbal IQ was also the strongest predictor of spelling and mathematics. ATNR played a significant role in the prediction of these academic areas, although to a lesser extent. When the 2002 baseline data was compared to the 2004 data, significant reductions were observed in ATNR levels for both year groups; significant improvements in reading and mathematics; but only a small effect on spelling. Effect sizes demonstrated that the magnitude of the treatment effect was relatively strong in relation to reading gains and ATNR, whilst very strong for mathematics. However, the study noted that the influence of other mediating factors cannot be ruled out on account that reassessment was conducted a full academic year post intervention.

The quasi-experimental group reported significantly larger reading and mathematical gains compared to the control group, although spelling did not improve significantly for either group. It was noted that even though significant improvements observed in the experimental group were greater than those seen in the controls, the experimental group were in fact further behind academically. As a result one cannot be sure whether improvements were due to group imbalances or treatment effects. A cross-over design may have been able to address the study's issue of imbalance.

In summary there is evidence that the rehearsal of specific movements intended to mimic and subsequently inhibit retained primary reflexes, may contribute to the reduction in continued reflex levels (specifically ATNR) and consequently facilitate progress in reading (McPhillips, Hepper, and Mulhern 2000, and Jordan-Black 2005) and mathematics (Jordan-Black, 2005). Although the positive results should not be dismissed, a review of the available evidence, which to date is sparse, has unanswered questions and limitations that cannot be overlooked when interpreting these results. For instance, the aforementioned movement studies (McPhillips, Hepper, and Mulhern, 2000, and Jordan-Black, 2005) are not transparent in their disclosures. The small sample sizes limit the degree to which these results can be generalised, and the small scale may have resulted in an overestimation of the strength of associations reported. And the lack of consistency between the studies makes it difficult to draw conclusions regarding the most effective way to deliver the intervention. On one hand significant improvements have been observed in reading, writing speed, spelling, spoonerisms, rapid naming speed and ATNR persistence when the movement programme is administered daily at daily home for a year (McPhillips, Hepper, and Mulhern, 2000), and significant progress has also been reported in reading, mathematics and ATNR levels when administered by a teacher, accompanied by action songs and rhymes, in a classroom environment, 5 days per week over one academic year (Jordan-Black). In contrast, when the Institute of Neuro-Physiological Psychology, who devised the movements for the Primary Movement programme, evaluated the effectiveness of the I.N.P.P. programme in primary schools, the impact on reading was small (Goddard-Blythe, 2005). Future research is needed to (1) determine the appropriate treatment dosage, frequency and duration, (2) to determine whether an upper age limit applies to the intervention's effectiveness, (3) to investigate the intervention's long-term efficacy, (4) to find out which population(s) are most likely to benefit from the intervention, and (5) to gain full disclosure of the intervention in order to allow the reader to make an informed decision.

Conclusion

Although the health benefits of physical activity are well established, its effectiveness in enhancing cognitive and academic performance remains unclear. Neuroscience is encouraged by research which has found that several days of running can enhance the production of proteins in the hippocampus of animals, as this may benefit cognitive functioning and learning in humans (Berg, 2010). Research into the neuroelectric changes underlying cognitive functioning have reported increased P3 amplitude and significant improvements in reading comprehension following an acute bout of aerobic exercise, compared to rest (Hillman, *et al.,* 2009). Tomporowski's (2003) review found that behaviour and cognitive functioning can improve post acute exercise, however the majority of populations included within the analysis were diagnosed with clinical disorders so this hampers the ability to generalise the findings to other populations. In considering the value and impact of PE in schools, while there remains uncertainty regarding what modes of physical activity benefit which areas of learning, it may be of comfort for those worried about the decline of PE in schools, that evidence has shown an increase in time allotted to PE does compromise academic performance (Ahamed, *et al.,* 2007; Carlson, *et al.,* 2008; Trudeau, and Shephard, 2008). In contrast to an emphasis on moderate intensity physical activity, movement based interventions have endeavoured to provide explanations and remedies for children struggling with learning difficulties. Reynolds, Nicolson, and Hambly (2003) maintain that the DDAT intervention is an effective means of improving cerebellar function, cognitive skills and literacy performance. However, this intervention has been heavily criticised for its methodological flaws (Snowling, and Hulme, 2003; McArthur, 2007, Rack, *et al.,* 2007). Further interventions based on the theory that the continuation of primary reflexes impedes the progression of learning in certain populations (Goddard-Blythe, 2005, Jordan-Black, 2005, and McPhillips, Hepper, and Mulhern, 2000) claim that the rehearsal of reflexes facilitates learning. Evidence has been presented to indicate that the inhibition of primitive reflexes may assist those struggling academically, however as detailed earlier, further research is needed before strong conclusions can be drawn.

Further research needs to be conducted in to the effectiveness of exercise on enhancing children's academic and reading ability. The differences in methodological rigour, outcome measures assessments, types of exercise and population characteristics, make it difficult to reach a strong conclusion. Much research has been based on theory, and trial and error. Future research needs to employ longitudinal designs to determine the long lasting effects of exercise, larger sample sizes, be more transparent in its reporting as there is still some uncertainty around what exercise duration, mode, dosage, frequency will benefit what type of academic area and population group.

References

Ahamed, Y., Macdonald, H., Reed, K., Naylor, P. J., Liu-Ambrose, T., and McKay, H. (2007). 'School-Based Physical Activity Does Not Compromise Children's Academic Performance.' *Medicine and Science in Sports and Exercise,* 39 (2), 371-376.

Audit Commission (2004). *Youth Justice 2004: A review of the reformed youth justice system.* London: Audit Commission.

Basterfield, L., Adamson, A. J., Parkinson, K. N., Maute, U., Li, P. X., Reilly, J. J., and the Gateshead Millennium Study Core Team. (2008). 'Surveillance of physical activity in the UK is flawed: validation of the Health Survey for England Physical Activity Questionnaire.' *Archives of Disease in Childhood,* 93, 1054-1058.

Berg, K. (2010). 'Justifying Physical Education Based on Neuroscience Evidence.' *The Journal of Physical Education, Recreation and Dance,* 81 (3), 24-31.

Borraccino, A., Lemma, P., Lannotti, R. J., Zambon, A., Dalmasso, P., Lazzeri, G., Giacchi, M., and Cavallo, F. (2009). 'Socioeconomic Effects of Meeting Physical Activity Guidelines: Comparisons among 32 countries.' *Medicine and Science in Sports and Exercise,* 41 (4), 749-756.

British Dyslexia Association (n.d.). *About Dyslexia: Frequently Asked Questions* [online] available from <http://www.bdadyslexia.org.uk/about-dyslexia/faqs.html> [21 November 2010].

Carlson, S. A., Fulton, J. E., Lee, S. M., Maynard, M., Brown, D. R., Kohl, H. W., and Dietz, W. H. (2008). 'Physical Education and Academic Achievement in Elementary School: Data From the Early Childhood Longitudinal Study.' *American Journal of Public Health,* 98 (4), 721-727.

Caterino, M. C., and Polak, E. D. (1999). 'Effects of two types of activity on the performance of second-, third-, and fourth-grade students on a test of concentration.' *Perceptual and Motor Skills,* 89, 245-248.

Centre for Longitudinal Studies (2008). ed. by Elliott, J., and Vaitilingam, R. *Key finding from the National Child Development Study* [online] available from < http://www.ncds.info/page.asp?section=000100010004andsectionTitle=Publications> [19 February 2011].

Colcombe, S. J., Kramer, A. F., Erickson, K. I., Scalf, P., McAuley, E., Cohen, N. J., Webb, A., Jerome, G. J., Marquez, D. X., and Elavsky, S. (2004). 'Cardiovascular fitness, cortical plasticity, and aging.' *Proceedings Of The National Academy Of Sciences Of The United States Of America,* 101 (9), 3316-21.

Cotman, C. W., Berchtold, N. C., and Christie, L. A. (2007). 'Exercise builds brain health: key roles of growth factor cascades and inflammation.' *Trends in Neurosciences,* 30 (9), 464-472.

Department for Children, Schools, and Families (2010). *Breaking the link between special educational needs and low attainment: Everyone's business.* Nottingham: Department for Children, Schools, and Families Publications.

Department for Education (2010). *Topic guide to: School and College Attainment Behaviour* [online] available from < http://www.statistics.gov.uk/hub/children-education-skills/school-and-college-education/school-and-college-attainment-and-behaviour > [1 March 2011].

Department of Health (2009). *Be Active, Be Healthy: A Plan for Getting the Nation Moving.* London: Department of Health.

Dollman, J., Boshoff, K., and Dodd, G. (2006). 'The relationship between curriculum time for physical education and literacy and numeracy standards in South Australian primary schools.' *European Physical Education Review,* 2 (2), 151-163.

Drenowatz, C., Eisenmann, J. C., Pfeiffer, K. A., Welk, G., Heelan, K., Gentile, D., and Walsh, D. (2010). 'Influence of socio-economic status on habitual physical activity and sedentary behaviour in 8- to 11- year old children.' *BMC Public Health,* 10,214-224.

Dwyer, T., Sallis, J. F., Blizzard, L., Lazarus, R., and Dean, K. (2001). 'Relation of Academic Performance to Physical Activity and Fitness in Children.' *Pediatric Exercise Science,* 13, 225-237.

Dyslexia Research Trust (n.d.). *About Dyslexia: What causes dyslexia?* [online] available from <http://www.dyslexic.org.uk/aboutdyslexia2.htm> [21 November 2010].

Gabbard, C., and Barton, J. (1979). 'Effects of Physical Activity on Mathematical Computation Among Young Children.' *The Journal of Psychology,* 103, 287-288.

Goddard Blythe, S. (2006). *The INPP Test Battery and Developmental Exercise Programme for use in Schools.* Chester: The Institute for Neuro-Physiological Psychology.

Goddard Blythe, S. (2005). 'Releasing Educational Potential Through Movement: A Summary of Individual Studies Carried Out Using the INPP Test Battery and Developmental Exercise Programme for use in Schools with Children with Special Needs.' *Child Care in Practice,* 11 (4), 415-432.

Hackshaw, A. (2008). 'Small studies: strengths and limitations.' *European Respiratory Journal,* 32 (5), 1141-1143.

Hardman, K., and Marshall, J. (2000). 'The state and status of physical education in schools in international context.' *European Physical Education Review,* 6 (3), 203-229.

Hillman, C. H., Pontifex, M. B., Raine, L. B., Castelli, D. M., Hall, E. E., and Kramer, A. F. (2009). 'The Effect of Acute Treadmill Walking on Cognitive Control and Academic Achievement in Preadolescent Children.' *Neuroscience,* 159, 1044-1054.

Holmes, G. (1939). 'The cerebellum of man.' *Brain,* 62 (1), 1-30.

Janssen, I., and LeBlanc, A. G. (2010). 'Systematic review of the health benefits of physical activity and fitness in school-aged children and youth.' *International Journal of Behavioural Nutrition and Physical Activity,* 7, 1-16.

Joly-Puttuz, B., Mercier, M., Leynaud, A., and Habib, M. (2008). 'Combined auditory and articulatory training improves phonological deficit in children with dyslexia.' *Neuropsychological Rehabilitation,* 18 (4), 402-429.

Jordan-Black (2005). 'The effects of the Primary Movement programme on the academic performance of children attending ordinary primary school.' *Journal of Research in Special Educational Needs,* 5 (3), 101-111.

Kamphaus, R. W. (2005). *Clinical Assessments of Child and Adolescent Intelligence.* 2nd edn. New York: Springer Science + Business Media Inc.

Kibby, M. Y., Fancher, J. B., Markanen, R., and Hynd, G. W. (2008). 'A Quantitative Magnetic Resonance Imaging Analysis of the Cerebellar Deficit Hypothesis of Dyslexia.' *Journal of Child Neurology,* 23 (4), 368-380.

Kolb, B., and Whishaw, I. Q. (2011). *An Introduction to Brain and Behavior.* 3rd edn. New York: Worth Publishers.

Kramer, A. F., Colcombe, S. J., McAuley, E., Scalf, P. E., and Erickson, K. I. (2005). 'Fitness, aging and neurocognitive function.' *Neurobiology of Aging,* 26 (1), 124-127.

May-Benson, T. A., and Koomar, J. A. (2010). 'Systematic Review of the Research Evidence Examining the Effectiveness of Interventions Using a Sensory Integrative Approach for Children.' *The American Journal of Occupational Therapy,* 64 (3), 403-414.

McArthur, G. (2007). 'Test-Retest Effects in Treatment Studies of Reading Disability: The Devil is in the Detail.' *Dyslexia,* 13, 240-252.

McNaughton, D., and Gabbard, C. (1993). 'Physical exertion and immediate performance of sixth-grade children.' *Perceptual and Motor Skills,* 77, 1155-9.

McPhillips, M., Hepper, P. G., and Mulhern, G. (2000). 'Effects of replicating primary-reflex movements on specific reading difficulties in children: a randomised, double-blind, controlled trial.' *The Lancet,* 355, 537-541.

Mitchell, M. L., and Jolley, J. M. (2010). *Research design explained.* 7th edn. Belmont, USA: Wadsworth.

National Literacy Trust (2005). *Every Which Way We Can: A Literacy and social inclusion position paper.* London: National Literacy Trust.

National Literacy Trust (2010). *Literacy: State of the Nation. A picture of literacy in the UK today.* London: National Literacy Trust.

Nelson, M. C., and Gordon-Larsen, P. (2006). 'Physical Activity and Sedentary Behavior Patterns Are Associated With Selected Adolescent Health Risk Behaviors.' *Pediatrics,* 117, 1281-1290.

Nicolson, R. I., Fawcett, A. J., and Dean, P. (2001). 'Developmental dyslexia: the cerebellar deficit hypothesis.' *Trends in Neurosciences,* 24 (9), 508-511.

Office for Standards in Education, Children's Services and Skills (2010). *Reading by six: How the best schools do it.* Manchester: The Office for Standards in Education, Children's Services and Skills.

Pallant, J. (2007). *SPSS Survival Manual: A step-by-step Guide to Data Analysis using SPSS version 15.* 3rd edn. Maidenhead: Open University Press.

Pate, R. R., Heath, G. W., Dowda, M., and Trost, S. G. (1996). 'Associations between Physical Activity and Other Health Behaviors in a Representative Sample of US Adolescents.' *American Journal of Public Health,* 86 (11), 1577-1581.

Raberger, T., and Wimmer, H. (2003). 'On the automaticity/cerebellar deficit hypothesis of dyslexia: balancing and continuous rapid naming in dyslexic and ADHD children.' *Neuropsychologia,* 41, 1493-1497.

Rack, P. J., Snowling, M. J., Hulme, C., and Gibbs, S. (2007). 'No Evidence that an Exercise-based Treatment Programme (DDAT) has Specific Benefits for Children with Reading Difficulties.' *Dyslexia,* 13, 97-104.

Raudsepp, L. (2006). 'The relationship between socio-economic status, parental support and adolescent physical activity.' *Acta Pædiatrica,* 95, 93-98.

Reynolds, D., Nicolson, R. I., and Hambly, H. (2003). 'Evaluation of an Exercise-based Treatment for Children with Reading Difficulties.' *Dyslexia,* 9, 48-71.

Reynolds, D., and Nicolson, R. I. (2007). 'Follow-up of an Exercise-based Treatment for Children with Reading Difficulties.' *Dyslexia,* 13, 78-96.

Sibley, B. A., and Etnier, J. L. (2003). 'The Relationship Between Physical Activity and Cognition in Children: A Meta-Analysis.' *Pediatric Exercise Science,* 15, 243-256.

Snowling, M. J., and Hulme, C. (2003). 'A Critique of claims from Reynolds, Nicolson and Hambly (2003) that DDAT is an Effective Treatment for Children with Reading Difficulties – 'Lies, Damned Lies and (Inappropriate) Statistics?' *Dyslexia,* 9, 127-133.

Stein, J., and Walsh, V. (1997). 'To see but not to read; the magnocellular theory of dyslexia.' *Trends in Neurosciences,* 20 (4), 147-152.

Taras, H. (2005). 'Physical Activity and Student Performance at School.' *Journal of School Health,* 75 (6), 214-218.

The NHS Information Centre (2010). *Statistics on obesity, physical activity and diet: England 2010* [online] available from < *http://www.ic.nhs.uk/webfiles/publications/opad10 /Statistics_on_Obesity_Physical_Activity_and_Diet_England_2010.pdf*> [11 October 2010].

Tomporowski, P. D. (2003). 'Cognitive and Behavioral Responses to Acute Exercise in Youths: A Review.' *Pediatric Exercise Science,* 15, 348-359.

Trudeau, F., and Shephard, R. J. (2008). 'Physical Education, school physical activity, school sports and academic performance.' *International Journal of Behavioural Nutrition and Physical Activity,* 5 (10), 1-12.

Vayman, S., Ying, Z., and Gomez-Pinilla, F. (2004). 'Hippocampal BDNF mediates the efficacy of exercise on synaptic plasticity and cognition.' *European Journal of Neuroscience,* 20, 2580-2590.

Vayman, S., Ying, Z., and Gomez-Pinilla, F. (2003). 'Interplay between brain-derived neurotrophic factor and signal transduction modulators in the regulation of the effects of exercise on synaptic-plasticity.' *Neuroscience,* 122, 647-657.

Walker, S. O., Petrill, S. A., and Plomin, R. (2005). ' A Genetically Sensitive Investigation of the Effects of the School Environment and Socio-economic status on Academic Achievement in Seven-Year-Olds.' *Educational Psychology,* 25 (1), 55-73.

Watkinson, C., Van Sluijs, E. M. F., Sutton, S., Hardeman, W., Corder, K., and Griffen, S. J. (2010). 'Overestimation of physical activity level is associated with lower BMI: a cross-sectional analysis.' *International Journal of Behavioral Nutrition and Physical Activity,* 7 (68), 1-9.

World Health Organisation (2010). *Global Recommendations on Physical Activity for Health.* Geneva: World Health Organisation.

World Health Organisation (2011). *Global Strategy on Diet, Physical Activity and Health: Childhood overweight and obesity* [online] available from < http://www.who.int/dietphysicalactivity/childhood/en/ > [23 February 2003].

Zeffiro, T., and Eden, G. (2001). 'The cerebellum and dyslexia: perpetrator or innocent bystander?' *Trends in Neurosciences,* 24 (9), 512-513.

In: Reviews in Pediatric Exercise Science
Editor: Michael Duncan, pp. 115-124
ISBN: 978-1-61470-978-7

Chapter VIII

The Relationship between Fundamental Movement Skills and Physical Activity in Primary School Children: A Short Review

Luke C. Baker, Samantha Birch and Michael J. Duncan
Coventry University, UK.

Introduction

Declines in Physical activity (PA) and increasing obesity levels in children have encouraged increasing interest in understanding children's PA behaviour. Currently in the United Kingdom (UK), an estimated 1 in 3 children in the age range of 4-11 are overweight (NCMP, 2010). Existing research in this field has related these statistics with the lack of PA children engage in (Gorely *et al.*, 2004; Mackett and Paskins, 2008) and the rise in sedentary behaviours such as video gaming or sustained periods watching television (Salmon *et al.* 2005).

PA tracking has identified a substantial decrease from childhood to adolescence (Malina *et al.*. 1990; Telama *et al.*. 1996). This is primarily related to movement skill refinement and the ability to move efficiently and perform these skills competently (Okely, Chey and Booth. 2001; Timmons *et al.*, 2007). Movement skills track at low-moderate levels during childhood, so greater motor proficiency may be predictive of later PA (Pate and Kann, 2002).

The mastery of fundamental movement skills (FMS) is a potential correlate of the involvement of children's PA participation (Welk, 1999). These movement skills form the prerequisites for sport competence and other forms of PA (Gallahue and Ozmun, 2002; Barnett et al., 2009), therefore acquiring these skills during early childhood may increase the likelihood for longer term PA. Young children who are equipped with movement skills are more likely to be successful in PA and will be able to seek greater opportunities to be physically active (Sallis *et al.*, 2002; Fisher *et al.*, 2005). Conversely, children without these skills lack the confidence in their ability and may therefore be more likely to drop out of sport, games and physical activity in the future (Gallahue and Ozmun, 2002).

With this in mind, the development of FMS in children could be important for PA promotion and the enhancement of public health. However, despite suggestions that the development of FMS in children leads to increased PA (Gallahue and Ozmun, 2002), few studies have actually examined the relationship between these two variables in primary and pre-school children since the majority of research has focussed on using older children and adolescents (McKenzie *et al.*, 2002; Wrotniak *et al.*, 2006). Such a focus on older children and adolescents arguably has little effect in improving PA habits as it may be too late for those children who have not yet already gained prerequisite mastery in the FMS to do so for wider activity benefit. Furthermore, during early childhood, the developing neuromuscular systems are at optimal readiness to learn these basic movement skills (Gallahue and Ozmun, 2003; Lubans el al., 2010). Prior research has also relied heavily on using subjective measures and non validated instruments such as self report measures (Fisher et al. 2005) to assess PA and its relationship with FMS (Duncan *et al.*, 2007), therefore future research may benefit from using objective measures of PA (Morgan *et al.* 2008). This short review will focus on the previous literature examining FMS and PA and various correlates of the two such as age, gender and weight status.

Physical Activity and Children

Active living and pursuing a life long engagement in PA provides many benefits to cardiorespiratory and muscular systems (Anderson and Butcher, 2006; Sallis and Patrick, 1994). PA is a key component of energy balance and PA is promoted in children and adolescents as lifelong positive health behaviour (Welk *et al.* 1999). Existing research currently shows children are not engaging in enough PA, which is primarily due to an increase in sedentary behaviours such as video gaming or sustained periods in front of the television (Salmon *et al.* 2005; Okely *et al.* 2004).

PA plays an important role for cognitive, social and physical development and it is well established in the literature that PA helps prevent obesity and other chronic diseases (Weiss and Dziura, 2004; Fisher *et al.*, 2005; Lubans *et al.*, 2010). Statistics from the UK state that only 1 in 3 children are currently meeting the minimum recommended exercise guidelines of 60 minutes of moderate-vigorous physical activity (MVPA) daily (ACSM, 1998; Gorely *et al.,* 2004). This is a major concern for children in the future since it is now recommended by the National Association of Physical Education (NASPE, 2010) that children should be engaging in 120 minutes of exercise daily, 60 minutes organised activity (Physical Education (PE) lessons etc) and 60 minutes unstructured activity (free play, break times).

Organised PA is an important aspect of the curriculum in primary schools, and provides a 'window of opportunity' for children to be physically active (Warburton et al. 1996). However, evidence from studies has found that children are not meeting the recommended guidelines of 2 hours quality PE and PA every week (Warburton *et al.,* 1996; Fairclough and Stratton, 2005). This is primarily due to schools not providing sufficient high quality PE specialists to carry out these lessons and schools focusing on other lessons such as Numeracy and Literacy, where they feel these lessons are of more importance (Warburton *et al* 1996).

This is an important concern as mastery of fundamental movement skills may be maximised in the school setting where PE lessons focusing on development of the motor skills and patterns that underlie all forms of PA are taught by subject specialists..

PA tracking has identified a substantial decrease in activity levels from childhood to adolescence (Malina *et al.*, 1990; Telama *et al.*, 1996), which shows that children prior to leaving school have developed more sedentary and less physically active behaviours. However, the extant literature in this area has tended to focus on older children and adolescents, therefore a research priority is to look at working with younger children, so researchers can fully understand the relationship between PA and age and identify some of the determinants for the reported age related decline in PA behaviour (Branta *et al.*, 1984; Malina *et al.*, 1990; Telama *et al.*, 1996).

Fundamental Movement Skills (FMS)

The mastery of fundamental movement skills (FMS) is widely regarded as an essential contributor to children's physical and cognitive development and research suggests that these FMS form the pre-requisites and foundations for further participation in sport and all other forms physical activity (Van Beurden *et al.*, 2003; Stodden *et al.*, 2008; Hardy *et al.*, 2010; Lubans *et al.*, 2010). FMS are classified into three major components 1) Locomotor skills, 2) Object control skills, and 3) Non-Locomotor skills (Gallahue and Ozmun, 2003; Lubans *et al.*, 2010). Locomotor skills refer to movement skills, these skills may include running, jumping, galloping or hopping.

Object control skills require the manipulation of an object, skills of this kind would include catching, kicking or throwing a ball. Finally non locomotor skills refer to body management skills; these may include balancing for example (Haubenstricker and Feldt, 1986).

The acquisition of FMS during early childhood has been identified as an important time to promote physical literacy (LTAD, 2008) and physical fitness. These skills during this period are critical for children's development, especially while neuromuscular systems are maturing (Gallahue and Ozmun, 2002). Furthermore, Stodden and colleagues (2008) suggest that the more time spent initially developing these movement skills will increase the likelihood of continued PA behaviour and also improve neuromotor development (Gallahue and Ozmun, 2002). Children without these basic skills are more likely to drop out of exercise and games, due to their incompetence and loss of confidence in their ability (Gallahue and Ozmun, 2002), therefore primary schools which provide a 'window of opportunity' for developing these fundamental skills should employ more programs and interventions to develop FMS (McKenzie *et al.*, 2002). This could potentially provide the best opportunity for children, given that PE is a compulsory part of education, therefore if pupils can be made active as possible and acquire these competencies in structured lessons, along with 'free play' (break times) this may influence the time spent being active.

Physical educators or PE specialists provide the catalysts for developing these skills and do more than just provide enjoyable activity for children. The activity children participate in during PE lessons must be made purposeful; therefore PE specialists should aim at mastering FMS and learning developmentally appropriate fitness concepts (Colvin, Markos and Walker,

2000; Olrich, 2002). If children miss the opportunity to develop FMS, it is likely they will refrain from pursing physically active lifestyles and will not enjoy sports activities (Wrotniak *et al.,* 2006). This most likely results in the use of withdrawal as a coping strategy (Wrotniak *et al.,* 2006). Although FMS plays a fundamental role in schools, these skills not only require reinforcement and good teaching, but assessing also. Assessment is important to ensure all children can competently move effectively and perform basic throwing and catching tasks before moving towards more specific sporting activities (Colvin, Markos and Walker, 2000; McKenzie *et al.*, 2002), and is a critical aspect of making sure children develop and progress. On the other hand, time constraints can be a problem in primary schools; therefore immediate focus could be to employ practical solutions to assessing FMS effectively (Olrich, 2002). This could be through after school classes, planning and making PE lessons more centred on mastering FMS, setting up community PA in a bid to develop FMS competencies.

Olrich (2002) also suggests using practical technology or the use of peer assessment to assess FMS in primary schools, however, the use of technology assessment methods can be expensive and require validation. Likewise, peer assessment may be time consuming and results are based on opinion (Colvin, Markos and Walker, 2000). In conclusion, more research is needed to look at ways of assessing FMS and employing interventions to improve movement skills (Wrotniak *et al.*, 2006; Morgan *et al.,* 2008).

A consistent body of research has looked at the benefits of FMS and its relationship with PA and evidence has positively associated FMS proficiency with subsequent PA (Lubans *et al.*, 2010; Wrotniak *et al.*, 2006; Fisher *et al.*, 2005; Barnett *et al.*, 2009). Although positive associations have been found between FMS and subsequent PA, these associations have been weak to moderate. Additionally, other studies have identified no interactions between FMS and PA (Reed *et al.*, 2004; McKenzie *et al.*, 2002). Despite the equivocal nature of past research on this issue it is logical to suggest that children leaving school with FMS difficulties are unlikely to pursue PA, as a result of their perceived incompetence. For example, a child who has difficulty catching may be less likely to engage in any form of sport or physical activity where this FMS is a component (e.g., basketball, rugby, cricket, baseball, etc) due to low physical self-efficacy for a given fundamental skill.

Moreover, FMS proficiency has been positively linked with increased motivation and self confidence (Sallis, 1994; Trost *et al.*, 2000). Having the ability to perform movement skills that form the building blocks for further participation in sport and games will increase enjoyment of PA (Okely and Booth, 2001) and will result in a greater likelihood of continuation of lifelong PA (Van Beurden *et al.*, 2003; Cairney *et al.*, 2005).

PA and FMS

Researchers often suggest that there are critical periods for the learning of FMS and that refining FMS prior to leaving primary school may be necessary for children and adolescents to enjoy recreational activities (Gallahue and Ozmun, 2003; Van Beurden *et al.*, 2003; Barnett *et al.*, 2009). These research studies have focussed on the hypothesis that children with poorer movement skills will withdraw from PA than those children with better movement skills (Graf *et al.*, 2004; Fisher *et al.*, 2005; Wrotniak *et al.*, 2006).To date there have been few findings in this field in relation to younger children (Early Years/Key Stage 1) and whether habitual activity is correlated with the ability to perform FMS (Hands, 2007) However, researchers have concluded that children with refined FMS are more physically active and vice versa (Van Beurden *et al.*, 2003; Okely *et al.*, 2004; Wrotniak *et al.*, 2006; Lubans *et al.*, 2010).

Although these conclusions have been made, the results from research studies investigating FMS and PA are inconclusive (Shephard, 2002; Fisher *et al.*, 2005). The differences in research design, FMS tests and most importantly methods of assessing PA have contributed to these equivocal findings. Research (Barnett *et al.*, 2009; Lubans *et al.*, 2010) has specifically suggested that children more proficient in object control skills are more likely to be active adolescents and, more specifically, are likely to engage in a greater proportion of PA at moderate-to-vigorous intensity. (Raudsepp, and Paasuke, 1995).

However, the associations that have been identified have been weak (Okely *et al.*, 2004; Fisher *et al.*, 2005). Other findings by McKenzie and colleagues (2002) and Reed (2004) actually found no relation between PA and FMS. Given this inconsistency in findings it could be suggested that additional research is required. One of the factors that may account for the inconsistency in the current body of research relating to FMS and PA is the accuracy of assessment used to assess PA in children (Morgan *et al.*, 2008; Duncan *et al.*, 2007). Self-report measures of PA have tended to be favoured due to their ease of administration, despite the shortcoming in validity of PA data gained using this method. Subsequently, there are still questions that have yet to be answered; firstly is there a relationship between movement skills and habitual PA? Furthermore, how strong is the correlation between these two variables? Finally, what effect to related variables such as gender, age and weight status play in any association between FMS and PA?

Gender and FMS

Numerous studies (Sallis et al., 1999; Okely et al., 2001; Van Beurden *et al.*, 2002; Fisher et al., 2005) have explored gender differences in FMS ability. It is well documented currently from these studies that males have a greater mastery of object control skills, and females to be more proficient at skills involving body management (balance) and movement (locomotor skills).

The research currently geared towards gender and FMS have linked these findings with more environmental factors, such as parental expectations and opportunity to practice (Sallis, 1999; Trost *et al.*, 2000), rather than biological factors. The assumption that boys are physically stronger and able to perform these skills better is incorrect, since boys and girls are very similar physically prior to puberty (Hardy *et al.*, 2010). This suggests that biological characteristics do not fully explain gender differences in FMS performance among young children. More recently, research has associated these differences with children's socialization (Barnett *et al.*, 2009), which are influenced by family, peers and teachers. Opportunities to practice FMS tend to be higher in boys, since fathers push their sons to be competitive and perform in sports such as football, rugby etc, where object control proficiency is required (Barnett *et al.*, 2009). Conversely, girls tend to participate in sports such as dance or gymnastics (Okely 2001; Hardy et al., 2010) which refine movement and postural control skills such as balancing (McKenzie, 1999; Okely and Booth, 2004).

Although these factors may explain gender differences in FMS, it is clear from research that boys are more physically active than girls. A number of studies support this and also commented that boys are more active than girls from preschool age through to adolescence (Baranowski *et al.*, 1993; Finn *et al.,* 2002; Jackson *et al.*, 2003; Kelly *et al.*, 2006). This leaves concern of potential risk for inactive lifestyles when compared to boys (Finn *et al.*, 2002) and could suggest that boys are more competent in performing FMS, since they engage in sport and games more often than girls giving them more time to refine skills like catching and running (Fisher *et al.*, 2005; Hardy *et al.*, 2010). Although there have been associations studies that have identified gender differences between skills, more research is a priority for us to find where these differences lie. A question that is yet to be answered is are boys more competent at FMS due to physical reasons (biological factors) or due to the quality and quantity of PA boys engage in compared to girls?

Weight Status and FMS

Weight status and FMS ability is an area of well documentation, and currently research has looked at the relationship between obese/non obese children and FMS proficiency (Okely *et al.*, 2004; Trost *et al.*, 2005; Wrotniak *et al.*, 2006). Current findings from these studies associate an inverse relationship between weight status and FMS proficiency. In general, studies have found children with a higher body mass index (BMI) to perform locomotor skills such as running and hopping less competently than children with a lowerBMI. Deforche and Colleagues (2008) performed a study looking at FMS and the differences in a sample of obese and non/obese children. From this study the findings demonstrated that children with higher mass perform locomotor and postural skills, such as balancing poorer than children with a lower mass. These differences have been linked to geometry changes, which larger children tend to have, as result causing postural constraints and impaired FMS performance (Deforche *et al.,* 2009). Okely, Booth and Chey (2004) also found relationships between weight status and FMS performance, nevertheless these associations were only weak-moderate, therefore further research is required to more fully determine the impact of weight status on FMS.

Another study by Hume and colleagues (2008) looked at the influence of weight status between children's FMS and PA and it was evident that children classified as obese in both boys and girls were potentially less competent and less active. Nevertheless, there was no significant interaction between the variables. From this it was concluded that future studies should examine a broader range of FMS and types of activity to better understand this relationship (Hume *et al.,* 2008). Other studies (Davies *et al.*, 1995; Sallis *et al.,* 2000) supported these findings, leaving a gap for future studies to investigate further the relationship between weight status, FMS and PA.

However, although BMI is a widely used method for assessing weight status in children and adolescents, there are limitations with its use. Firstly, BMI is a simplistic method and is determined by height and weight (kg/m^2). Secondly, and most importantly the method is not a true measure of adiposity and does not determine the difference between fat mass and lean body tissue (Dietz and Bellizzi, 1999; Cole *et al.*, 2000). Therefore, the accuracy of this instrument can be questioned (Dietz and Bellizzi, 1999; Cole *et al.*, 2000). Consequently, future research would benefit from using more accurate techniques such as skinfold measurement, air displacement plethysmography or hydrostatic weighing to more accurately determine weight status in children and adolescents.

Age and FMS

Data tracking PA over time has clearly shown a decline in quality and quantity of PA during childhood and adolescence (Malina, *et al.*, 2004). During early childhood the fundamental motor phase (Gallahue and Ozmun, 2003) reflects the phase which young children should competently be able to move effectively and demonstrate competency in FMS, such as running, hopping and jumping. Through Primary school years these movement skills should be able to develop and consistently improve as children's bodies mature and grow (Okely and Booth, 2004). However studies (Okely and Booth,2004; Branta *et al.*, 1996) have shown there is a negative association with age and FMS, showing very little development and even declines in performance in each of the movement skills. The study by Okely and Booth (2004) focussed on years 1-4 and found that FMS did not change as such as children matured. There was a slight change in skill differences by a maximum of 35% for each of the skills, however the prevalence of FMS mastery is low and shows need for improvement. From this, it could be suggested that primary schools, that provide the opportunity for children to develop their FMS should employ more programs and supply more time with focussing on developing these movement skills before working on more sport specific games/activities. Furthermore, it was identified from the study by Okely and Booth that object control skills, particularly the throw was mastered more slowly than the locomotor skills (running, jumping) through years 1 and 4 (Okely and Booth, 2004), suggesting that programs should maybe emphasise object skill mastery into these programs, given that object control proficiency has previously been found to predict long term PA in children and adolescents (Van Beurden *et al.*, 2009).

Conclusion

A range of research studies have identified proficiency in fundamental movement skills (FMS) as important factors in enabling young people to lead physically active lifestyles. There is some robust evidence that FMS is related to current levels of physical activity and weight status and suggestions that become proficient in FMS during childhood will lead to greater levels of physical activity throughout life. However, data supporting the latter claim are unavailable and longitudinal research is needed to verify this suggestions. Moreover, while it is logical to assume that children who are not proficient in one or more fundamental motor skills will be less inclined to participate in activities where those skills are required, the current body of knowledge in relation to FMS is not without its limitations. The majority of prior research on this topic has focused on older children and adolescents, used proxy measures of weight status and physical activity behaviour, which are questionable in terms of validity and accuracy and finally, have not fully considered factors such as age, gender and ethnicity in their analysis. Future research is therefore needed taking these issues into account and employing objective measures of physical activity behaviour in order to more fully understand the association between FMS and physical activity.

References

American College of Sports Medicine (ACSM) 1998.The list of references illustrated [online] available from >*http://www.acsm.org*< [6th February 2011].

Anderson, P.M., and Butcher (2006). Childhood obesity, trends and potential causes. *The Future of Children,* 16, 19-45.

Barnett, L.M., Van Beurden, E., Morgan, P.J., Brooks, L.O., and Beard, J.R. (2009). Childhood Motor Skill Proficiency as a predictor of adolescent physical activity. *Journal of Adolescent Health*, 44, 3, 252-259.

Bouffard, M., Watkinson, E. J., Thompson, L. P., Dunn, J. L. C., and Romanow, S. K. E. (1996). A test of the activity deficit hypothesis with children with movement difficulties. *Adapted Physical Activity Quarterly*, 13, 61-73.

Branta., C, Haubenstricker, J., and Seefeldt, V. (1984). Age changes in motor skills during childhood and adolescence. *Exercise and Sports Science Reviews*, 12, 467-520.

Cairney, J. Hay,. A., Faught, B.E., and Hawkes, R. (2005). Detrimental coordination disorder and overweight and obesity in children aged 9-14 years. *International Journal of Obesity*, 29, 369-372.

Cole, T. J., Bellizzi, M. C., Flegal, K. M., Dietz, W. H. (2000). Establishing a standard definition for child overweight and obesity worldwide: international survey, *British Medical Journal,* 320, 1–6.

Colvin, A., Markos, N., Walker, P. (2000). *Teaching the nuts and bolts of physical education.* Champaign. IL: Human Kinetics.

Deforche, B., Hills, P.A., Worringham, J.C., Davies, P. and Murphy, J.A (2009). Balance and postural skills in normal-weight and overweight prepubertal boys. *International Journal of Pediatric Obesity,* 4, 3, 175-182.

Dietz, H.W., and Bellizi, C.M. (1999). Introduction: the use of body mass index to assess obesity in children. *American Journal of Clinical Nutrition*, 70, 1, 123-125.

Duncan, M.J., Nakeeb-Al, Y., Woodfield, L., and Lyons, M. (2007). Pedometer determined physical activity levels in primary school children from central England. *Preventative Medicine,* 44 (5) 416-420.

Fisher, A. Reilly, J.J., Kelly, L.A, Montgomery, C., Williamson, A., Paton, J.Y., Grant, S. (2005) Fundamental movement skills in habitual physical activity in young children. *Medicine and Science in Sports and Exercise*, 37, 684-688.

Gallahue, D. L., and Ozmun, J. C. (2002). *Understanding motor development: Infants, children, adolescents, adults* (5th ed.). New York: McGraw-Hill.

Graf, C. (2003). Das CHILT-PROJEKT (The CHILT PROJECT). *Deutsche Zeitschrift for sportmedizin*, 54, 247 (In German, English Abstract).

Gorely, T., Biddle, S., Stensel, D.J. (2004). Health-enhancing physical activity and sedentary behaviour in children and adolescents. *Journal of Sports Sciences,* 22 (8), 679-701.

Hands, B. (2007). Changes in Motor Skill and Fitness Measures Among Children with High and Low Motor Competence: A Five Year Longitudinal Study. *Journal of Science and Medicine in Sport,* 11, 155-162.

Haubenstricker, J. and Seefeldt, V. (1986) Acquisition of motor skills during childhood. In Reston, V. editor. *Physical activity and well-being.* AAHPERD, 41-92.

Hardy, L.L. (2010). Fundamental movement skills among Australian preschool children. *Journal of Science and Medicine in Sport,* 13, 505-508.

Hume, C., Okely, A., Bagley, S., Telford, A., Booth, M.M, Crawford, D., Salmon, J. (2008). Does weight status influence associations between children's fundamental movement skills and physical activity? *Research Quarterly for Exercise and Sport,* 79 (2), 158-165.

Kohl, W.H., and Hobbs, E.K (1998). Development of Physical Activity Behaviours Among Children and Adolescents. *Pediatrics,* 101, 549-554.

LTAD (2008) Long-Term Athlete Development – Canadian Sport for Life. The list of references illustrated [online] available from: https://vle.coventry.ac.uk/webct/urw/lc4130011.tp0/cobaltMainFrame.dowebct [2nd December 2010].

Lubans, R.L., Morgan, J.P., Cliff, P.D et al. (2010). Fundamental Movement Skills in Children and Adolescents. Review of Associated Health Benefits. *Sports Medicine,* 40 (12): 1019-1035.

Mackett, R.L., and Paskins, J. (2008). Children's physical activity: The contribution of playing and walking. *Children and Society,* 22, 345-357.

Malina, R.M. (1990). Tracking of physical fitness and performance during growth. In: Buenen G, Hesquiere J.G, Reybroock T, Claessens Al, eds. *Children and exercise,* Stuttgart, Germany: Ferdinand Enke, 1-10.

Malina, R. M., Bouchard, C., Bar-Or, O. (2004). *Growth, Maturation and Physical Activity.* Champaign, Ill: Human Kinetics.

McKenzie, L.T., Alcaraz, J.E., Sallis, J.F., and Faucette, F.N. (1998). Effects of a physical education program on children's manipulative skills. *Journal of Teaching Physical Education,* 17, 327-341.

McKenzie, T. L., Sallis, J. F., Broyles, S. L., Zive, M. M., Nader, P. R., Berry, C. C., et al. (2002). Childhood Movement Skills: Predictors of Physical Activity in Anglo American and Mexican American Adolescents? *Research Quarterly for Exercise and Sport,* 73(3), 238-244.

Morgan, J.P., Okely, A. D., Cliff, D. P., Jones, R. A., Baur, L. A. (2008). Correlates of Objectively Measured Physical Activity in Obese Children. *Obesity,* 16, 2634-2641.

NASPE (2010) The list of references illustrated [online] available from < http://www.naeyc.org/files/yc/file/200605/NASPEGuidelinesBTJ.pdf> [1st December 2010].

NCMP (NHS Health and Social Information Centre: National Child Measurement Programmme) (2008) The list of references illustrated [online] available from <http://www.ncmp.ic.nhs.uk/newresults.aspx> [5th December 2010].

Okely, A.D., Booth, M.L. and Patterson, J.W (2001a). Relationship of physical activity to fundamental movement skills among adolescents. *Medicine and Science in Sports and Exercise,* 33 (11), 1899-1904.

Okely, A. D., Booth, M. L., and Chey, T. (2004). Relationships between body composition and fundamental movement skills among children and adolescents. *Research Quarterly for Exercise and Sport,* 75(3), 238-237.

Olrich, T. (2002). Assessing Fundamental Motor Skills in the Elementary School Setting Issues and Solutions, *JOPERD,* 73 (7), 26-28.

Raudsepp, L. and Paasuke, M. (1995). Gender differences in fundamental movement patterns, motor performances, and strength measurements of prepubertal children. *Pediatric Exercise Science*, 7(3), 294-304.

Reed, J. A., Metzker, A., and Phillips, D. A. (2004). Relationships between physical activity and motor skills in middle school children. Perceptual and Motor Skills, 99, 483-494.

Sallis, J.F., and Patrick, K. (1994). Physical activity guidelines for adolescents consensus statement. *Pediatric Exercise Science*, 6, 302-314.

Sallis, J. F., Prochaska, J. J., and Taylor, W. C. (2000). A review of correlates of physical activity of children and adolescents. *Medicine and Science in Sports and Exercise*, 32(5), 9

Salmon, J., Ball, K., Crawford, D., Booth, M., Telford, A., Hume, C., Jolley, D., and Worsley, A. (2005). Reducing sedentary behaviour and increasing physical activity among 10 year old children: overview and process evaluation of the 'switch-play' intervention. *Health Promotion International*, 20, 7-17.

Shephard, R. J. (2002). Limits to the measurement of habitual physical activity by questionnaires. *British Journal of Sports Medicine*, 37, 197-206.

Stodden, D.F., Goodway, J.D., Roberton, M.A., Rudisill, M.E., Garcia, C., and Garcia L.E. (2008). A development perspective on the role of motor skill competence in physical activity: An Emergent Relationship. *Quest,* 60, 290-306.

Telama, R., Leskinen, E., Yang, X. (1996). Stability of habitual physical activity and sport participation: A longitudinal tracking study. *Scandinavian Journal of Medicine and Science in Sports,* 61, 371-378.

Trost, S. G., Pat, R. R., Freedson, P. S., Sallis, J. F. and Taylor, W. C. (2000). Using objective physical activity measures with youth: how many days of monitoring are needed? *Medicine and Science in Sports and Exercise*, 32, 426–431.

Warburton, P., and Woods, J. (1996). Observation of children's physical activity levels during primary school PE lessons. *Physical Education and Sport Pedagogy*, 1, 56-65.

Weiss, R., and Dziura, J. (2004). Obesity and the metabolic syndrome in children and adolescents. *Journal of Public Health*, 350: 2362-2374.

Welk, G. J. (1999). The Youth Physical Activity Promotion Model: A Conceptual Bridge Between Theory and Practice. *Quest,* 51, 5-23.

Wrotniak, H.B., Epstein, H.L., and Jones, E.K (2006). Relationship between motor proficiency and physical activity in children. *Paediatrics,* 118, e1758-e1765.

Van Beurden, E., Zask, E., Barnett, L.M., andDietrich, U.C. (2002). Fundamental Movement Skills- How do primary school children perform? The 'Move it Groove it' program in Rural Australia. *Journal of Science and Medicine in Sport*, 5, 244-252.

In: Reviews in Pediatric Exercise Science
Editor: Michael Duncan, pp. 125-146
ISBN: 978-1-61470-978-7

Chapter IX

Physical Activity Patterns in Children from Different Ethnic Backgrounds

Emma Lisa Jane Eyre and Krystyna Anna Matyka
The University of Warwick, UK.

Introduction

Patterns of cardiovascular and metabolic disease vary in ethnic groups. British South Asian adults have an increased risk of type 2 diabetes mellitus which is associated with increased cardiovascular disease (CVD) death rates (Mckeigue, Shah and Marmot, 1991; Balarajan, 1996; Bhopal, Unwin, White, Yallop, Walker, and Alberti , 1999). People from Afro Caribbean descent experience lower CVD mortality rates but are at higher risk of type 2 diabetes mellitus and hypertension compared to White Europeans (Cruickshank, Cooper, Burnett, Macduff and Drubra, 1991; Chaturvedi, Mckeigue and Marmot, 1994; Cappucio, Cook, Atkinson and Strazullo, 1997; Lane, Beevers and Hip, 2002; Thom et al, 2006).

Growing evidence suggests that early markers of metabolic disease risk emerge in childhood which is strongly related to ethnicity and obesity (Berenson, Srinivasan, Bao, Newman, Tracy and Wattigney 1998; Ehtisthan, Barrett, and Shaw, 2000; Whincup , Gilg, Owen, Odoki, Alberti and Cook, 2002; Whincup, Owen, Orfei, McKay and Cook, 2007). Higher levels of fasting insulin are evident in South Asian and Black children compared to white children (Whincup et al, 2010). Insulin levels have been found to track well into adulthood and are positively related to measures of obesity, systolic and diastolic blood pressure, triglyceride and cholesterol levels. Children from ethnic minorities have also been found to have differences in body composition which have been demonstrated in the neonatal period suggesting that some of this risk is likely to be inherited rather than related to lifestyle (Yajnik et al, 2002).

Physical inactivity is identified as the fourth leading modifiable risk factor for global mortality (WHO, 2010). The metabolic benefits of physical activity are well described both in adults and children (Powell, Thompson, Caspersen, and Kendrick, 1987; Strazzullo et al, 1988; Berlin and Coldwitz, 1990; Brage et al, 2004). Studies have shown low levels of objectively measured activity in childhood to be associated with increased adiposity and insulin resistance (Ekelund et al, 2004; Ekelund, Neovius, Linné, Brage, Wareham and Rössner, 2005; Sardinha et al 2008; Wittmeir, Mollard, and Kriellaars, 2008; Riddoch et al, 2007). However, little is known about differences in physical activity patterns between ethnic groups and the possible contribution to CVD risk.

The aim of this review is to examine the objective evidence of patterns of physical activity in children from differing ethnic backgrounds.

Method

The electronic databases Pubmed, Embase, and Cochrane database of systematic reviews were searched for articles published from January 1990 until December 2010. Childhood was defined as a subject who was less than 18 years of age. The search terms used included: physical activity, inactivity, sedentary time, exercise, active commuting, energy expenditure, fitness, ethnicity, race, ethnic minority and children. Studies were included if they made ethnic comparisons for: Black, African American, non Hispanic black, black African, afro Caribbean, Hispanic, Mexican American, Latino, South Asian, Indian, Pakistani, Bangladeshi, non Hispanic white, White European, Caucasian, European American, or white children. They also had to include an objective measure of activity, fitness or energy expenditure and which reported descriptions of activity patterns, energy expenditure calculations or fitness levels results for ethnic groups separately. Subjective measures including questionnaires, interviews and parental report and studies of adults were excluded. Searches were limited to those published in the English language.

One thousand two hundred and seventy nine abstracts were identified by initial searches. Results from the different search engines were compared and any duplicates removed (n=7). Titles and abstracts were scanned and removed if they failed to measure physical activity between ethnic groups (N= 1219). Full text articles were obtained for the remaining articles (N=53) which were assessed for eligibility. 28 articles were excluded for using only subjective measures of activity, fitness or energy expenditure (see Figure 1). A total of 25 studies were included in the review of objective measures of physical activity levels in ethnic children (see Table 1).

Data Extraction

The following data were extracted from each paper: study design, country of origin, sampling method, instrument for gathering ethnic information, population characteristics, measuring instrument, outcomes measured and results.

For the purpose of this report people are referred to as Black if their ethnicity descends from Black, African American, non-Hispanic black, black African, Afro Caribbean descent. White ethnic origin was used to describe people from Non Hispanic white, White European, Caucasian, European American, Anglo Saxon, or white backgrounds. South Asian ethnicity was defined as people with ancestral origins in India, Pakistan or Bangladesh. Finally Mexican American/Hispanic was defined as Hispanic, Mexican American, Latino, and Hispanic American descent.

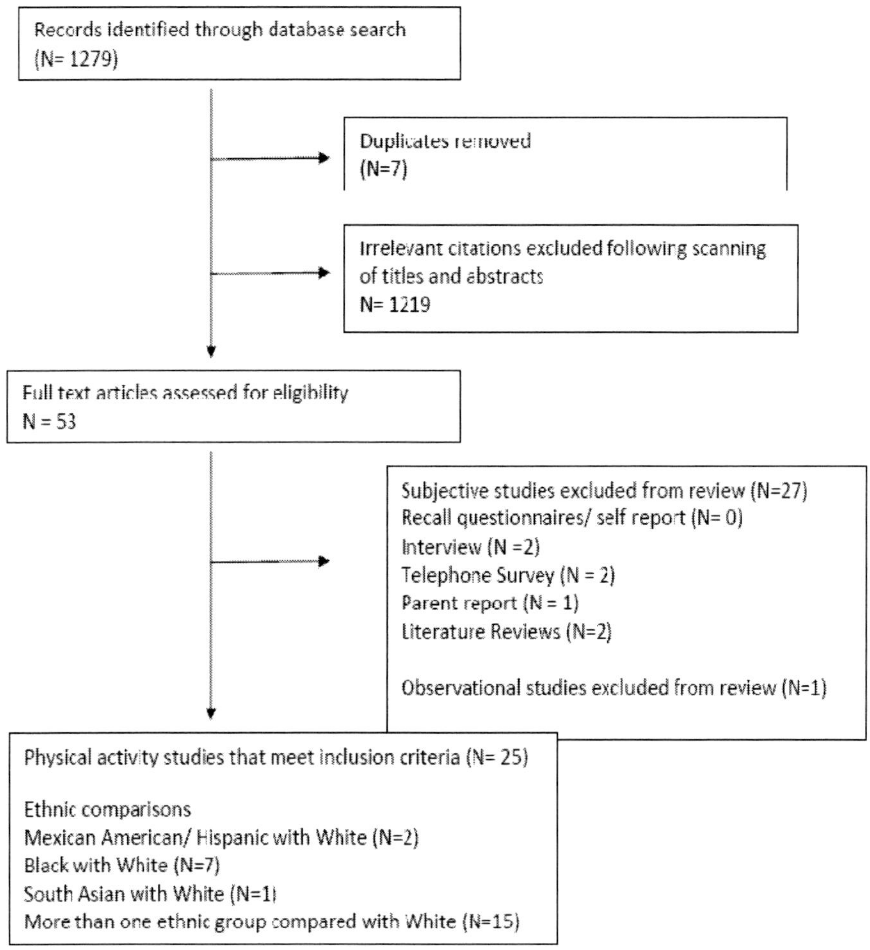

Figure 1. Flow chart of processes to obtain articles on physical activity patterns between ethnic groups from January 1990 to December 2010.

Results

A total of 25 studies were found, 21 studies were from North America, three studies from the UK and one from New Zealand (Table 1). The sample sizes varied widely from 23- 4372 participants. Nine of the studies used a sample population above 1000 subjects. 12 studies reported using a cross sectional design. Results are presented under ethnic groupings but some studies did multi-ethnic comparisons (n = 15).

Table 1. Objective studies making ethnic comparisons in physical activity levels

Author	Total Number, Age and Ethnic group	Instrument	Outcome measures	*Results*
Mexican American/Hispanic				
Byrd-Williams et al 2007 [1] US	Total = 169 (Mean age 9.4 years) Hispanic (63%) Non Hispanic White (37%)	Actigraph	Activity counts per minute Hours spent in MET levels	Physical activity: Significant correlation between Gender, ethnicity and overweight for total PA and MVPA ($p>.01$). MVPA and counts per minute were lower in overweight white girls and Mexican American/ Hispanic boys ($p<0.05$).
Dugas et al 2008 [2] US	Total = 47 (Age 6-10 years) Mexican American 20 EU American 27	Doubly labelled water	Total Energy Expenditure TEE/REE= PAL	Energy expenditure: Mexican American/Hispanic and White boys did not differ in TEE, AEE or PAL. Mexican American/Hispanic girls had significantly lower TEE, AEE and PAL than White girls of comparable size ($p<0.005$) (controlled for age, body fat, fat free mass).
Black				
Andreacci et al. 2004 [3] US	Total = 87 *Prepubertal (Age 8-11 years)* White 22 Black 23 *Pubertal (Age 11-13years)* White 20 Black 22	$V0_{2\,max}$ test-Bruce multistage fitness Body composition-DXA	$V0_{2\,max}$ $V0_{2max}$ adjusted for Fat free mass	Fitness: Black prepubertal children and pubertal children had lower VO_{2max} values compared to white children (22.8±7.8 vs. 35.0±6.5ml.kg-1.min-1, $p<0.01$: prepubertal: 33.7±6.4 vs. 40.4±10.2 ml.kg-1.min-1, $p<0.05$, pubertal; black vs. white respectively). No difference in $V0_2$ when expressed in absolute terms (ml/min) (matched for age, puberty and BMI) Both race ($p<0.01$) and gender ($p<0.001$) were significant predictors of $V0_2$ max, explaining 60% of variance for prepubertal and 55% for pubertal.
Andreacci et al. 2005 [4] US	Total = 44 (Mean age range 10.9-16.8 years) 23 black 21 white	$V0_{2\,max}$- Bruce treadmill tests Body composition-DXA	$V0_{2\,max}$ Respiratory exchange	Fitness: Black obese adolescents had lower $V0_2$ max (26.1±4.2 vs. 29.9±3.1) and $V0_2$ adjusted for fat free mass (48.3±8.8 vs. 55.6±5.2) compared to white adolescents ($p<0.05$)- matched for age No difference between maximal heart rate (189±9vs. 193±6) or maximal respiratory exchange (1.05±0.08 vs. 1.08±0.8) ($p>0.05$).

Author	Total Number, Age and Ethnic group	Instrument	Outcome measures	*Results*
Arslanian et al 1997[5] US	Total = 23 (Age 8-12years) Black 12 White 11	V02 max-Treadmill Indirect calorimetry	$VO_{2\,Max}$ REE	Energy expenditure REE lower in blacks than whites-adjusted for body weight ($p=0.03$) Fitness $VO_{2\,max}$ lower in blacks than whites ($p=0.0005$)
Ku et al 1999 US [6]	Total = 68 (Age 5-11 years) African American 34 White 34	Fasted testing $V0_{2\,max}$- Treadmill	$V0_{2\,max}$	Fitness No differences between gender or racial groups were evident for body weight, and lean mass. $V0_{2\,max}$ significantly lower in Blacks ($p<0.05$).
McMurray et al 2003 [7] US Abstract only	Total = 1540 (Age 8-16 years) African American 21.4% Caucasians 78.6%	Cycle ergometer	Aerobic power ($_PVO_2$ max)	Fitness: Blacks have lower relative aerobic power than whites (controlled for weight and skinfold thickness).
Pivarnik et al 1995 [8] Us	Total = 93 (Mean age 13.5 years) Black 40 White 53	V02 max-Bruce test, Treadmill	VO_{2Max}	Fitness $V0_{2\,max}$ lower in black girls vs. white girls (31.8±5.8 vs. 38.5±6.8; $p<0.01$) - adjusted for fat free mass. Time to exhaustion was lower in blacks (8.49±1.30min vs. 9.41±1.60; $p<0.01$).
Trowbridge et al 1997[9] Us	Girls only Total = 94 (Age 5-10 years) African American 60 Caucasian 34	Doubly labelled water $VO_{2\,max}$ test-treadmill	TEE, REE and AEE Peak VO_2	Energy expenditure No difference in adjusted means for TEE, REE and AEE between groups Fitness Significant effect of ethnicity and $V0_2$ max ($p<0.01$). Black absolute peak values 15% lower than white children ($p<0.01$). Difference still evident when adjustments made for lean tissue mass.
SA				
Hardy , Eston 1985 [10] UK	Total = 57 Anglo Saxon 32 (Age 16-18 years) Indian 27 (Age 16-23 years)	VO_{2max} - Ergometer test (Tunturi) Body composition-skinfold callipers	VO_2max-estimated by indirect linear relationship between HR, oxygen uptake and workload at sub maximal levels.	FITNESS: white have higher maximal oxygen uptake values when adjusting for fat free mass (49.1±6.9 vs. 43.2±7.9 l.kg-1min-1; p=<0.01). Other measures: No difference body fat % ($p>0.05$). Whites had higher lean body mass compared to Indians (55.9±7.0 vs. 51.6±4.5, $p<0.01$).

Table 1. (Continued).

Author	Total Number, Age and Ethnic group	Instrument	Outcome measures	*Results*
Mixed				
Belcher et al. 2010[11] US	Total = 3106(Boys1508/Girls 1598) (Age 6-19 years) Non Hispanic black 605/522 Non Hispanic white 416/428 Mexican American 548/1587	Actigraph	Mean counts per minute Minutes spent in MVPA Inclusion: 4 days, 10 hours minimum per day of data collection.	Physical activity *Overall:* Whites had lower mean counts than blacks and Mexican American/Hispanics (p=0.05). Overweight black children had higher counts per minute than whites (p=0.002). Black children 16-19 years were most active. Mexican American/Hispanic boys spent more time in MVPA and vigorous PA than White boys (P<0.05). No differences between ethnic groups and girls sedentary, MVPA and vigorous activity. *6-11 years:* Black children and Mexican American/Hispanic were more sedentary than white (p<0.05). No difference between Whites and Mexican American/Hispanics in moderate, vigorous or MVPA. Black spent more time in moderate activity, vigorous activity and MVPA than Whites (p= 0.05). *12-15years:* Whites less sedentary than Blacks and Mexican American/Hispanics (p=0.05). Blacks spent more minutes in moderate activity, vigorous activity and MVPA than White. Mexican American/Hispanics spent more minutes in moderate, vigorous and MVPA than White. *16-19 years:* Whites less sedentary than Blacks. No difference between Whites and Mexican American/Hispanics. Blacks spent more time in moderate activity than whites.
Bettiol et al 1999 [12] Uk	Total = 711 (Age 9 years) White English 317 White Scottish 152 White inner city 87 Afro Caribbean 38 Indian subcontinent 81 Others 36	Ergometer test (PWC85%)- physical work capacity	PWC85% - power output against load at 85% of maximum heart rate (watt/kg). Ability to finish test	Fitness: South asian boys and girls were less likely to finish the test (South Asian boys vs. White boys = 34.6% vs. 11.7% children did not finish the and South asian girls vs. White girls = 35.7% vs. 12.1% did not finish the test; p=016 and p<0.001, respectively). PWC85% lower in SA girls compared to White (2.17 vs. 1.89 watts/kg p<0.001). No significant difference in SA

Author	Total Number, Age and Ethnic group	Instrument	Outcome measures	*Results*
				boys. Black children were less likely to finish the test compared to White children (Black boys vs. White boys = 13.2% vs. 11.7% and Black girls vs. White girls = 17.9% vs. 12.1%; p=0.016 and p<0.001 respectively).
Casazza et al. 2009 [13] US	Total = 202 (Age 7-12 years) White 68 African American 79 Hispanics 55	Actigraph Body composition-DXA	Counts per minute Minutes in MVPA, vigorous , sedentary and moderate activity Inclusion: 1 minute epochs, Wake hours.	Total PA/Sedentary: No significant difference in daily minutes of total activity or sedentary activity between ethnic groups (Total PA= White 670.88±16.4, Black 670.94±16.9, Mexican American/ Hispanic 661.08±18.8 (min/d), Sedentary= white 438.07±9.2, Black 423.97±10.4, Mexican American/ Hispanic 431.53±10.8 (min/d)) (P>.0.05). MVPA: No difference between Blacks or Mexican American/ Hispanics and Whites (MVPA= White 69.22 ±4.5, African 59.87±4.4, Hispanic 51.07±4.9 (min/d) (p>0.05).
Casazza et al. 2009 [14] US	Total = 215 (Age 7-12 years) African American 68 European American 92 Hispanic American 55	MTI Actigraph Fitness-Indirect calorimetry on treadmill (VO_2-170) Body composition-DXA	VO_2-170= VO_{2Max} at 170bpm Daily counts Minutes in METS Measured: 7 days, 1minute epoch	Fitness: Black children had lower fitness than white and Mexican American/ Hispanic after adjustments for Body weight and lean mass. Mexican American/ Hispanic children were the fittest when assessed by VO_2-170 (p<0.05) PA/Sedentary behave: No difference in total PA or sedentary activity between racial/ethnic groups (p<0.05) *Total MVPA:* White children engaged in more moderate and hard activity than Mexican American / Hispanic (p<0.05). *Daily MVPA:* No difference between white, Black and Mexican American and Hispanic. No difference in sedentary behaviour. Pubertal status assessed
Duncan et al. 2008[15] New Zealand	Girls only Total = 1213 (Age 6 – 16 years) 637 EU 272 pacific island 207 East Asian 179 Maori 142 South Asian 76 other ethnic groups	Pedometer (NL-2000)	steps per day	No difference in pedometer compliance between ethnic groups. PA: South Asian girls were the least active ethnic groups during weekdays and weekend, P<.0.005)

Table 1. (Continued).

Author	Total Number, Age and Ethnic group	Instrument	Outcome measures	*Results*
Johnson et al. 2010 [16] US	Total = 582 (mean age 10.37±0.48 years) Hispanic 307 Caucasian 150African American 125 Urban, rural, suburb	Pedometer (yamax digi walker)	Steps per day Inclusion: 3 days	PA: White girls averaged more steps per day than Mexican American/Hispanic and Black ($p<0.05$). No significant differences between boys
Kelly et al 2010 [17] Us	Girls Only Total = 1180 (Age 12 years) Black 24.5% Hispanic 15.7% White 59.8%	Actigraph	MVPA time	MVPA: No significant difference in Mexican American/ Hispanic girls and Black girls MVPA compared to White (Mexican American/Hispanic= 21.7minutes per day, Black 19.5 minutes per day and White 22.8 minutes per day, P=0.100).
Matthews et al. 2007 [18] US	Total = 1612 *6-11 years Boys 360 (Girls 404)* Non Hispanic white 104 (117) Non Hispanic blacks 138 (149) Mexican Americans 118 (138) *12-15 years Boys 447 (Girls 401)* Non Hispanic whites 121 (105) Non Hispanic blacks 180 (145) Mexican Americans 146 (151)	Actigraph	Amount of time spent in sedentary behaviour (hours/day) Inclusion: 7 days, 1 minute epochs, 10 hours of data collection.	Sedentary activity: 6-11yrs: Black girls less sedentary (5.88±0.06) than White (6.18±0.06) or Mexican Americans/Hispanic (6.02±0.08) ($p<0.05$). Mexican American/Hispanic less sedentary than white ($p<0.05$)
Owen et al. 2009 [19] Uk	Total = 2144 (Age 9-10 years) White EU 565 SA 494 Black African 607 Other 408	Actigraph	Mean daily activity (counts per minutes, daily steps) Time spent in MET levels Mean registered time Measured: 30sec Inclusion: >600 minutes data collection.	Physical activity: South Asian children recorded fewer minutes in moderate and vigorous levels of physical activity ($p=0.02$). South Asians spent more time in sedentary activities and recorded fewer counts per minute, daily steps and time in MVPA ($p<0.0001$) compared to White. Black children spent more time in sedentary, light activities, MVPA and vigorous PA ($p<0.0001$) and recorded fewer steps compared to White EU ($p<0.0001$). *60mins day MVPA (government recommendations):* lower proportion of South asians achieved 60minutes of MVPA (54%) compared to white (70%) and blacks (69%) but gender differences were not modified by

Author	Total Number, Age and Ethnic group	Instrument	Outcome measures	*Results*
				ethnicity (p>0.07). Patterns of PA in South Asian were similar among Indians, Pakistanis and Bangladeshis and between black African and black Caribbean.
Pate et al. [20] 2006 Us	Girls only Total = 1578 (Mean age 11.7±0.4 to 12.3±0.7 years) 706 White 344 African American 343 Hispanic 61 Asian American	Actigraph	Compliance to 30 minutes a day recommendation Inclusion: 6 days, 30 sec, 12 hours data collection.	PA: White girls were more active (MVPA) than other ethnic groups (Black, Mexican American /Hispanic, (p=0.01)).
Pate et al. 2006 [21] US	Total = 4372 (Age 12-19 years) Non Hispanic white Non Hispanic black Mexican American	Estimated $V0_2max$ by sub maximal treadmill test	$V0_{2max}$	Fitness: Male $V0_{2max}$: no ethnic difference (p=0.27, means 46.7, 46.9, 46.1ml.kg.min-1 for White, Black and Mexican American/Hispanic respectively). Female VO_{2max}: no significant ethnic difference (p=0.15, mean 39.0, 37.9, 39.3ml/kg/minute respectively).
Pfeiffer et al. 2009 [22] US	Total = 331 (Age 3-5) White 40.2% African American 51.4% Other 8.5%	Actigraph	MVPA min.hr Non sedentary activity Measured: 15 second intervals, 5 days Inclusion: >5hours and <18hours data collection	Physical Activity: Black children were more active than white children (MVPA= 7.9 vs. 7.3min/hr, p<0.05). Black males more active than white males (MVPA=8.5 vs. 7.8 min/hr p=.0.05)
Roberts et al. 2010 [23] US	Total = 1989 (5th-9th grade) Non Hispanic white (59%) Hispanic 27% African American 7% Asian/pacific islander 6%	Aerobic fitness- Fitness gram (1 mile run test)	$VO_{2\ MAX}$	Fitness: Black students were less likely to achieve California fitness standards than White students (p=0.04, p.005). Mexican American/Hispanic were less likely to meet standards than Whites (p<.005).
Shaibi et al. 2006 [24] Us	Total = 73 (Age 7-14 years). Caucasian 18 African American 19 Latino 36	$V0_2$ peak – treadmill test Body composition-DXA	$V0_2$ peak Peak Heart rate Respiratory Exchange Ratio	Fitness: VO_2 peak relative to body mass was significantly lower in Latino Mexican American/Hispanic compared to White – adjusted for gender, maturation and body composition (p<0.05). Mexican American/ Hispanic children had lower VO_2 peak than white- adjusted for fat free mass. Black children had lower VO_2 peak than white (p=.001) No ethnic difference in peak heart rate or respiratory exchange ratio (P>0.05)

Table 1. (Continued).

Author	Total Number, Age and Ethnic group	Instrument	Outcome measures	*Results*
Treuth et al 2000 [25] US	Girls only Total = 101 (Age 8-9 years) White 52 Black 30Hispanic 19 Lean (30) Lean- Obese (44) Obese (27)	Heart rate monitoring $V0_{2\ max}$- treadmill Doubly Labelled water	Total minutes recorded for which heart rate was >125% of basal heart rate (BHR) and > 150% of BHR Recorded: 24 hours, 1000 minutes inclusion.	Physical activity Black girls spent less time than white girls in >125% of BHR (159±126 min vs. 268±192) week and weekend ($p<0.05$). No difference between Mexican American/ Hispanic and White. No ethnic difference in mean heart rate. Energy expenditure No ethnic difference in physical activity level. Free living TEE lower in blacks than in white girls ($p<0.05$). Fitness No significant differences between Black girls or Mexican American/Hispanics and White girls ($p=0.12$ and $P=0.06$ respectively) - after adjustment for fat free mass.

Abbreviations: V02 max- maximal oxygen consumption, MVPA- Moderate – vigorous physical activity,DXA- Dual x ray absorptiometry, TEE- total energy expenditure, PAL- physical activity level, AEE- activity energy expenditure, REE- resting energy expenditure, PA- physical activity, BHR- basal heart rate, PWC85%- power output against load at 85% of maximal heart rate.

Black vs. White European

Study Information

A total of 21 studies included black children. Nineteen of these were conducted in the US with only two conducted in the UK (Table 1 references: 12, 19). Six of the US Studies were multicentre studies (Table 1 references: 11, 16, 17, 18, 20, 21) and the rest were single centre. Both UK studies were multicentre.

Age and Gender

Seventeen studies recruited mixed groups of boys and girls and four studies used girls only (Table 1 references: 9, 17, 20, 25). Eight studies included children 11 years or younger and six studies included young people aged 11-18 years. The remaining studies used a wide age range of participants including both pubertal and pre-pubertal subjects.

Collection of Ethnic Information

Nine studies gathered ethnic information using parent report or self-report (Table 1 references: 1, 11, 13, 19, 20, 21, 22, 23, 24). Nine studies reported their criteria for defining ethnic grouping (Table 1 references: 1, 11, 13, 17, 19, 20, 21, 23, 24). A final 14 studies failed to describe how they gathered information on ethnic background.

Method of Measurement

Physical Fitness

Thirteen studies examined physical fitness. Twelve studies measured fitness levels using either a treadmill (Table 1 references: 3, 4, 5, 6, 8, 9, 14, 21, 24, 25) or ergometer exercise test to measure oxygen uptake (Table 1 references: 7, 12). Pate et al's study (Table 1 reference: 21) was the only treadmill test which used a sub-maximal protocol to estimate VO_2max. From the studies using ergometer protocols Arslanian et al (Table 1 reference: 5) was the only study which measured VO_2 max. Bettiol, Rona and Chinn (Table 1 reference: 12) assessed power output against load at 85% of maximum heart rate (PWC85%) and Casazza, Gower, Willig, Hunter and Fernandez (Table 1 reference: 14) measured $V0_2$ at a heart rate of 170 beats/minute via indirect calorimetry ($V0_2$-170) instead of $V0_2$ max test. Roberts, Freed and McCarthy (Table 1 reference: 23) was the only study to determine physical fitness by the amount of time it took each child to complete the 1 mile run test for the fitness gram assessment.

Twelve of these studies reported that aerobic fitness was lower in blacks across a range of age groups varying from 5 to 18 years. The remaining study reported no significant difference but this could be explained by the method of assessment chosen (Table 1 reference : 21). This study used a six-minute sub-maximal treadmill test to measure estimated VO_2 max based on linear assumptions of heart rate, oxygen consumption and treadmill exercise. This methodology is less accurate than maximal exercise tests which could explain the differing results.

Physical Activity

Physical activity was assessed in 10 studies, eight studies used actigraph accelerometers (Table 1 reference: 11, 13, 14, 17, 18, 19, 20, 22) six described cut off criteria to define sedentary activity, moderate or vigorous activity (Table 1 references: 11, 13, 17, 18, 19, 22). One study used heart rate monitoring (Table 1 reference: 25) and another assessed physical activity by a pedometer (Table 1 reference: 16).

Findings were different between studies. Two studies using small sample sizes suggested that there was no difference in physical activity patterns (Table 1 references: 13, 14). Three studies reported that black girls were less active, spending less time in moderate and/or vigorous activity (Table 1 references: 20, 25) or recorded fewer steps (Table 1 reference: 16). One study suggested that black girls were less sedentary (Table 1 reference: 18) and a further study found no difference between black and white girls (17). Studies also reported that black children were *more* active spending more minutes in MVPA (Table 1 reference: 11, 19, 22) and recording more counts per minute in 3-5 years (Table 1 reference: 22) 9-10 years (Table 1 reference: 19) 6-18 year old children (Table 1 reference: 11). All of these three studies used activity monitors to measure activity levels and thus are comparable in methodology but not age. Two of these studies also reported that black children were more sedentary (Table 1 references: 11, 19) when considering age differences. Two of these studies used large sample sizes consisting of an even distribution of black to white participants and are part of large ongoing multi centre studies – NHAMES and CHASE (11, 19). The results from larger studies would therefore suggest that Black children may be both more active but also more sedentary than white children i.e. their time is spent at the extremes of activity levels.

Energy Expenditure

Energy expenditure was assessed in three studies: two studies used doubly labelled water (DLW) (Table 1 reference: 9, 25) and one study used indirect calorimetry to measure energy by respiratory gases (Table 1 reference: 5). Studies using the gold standard for measuring energy expenditure (DLW) found no differences in physical activity level (PAL) (Table 1 references: 9, 25) or resting energy expenditure (REE) and activity energy expenditure (AEE) (Table 1 reference: 9). There were inconsistencies in data for total energy expenditure (TEE). Arslanian , Suprasongsin and Janosky (Table 1 reference: 5) study using indirect calorimetry suggested REE energy was lower in blacks however the study failed to consider differences in body mass such as fat free mass, which might explain some of the differences. Further studies are needed before conclusions can be made.

Mexican American/Hispanic vs. White European

Study Information

A total of 13 studies included participants from Mexican American/Hispanic descent (Table 1 references: 1, 2, 11, 13, 14, 16, 17, 18, 20, 21, 23, 24, 25). All these studies were conducted in the United States. Of these 5 studies included multicentre sites of recruitment (Table 1 reference: 11, 17, 18, 20, 21).

Age and Gender

Studies recruited participants from 6-19 years: of these studies four looked at children from 9-11 years (Table 1 reference: 1, 2, 16, 25), three at young people 11-19 years (Table 1 references: 17, 20 , 21) and six reported combined aged groups (Table 1 references: 11, 13, 14, 18, 23 24). Ten studies included boys and girls together and three considered girls only (Table 1 reference: 9, 21, 25).

Ethnic Information

Seven studies reported the method of gathering ethnic information. This was from either parent or self reported (Table 1 references: 1, 11, 13, 20, 21, 23, 24). These all reported their criteria for definition for ethnic grouping.

Measuring Method

Physical Fitness

Five studies measured physical fitness; four of these used treadmill protocols. Two studies assessed VO_2 max using maximal treadmill protocols (Table 1 references: 24, 25) another study estimated $V0_2$ max via sub maximal testing (Table 1 reference: 21). The final study used indirect calorimetry to quantify $V0_2$ at 170 beats/minute (Table 1 reference: 14). Fitnessgram was also used in one study to assess physical fitness in children (Table 1 reference: 23).

The findings from these studies were inconsistent. One study reported Mexican American/Hispanic children to have higher fitness levels with higher oxygen consumption at 170bpm (Table 1 reference: 14) and another reported that Hispanic children were less likely to meet aerobic fitness standards than non-Hispanic white (Table 1 reference: 23). These conflicting results may be due to various reasons. Firstly, the method of measuring fitness was different between the two studies. Roberts et al (Table 1 reference : 23) study used school records to obtain information on the amount of time taken to complete a one mile run and compared them to national standards. This is unlikely to be a robust measure as the method of assessment will not have been rigorously standardised despite the sample size being large. Population sampling methods used for both studies were not reported and so this may influence the representation and generalisability of the results.

Shaibi (Table 1 reference: 24) used maximal fitness testing in children and supported Roberts et al (Table 1 reference : 23) findings suggesting peak VO_2 was lower in Mexican American/Hispanic children when compared to white, after accounting for fat free mass. Another large study of 4372 children found no difference in $V0_2$ max between Mexican American and white boys and girls (Table 1 reference: 21) aged 12-19 years. This study may have been limited by the use of a sub maximal testing to estimate $V0_2$ max, which allowed the study of a larger group but is a less robust measure of fitness.

The results from these studies are inconsistent and this may be due to some of the differences already described. In addition, the studies used wide age samples reporting results in 10-15 year olds (Table 1 reference: 23), 7-12 years old (Table 1 reference: 14), 7-14 years old (Table 1 reference: 24), and 12-19 years old (Table 1 reference: 21). Objective research on 2185 children from Denmark, Portugal , Estonia and Norway has reported differences in physical activity levels between children of 9 years compared to children 15 years (Riddoch, 2004) suggesting that children are less active as they get older, thus physical activity may be influenced by developmental changes. These studies however fail to consider these differences when reporting ethnic differences between groups and this is likely to affect the results obtained. Casazza et al (Table 1 reference: 14) study controlled for pubertal status and this is likely to strengthen the results obtained. However, more studies that control for developmental changes in children is needed to confirm whether Mexican American/Hispanic children are more or less active than White children through the age course.

Physical Activity

Nine studies collected objective data on physical activity using accelerometers, pedometers or heart rate monitoring (Table 1 reference: 1, 11, 13, 14, 16, 17, 18, 20 25). Of the studies using accelerometers, four studies reported the threshold used for determining metabolic equivalent levels (METS) (1, 14, 11, 18).

None of the studies that examined prepubertal children (5-11years) found Mexican American/Hispanic children to be more active. Studies reported that Mexican American/Hispanic children were less active, engaging in fewer minutes in moderate and/or vigorous physical activity (Table 1 references: 1, 14, 20) and fewer total step counts per day (Table 1 references: 16). Three studies found no differences in time engaged in moderate or vigorous activity (Table 1 references: 13, 17, 25).

Studies using larger sample sizes of boys and girls suggest Mexican American/Hispanic children spend more minutes in MVPA and less time in sedentary activities (Table 1 reference: 11). Studies using mixed groups of children across pubertal and prepubertal stages also supported these results (Table 1 reference: 14, 18). Belcher et al (Table 1 reference: 11) also reported results for boys and girls separately but found no significant difference in Hispanic/Mexican American girls vs. white Girls engagement in sedentary, moderate, vigorous and moderate to vigorous activity but found that Mexican American/ Hispanic boys spent more time in MVPA and vigorous activity. They reported results separately for age groups as well suggesting differences in activity patterns between Hispanic/Mexican American and white exist in 6-11 year and 12-15 year old children but that there were no differences found in children 16-19 years. The results suggest that ethnic differences in activity patterns are likely to be dependent on age and gender and may also be due to socio-environmental influences rather than ethnicity perse

Energy Expenditure

Two studies examined energy expenditure measured by double-labelled water (Table 1 references: 2, 25). One study looked at Mexican American/Hispanic boys and girls combined (Table 1 reference: 2) the other considered Hispanic girls only (Table 1 reference: 25). Dugas et al (Table 1 reference: 2) examined boys and girls together and found no difference in total energy expenditure (TEE), activity energy expenditure (AEE) and physical activity level (PAL) (PAL= TEE/AEE) in boys from Mexican American/Hispanic descent and white. Treuth (Table 1 reference: 25) also found no difference between ethnicity and PAL in girls

South Asian vs. White European

Despite South Asians experiencing the highest risk of metabolic disease there were few studies examining physical activity patterns in this ethnic group. A total of four studies included South Asian children, two studied Indian children (Table 1 reference: 10, 12), one studied a mix of Indian, Pakistani or Bangladeshi (Table 1 reference: 19) and the other study included predominantly Indian (91.5%) Sri Lankan, Bangladeshi and Nepalese (Table 1 reference: 15). These studies combined ethnic subgroups. Owens et al (Table 1 reference : 19) considered the affect of ethnic subgroups but did not report statistical information for this.

Measuring Instrument

Physical Fitness

Two studies have analysed physical fitness differences in children from Indian descent. Both these studies used ergometer tests in either male adolescents (Table 1 reference: 10) or a mixed gender group of pre-pubertal children (Table 1 reference: 12). Hardy and Eston's (1985) study used a small sample of adolescent college males to examine VO^2max by estimating the relationship between heart rate, oxygen uptake and workload at sub maximal levels of exercise. The study found that white adolescents had higher maximal uptake values when adjustments were made for fat free mass. Bettiol et al (Table 1 reference: 12) studied a larger sample of pre-pubertal children (n=711) to study power output against maximum heart rate (85%). They found that children from Indian backgrounds were less likely to be able to finish the ergometer test. Higher numbers of both Indian boys and Indian girls were unable to complete the ergometer test compared to white boys and girls (34.6% and 35.7% vs. 11.7% and 12.1%, $p= 0.016$ and $p<0.001$ respectively). For girls who managed to complete the test, the power output against load at 85% of maximum heart rate (PWC85%) was lower in Indian girls compared to white girls (2.17 vs. 1.89 watt/kg, $p<0.001$). However, no significant differences were found between Indian and white boys PWC85%.

Physical Activity

Two studies have examined physical activity patterns in south Asian children. One study examined only prepubertal children, both boys and girls, using accelerometers (Table 1 reference: 19). The other studied a wide age range of girls using pedometers (5-16years) (Table 1 reference: 15). Both studies found that children from south Asian descent were less active than White European children. Owen (Table 1 reference: 19) reported that SA children recorded fewer daily steps, less counts per minute, less time in MVPA ($p<0.0001$) less time in moderate or vigorous activity ($p=0.02$) and spent more time in sedentary activity ($p<0.001$) compared to White children. In addition, Owens et al (2009) study considered within-ethnic differences in the South Asian sample and although South Asians did have lower levels of physical activity as a whole there were no differences between Indians, Pakistanis and Bangladeshis.

Discussion

There have been a reasonable number of studies that have examined both physical activity and physical fitness in children from different ethnic backgrounds. Most of these studies have taken place in North America where the ethnic groupings are different to those seen in Continental Europe. There do appear to be many studies that have included black children. These studies have predominantly considered fitness and physical activity differences but there were limited studies examining energy expenditure differences between black and white children. The results appear to suggest that black children at all different ages have lower fitness levels than white children (Table 1 references: 3, 4, 5, 6, 7, 8, 9, 12, 14, 23, 25) . Large multicentre studies suggest that black children were also more active and more sedentary than white children i.e their data seemed to polarise at one or other extreme (Table

1 references: 11, 19). Physical activity is believed to be associated with increased physical fitness and thus this relationship of high physical activity yet low fitness needs exploring further in Black children.

There were also a number of studies that have considered physical activity differences in Hispanic/ Mexican American children compared to White. These studies have focused on physical activity patterns mainly, followed by assessments of fitness and energy expenditure. The results were most conflicting within this group of ethnic children. Some of this may be explained by methodological limitations and failure to account for influential factors such as age and gender, which made it impossible to conclude whether there were genuine differences in fitness between Hispanics and White Europeans. Physical activity patterns were likely to differ depending on age or gender. Limited information regarding energy expenditure differences also made it difficult to conclude whether differences existed and thus further studies are needed. There were limited studies in children from South Asian descent and this was due to a lack of data from European centres. Studies consistently reported that South Asian children were both less fit and less active (Table 1 references: 10, 12, 15, 19). Of these two were large studies with robust data collection (Table 1 references: 12, 19).

Methodological Limitations

There were a number of methodological differences among the studies making it difficult both to analyse the results and also to be able to compare study findings: certainly it was felt that some of the inconsistencies between studies were likely to be due to methodological differences. Most of the studies measuring fitness did use reliable and valid measures. However, the measurement of physical fitness in childhood is not without limitations. Peak VO_2, as opposed to maximum, is normally assessed in childhood as children lack the physiological mechanisms to continue beyond limits of maximal effort to achieve a plateau (Wellsman and Strong, 1995). However it is not clear whether an assessment to continue to exhaustion would be valid based on ethnicity. Children of different ages from different ethnic groups may be hindered by motivation and cognition, rather than physiological variables in their approach to such an assessment. Results are also influenced by age, growth, maturation and body size: factors which were not always considered in these studies and must be considered in future studies (Wellman and Strong, 1995).

The measurement of physical activity is a complex phenomenon. Physical activity can be assessed in many different ways including mechanical movement, metabolic components, intensity, frequency of activity or time spent in activity and thus presenting accurate and reliable measures of physical activity can be challenging (Haskell and Kiernan, 2000). The studies presented here have used predominantly accelerometers (actigraphs) to measure physical activity, which make it possible to measure both intensity and frequency whilst eliminating human error, but they do not capture all types of physical activity for example, swimming or cycling which are non weight bearing activities (Trost et al, 2002) and thus combining activity monitoring with self-report may provide additional information. In addition, different studies have also used different methods to analyse the data gathered for physical activity. Physical activity is measured as registered counts per minute or steps per day which is converted to time spent in sedentary activity, moderate activity, moderate to vigorous activity or vigorous activity using cut off point thresholds to make the results more meaningful when compared to health recommendations. However, there has been inconsistency in the types of cut off points used and this is due to a lack of a standardised measure of assessment. This has made it difficult to determine whether physical activity differences do exist or whether differences are due to differences in the criteria used. A recent systematic review of objective measures of physical activity measurement reanalysed all physical activity data in children using the three most popular cut off points (Reilly, Penpraze, Hislop, Davies, Grant and Paton, 2008). They found significant differences in the amount of sedentary behaviour and MVPA when these different cut off points were used suggesting that the assessment of engagement in physical activity is dependent on the cut off points which are applied to the data (Reilly et al, 2008). Global criterion measures are needed for consistency between studies.

The studies also varied in the choice of epoch used to count periods of activity. Studies used mainly 1 minute epochs followed by 30 second intervals or 15 second intervals. The nature of children's physical activity is intermittent and thus using longer epochs may fail to describe the true nature of these patterns. The same systematic review reanalysed physical activity data in children using 15, 30, 45 and 60 second intervals. The study found that there was a small significant difference in the results using different intervals but concluded that there was still limited evidence concerning the use of long of short epochs (Reilly et al, 2008). The study made recommendations that moderate and vigorous physical activity should be analysed together in order to reduce misclassification from epoch lengths. It is clear that consistency is needed when comparing results from ethnic groups. The studies also varied in the number of days used for monitoring ranging from 1 day to 7 days. The period of data collection that has been included has also varied from over 5 hours to less than 18 hours. This has important implications as data reliability is reported to increase with an increased number of days of monitoring. Seven days monitoring with an inclusion criteria of 10 hours per day of data is reported to be the most reliable (Penpraze, Reilly, Maclean, Montgomery and Kelly, 2006).

It is also important for studies to gain a whole picture when examining physical activity patterns. For example, studies in black children found that Black children were more sedentary. This would suggest that they are less active. However, studies have also reported that black children were more active. Thus by considering only one component of physical activity, it can cause overgeneralization about physical activity patterns which might not be a true indication of activity patterns. By gaining the whole picture it is possible to conclude that Black children can be both more active and more sedentary than other ethnic groups and thus their activity patterns lie at both extremes.

Age and gender are other important variables for physical activity and fitness. Studies have shown that males are more active/fitter and that physical activity/fitness declines with age in both sexes (Riddoch 2004; 2007; Trost et al, 2002). It is likely that some of the decline in physical fitness over time is related to declines in amounts of physical activity but there may be effects of the physiological changes of puberty, especially in girls. The studies included in this review used wide age ranges and some of these studies failed to report results separately for prepubertal and pubertal children or for boys and girls. It is likely that reporting these results separately for gender and age groups would yield different results.

Many studies used self-report measures or parental report measures to determine ethnicity. However, not all studies reported how they gained information about ethnic group or the criteria used to determine this. Studies should report ethnic criteria in depth for valid comparisons to be made. Although there were few studies of South Asians these data do also need to be reported separately for different South Asian populations - only Owens et al (2009) study considered this. This does significantly increase the size of the sample that needs to be examined. Finally, it is understood that gaining nationally representative information in ethnic groups is a challenge. Ethnic groups tend to cluster in sociodemographically deprived areas and thus recruitment from clustered areas becomes difficult to generalise to a wider population. The reasons for differences in patterns of physical activity may thus be more complex with environmental factors (e.g. safety issues, racism) becoming more important barriers to being active (Rai and Finch, 1997).

This review does suggest that there are ethnic differences in both physical activity and physical fitness in childhood. It is not clear whether these differences are due to physiological, ethnic, cultural or environmental differences or a combination of a number of these factors. Given the public health importance of managing cardiovascular disease risk in ethnic minorities more research is necessary to examine both the implications of different patterns of activity in children from different ethnic backgrounds and whether there may be any interventions which can improve activity and thus cardiovascular fitness in these groups.

References

Andreacci, J.L., Robertson, R. J., Dubé, J. J., Aaron, D. J., Balasekaran, G., and Arslanian, S. A. (2004). Comparison of maximal oxygen uptake consumption between black and white prepubertal and pubertal children. *Paediatric Research,* 56, 706-713.

Andreacci, J. L., Robertson, R. J., Dubé, J. J., Aaron, D. J., Dixon, C. B., and Arslanian, S. A. (2005). Comparison of Maximal oxygen consumption between obese Black and White adolescents. *Paediatric Research*, 58(3), 478-482.

Arslanian, S., Suprasongsin, C., and Janosky, J.E. (1997). Insulin secretion and sensitivity in Black versus White prepubertal healthy children. *Journal of Clinical Endocrinology and Metabolism*, 82(6), 1923- 1927.

Balarajan, R. (1996). Ethnicity and Variations in mortality from coronary heart disease. *Health Trends*, 28, 45-51.

Belcher, B. R., Berrigan, D., Dodd, K. W., Emken, A., Chou, C., and Spruijt-Metz, D. (2010). Physical activity in US youth: effect of race/ethnicity, age, gender, and weight status. *Medicine and Science in Sports and Exercise*, 42(12), 2211-21.

Berenson, G. S., Srinivasan, S. R., Bao, W., Newman, W. P., Tracy, R. E., and Wattigney, W. A. (1998). Association between multiple cardiovascular risk factors and atherosclerosis in children and young adults. *The New England Journal of Medicine*, 338, 1650-6.

Berlin, J. A., and Colditz, G.A. (1990). A meta-analysis of physical activity in the prevention of coronary heart disease. *American Journal of Epidemiology*, 132, 612-628.

Bettiol, H., Rona, R. J., and Chinn, S. (1999). Variation in physical fitness between ethnic groups in nine year olds. *International Epidemiological Association*, 28, 281-286.

Bhopal, R., Unwin, N., White, M., Yallop, J., Walker, L., Alberti, K. G. M. H.(1999). Heterogeneity of coronary heart disease risk factors in Indian, Pakistani, Bangladeshi, and European origin populations: cross sectional study. *British Medical Journal*, 319, 215-20.

Brage, S., Wedderkopp, N., Ekelund, U., Franks, P. W., Wareham, N. J., and Andersen, L. B., et al. (2004). Features of the metabolic syndrome are associated with objectively measured physical activity and fitness in Danish children: the European Youth Heart Study (EYHS). *Diabetes Care*, 27, 2141- 48.

Byrd-Williams, C., Kelly, L. A., Davis, J. N., Spruijit-Metz, D., and Goran, M. I. (2007). Influence of gender, BMI, and Hispanic ethnicity on physical activity in children. *International Journal Pediatric Obesity,* 2, 159-166.

Cappucio, F. P., Cook, D. G., Atkinson, R. W., and Strazullo, P. (1997). Prevalence, detection, and management of cardiovascular risk factors in different ethnic groups in south London. *Heart*, 78, 555-63.

Casazza, K., Dulin-Keita, A., Gower, B. A., and Fernandez, J. R. (2009). Differential influence of diet and physical activity on components of metabolic syndrome in a multiethnic sample of children. *Journal of American Diet Association*, 109, 236-244.

Casazza, K., Gower, B. A., Willig, A. L., Hunter, G. R., and Fernández, J. R.(2009). Physical fitness, activity, and insulin dynamics in early pubertal children. *Pediatric Exercise Science*, 21(1), 63-76.

Chaturvedi, N., McKeigue, P. M., and Marmot M. G. (1994) Relationship of glucose intolerance to coronary risk in Afro-Carribeans compared to Europeans. *Diabetologia*, 37,765-72.

Cruickshank, J. K., Cooper, J., Burnett, M., Macduff, J., and Drubra, U. (1991). Ethnic differences in fasting plasma C-peptide and insulin in relation to glucose tolerance and blood pressure. *Lancet,* 338, 842-47.

Dugas, L. R., Ebersole, K., Schoeller, D., Yanovski, J. A., Barquera, S., and Rivera, J., et al. (2008). Very low levels of energy expenditure among pre-adolescent Mexican-American girls. *International Journal Pediatric Obesity*, 3(2), 123-126.

Duncan, E. K., Duncan , J. S., and Schofield, G. (2008). Pedometer-determined physical activity and active transport in girls. *International Journal of Behavioural Nutrition and Physical Activity*, 5(2).

Ehtisthan, S., Barrett, T. G., and Shaw, N. J. (2000). Type 2 diabetes mellitus in UK children – an emerging problem. *Diabetic Medicine* , 17, 867-71.

Ekelund , U., Sardinha, L. B., Anderssen , S. A., Harro, M., Franks, P.W., and Brage, S., et al. (2004). Associations between objectively assessed physical activity and indicators of body fatness in 9-to 10-y-old European children: a population-based study from 4 distinct regions of Europe (the European Youth Heart Study). *American Journal of Clinical Nutrition*, 80, 584-90.

Ekelund, U., Neovuis, M., Linné, Y., Brage, S., Wareham, N. J., and Rössner, S. (2005) Associations between physical activity and fat mass in adolescents; the Stockholm weight development study. *American Journal of Clinical Nutrition*, 81, 355-60.

Hardy, C. P., and Eston, R. G. (1985). Aerobic fitness to Anglo-Saxon and Indian students. *British Journal of Sports Medicine*, 19, 217-218.

Haskell, W. L., and Kiernan, M. (2000). Methodological issues in measuring physical activity and physical fitness when evaluating the role of dietary supplements for physically active people [1-3]. *American Journal of Clinical Nutrition,* 72(supplement), 541s-50s.

Johnson, T. G., Brusseau, T. A., Graser, S.V., Darst, P.W., and Kulinna, P.H. (2010). Step counts of 10-to 11-year-old children by ethnicity and metropolitan status. *Journal of Physical Activity and Health*, 7, 355-363.

Kelly, E. B., Parra-Medina, D., Pfeiffer, K.S., Dowda, M., Conway, T. L., and Webber, L. S., et al. (2010). Correlates of physical activity in Black, Hispanic and White middle school girls. *Journal of Physical Activity and Health*, 7, 184-193.

Ku, C., Gower, B. A., Hunter, G. R., and Goran, M. I. (2000). Racial differences in insulin secretion and sensitivity in prepubertal children: role of physical fitness and physical activity. *Obesity Research*, 8(7), 506-515.

Lane, D., Beevers, D. H., and Lip, G. Y. (2002). Ethnic differences in blood pressure and the prevalence of hypertension in England. *Journal of Human Hypertension*, 16, 267-73.

Matthews, C. E., Chen, K.Y., Freedson, P.S ., Buchowski, M. S., Beech, B. M., Pate, R. R., (2007). Amount of time spent in sedentary behaviours in the United States, 2003-2004. *American J of Epidemiology*, 167(7), 875- 881

McMurray, R. G., Harrell, J. S., Bradley, C. B., Deng, S., and Bangdiwala, S. I., (2002). Predicted maximal aerobic power in youth is related to age, gender and ethnicity. Medicine and Science in Sports and Exercise, 34(1), 145-151.

McKeigue ,P. M., Shah, B., and Marmot, M.G., (1991). Relation of central obesity and insulin resistance with high diabetes prevalence and cardiovascular risk in South Asians. *Lancet*, 1337,382-86.

Owen, C. G., Nightingale, C. M., Rudnicka, A. R., Cook, D. G., Ekelund, U., and Whincup, P. H. (2009). Ethnic and gender differences in physical activity levels among 9-10-year-old children of White European, South Asian and African-Caribbean origin: the Child Heart Health Study in England (CHASE Study). *International Journal of Epidemiology*, 38, 1082-1093.

Pate, R. R., Stevens, J., Pratt, C., Sallis, J. F., Schmitz, K. H., and Webber, L. S., et al. (2006) Objectively measured physical activity in sixth-grade girls. *Archives of Pediatric Adolescent Medicine*, 160, 1262-1268.

Pate, R. R., Wang, C., Dowda, M., Farrell, S. W.,O' Niell, J. R., (2006). Cardiorespiratory fitness levels among US youth 12 to 19 years of age. *Archives of Pediatric Adolescent Medicine*, 160, 1005-1012

Penpraze, V., Reilly, J. J., Maclean, C. M., Montgomery, C., and Kelly, L. A. (2006). Monitoring of physical activity in young children: how much is enough? *Pediatric Exercise Science*, 18, 483-491.

Pfeiffer, K.A., Dowda, M., Mclver, K. L., and Pate, R, R., (2009). Factors related to objectively measured physical activity in preschool children. *Pediatric exercise science,* 21(2), 196-208.

Pivarnik, J.M., Bray, M. S., Hergenroeder, A.C., Hill, R. B., and Wong, W.W. (1995). Ethnicity affects aerobic fitness in US adolescents girls. *Medicine Science Sports Exercise* , 27, 1635-1638.

Powell, K. E., Thompson, C. J., Caspersen, C. J., and Kendrick, J. S. (1987). Physical activity and the incidence of coronary heart disease. *Annual Review of Public Health*, 8, 253-287.

Rai, D. K., and Finch, H. (1997). Physical activity 'from our point of view;: qualitative research among South Asian and black communities. London, HEA.

Reilly, J. J., Penpraze, J., Hislop, J., Davies, G., Grant, S., and Paton, J. Y., (2008). Objective measurement of physical activity and sedentary behaviour: review with new data. *Archives of Disease Childhood* , 93, 614-619.

Rice, M. H., and Howell, C. C. (2000). Measurement of physical activity, exercise, and physical fitness in children: issues and concerns. *Journal of Pediatric Nursing*, 15(3), 148-156.

Riddoch, C. J., Bo Andersen, L., Wedderkopp, B., Harro, M., Klasson- Heggebø, L., and Sardinha, L. B., et al. (2004). Physical activity levels and patterns of 9-and 15-yr-old European children. Medicine and Science in Sport and Exercise, 36(1), 86-92.

Riddoch, C. J., Mattocks, C., Deere, K., Saunders, J., Kirkby, J., and Tilling, K., et al. (2007). Objective measurement of levels and patterns of physical activity. *Archives of Disease in childhood*, 92, 963-969.

Roberts, K. A., Freed, B., and McCarthy, W. J., (2010). Low aerobic fitness and obesity are associated with lower standardized test scores in children. *The Journal of Paediatrics*, 156, 711-8.

Sardinha, L.B., Andersen, L.B., Anderssen, S.A ., Quiterio, A. L., Ornelas, R., and Froberg, K., et al. (2008). Objectively measured time spent sedentary is associated with insulin resistance independent of overall and central body fat in 9-10-year-old Portuguese children. *Diabetes Care*, 31, 569-75.

Shaibi , G. Q., Ball, G. D. C., and Goran, M. I., (2006). Aerobic fitness among Caucasian, African – American, and latino youth. *Ethnicity and Disease*, 16, 120 – 125.

Strazzullo, P. Cappucio, F. P., Trevisan, M., et al.(1988). Leisure time physical activity and blood pressure in schoolchildren. *Am J epidemiol* , 127, 726-33.

Thom, T., Haase, N., Rosamond, W., Howard, V. J., Rumsfield, J., and Manolio, T., et al.(2006). Heart disease and stroke statistics- 2006 update. *Circulation* , 113, e85-e151

Trost, S. G., Pate, R. R., Sallis, J. F., Freedson, P. S., Taylor W. C., and Dowda, M., et al. (2002). Age and gender differences in objectively measured physical activity in youth. *Medicine and Science in Sports and Exercise*, 34(2), 350-5.

Trowbridge, X., Gower, B.A., Nagy, T.E., Hunter, G. R., Treuth, M. S., and Goran, M. I. (1997). Maximal aerobic capacity in African- American and Caucasian children. *American Journal of Physiology* 36, E809-E814.

Treuth, M. S., Butte, N.F., Puyau, M., and Adolph, A. (2000). Relations of parental obesity status to physical activity and fitness in prepubertal girls. *Pediatrics* , 106, e49

Wellsman, J. R,. and Strong, N. (1996). The measurement and interpretation of aerobic fitness in children: current issues. *Journal of the Royal Society of Medicine*, 89, 281p-285p.

Wittmeier, K. D., Mollard, R. C., and Kriellaars, D.J. (2008) Physical activity intensity and risk of overweight and adiposity in children. *Obesity*, 16, 415-20.

Whincup, P., Gilg, J., Papacosta, O., Seymour, C., Miller, G. J.,and Alberti, K. G. M. M., et al. (2002). Early evidence of ethnic differences in cardiovascular risk: Cross sectional study comparison of British South Asian and White Children. *British Medical Journal*, 324, 1-6

Whincup, P. H., Gilg, J. A., Owen, C. G., Odoki, K., Alberti, K. G., and Cook, D. G. (2005). British South Asians aged 13-16 years have higher fasting glucose and insulin levels than Europeans. *Diabetic Medicine*, 22, 1275-77.

Whincup PH, Owen CG, Orfei L, McKay, C., and Cook, D. G. (2007). Ethnic differences in risk factors for chronic disease have their origins in early life: evidence for the CHASE study. *Early Human Development* , 83, S63.

Whincup, P. H., Nightingale, C. M., Owen, C. G., Rudnicka, A. R., Gibb, I., and McKay, C. M., et al. (2010) Early emergence of ethnic differences in type 2 diabetes precursors in the UK: The child heart and health study in England (CHASE study). *PloS Med*, 7(4), 1-10.

WHO.(2010) Global recommendations on physical activity for health. WHO. Available from: http://www.who.int/dietphysicalactivity/factsheet_recommendations/en/index.html. Accessed on: 8th December 2010.

Yajnik, C. S., Lubree, G. G., Rege, S. S., Naik, S.S. Despande, J.A., and Deshpande, S. S., et al. (2002). Adiposity and hyperinsulinaemia in Indians are present at birth. *Journal of Clinical Endocrinology and Metabolism*, 87, 5575-5580.

In: Reviews in Pediatric Exercise Science
Editor: Michael Duncan, pp. 147-160
ISBN: 978-1-61470-978-7

Chapter X

Heart Rate Variability, Weight Status and Physical Activity in Children: A Short Review

Craig Franklin, Samantha Birch and Michael J. Duncan
Coventry University, UK.

Introduction

Heart Rate Variability (HRV) is defined as an index of tonic autonomic activity (Blom et al., 2009) which in layman's terms is the fluctuations between consecutive heart beats. These fluctuations represent the changing levels of the activity of sympathetic and parasympathetic nerves, known collectively as the autonomic nerves, and modulate the intrinsic sinus node firing rate (Yutaka et al., 1989). The normal rhythm of the heart is controlled by the membrane processes of the sinoatrial node (SA node) which are controlled by the divisions of the sympathetic and parasympathetic nerves of the autonomic system (ANS) (Berntson et al., 1997). At rest the parasympathetic nerve systems dominates the heart rate (Goldberger et al., 2001). HRV is a non-invasive tool that measures the autonomic control of the heart (Leicht, Sinclair, and Spinks 2008), and has considerable potential to assess the role of autonomic system fluctuations in normal individuals and in patients with cardiovascular disorders (Task Force, 1996).

Reduced beat-to-beat variability is a predictor of mortality and arrhythmic complications and is found in individuals with a variety of cardiac abnormalities (Bigger et al., 2007). The risk of mortality has been proposed to be significantly greater in individuals with HRV less than 50ms (Kleiger et al., 1987; Martin et al., 1987). A reduced HRV positively correlates with obesity (Nagai et al., 2004), poor aerobic fitness (Aubert et al., 2001), low habitual physical activity (Blom et al., 2009), and increasing age (Silvetti et al., 2001), as well as racial differences (Reed et al 2006). However, although the literature on HRV contains is considerable, it has predominantly focused on the adult population while little research exists for children.

HRV measures are split into two categories; time domain indices, and frequency domain indices. There are two main groups of time domain variable measures (Stein and Kleiger, 1999). The first of which include; mean R-R intervals (the differences between successive R-R intervals) and SDRR (average standard deviation of all R-R intervals), which are known to reflect the circadian rhythms and therefore total variability (Stein and Kleiger, 1999). The second group includes pNN50 (the percentage of adjacent cycles that are >50 ms apart) and RMSSD (the root mean square of successive differences) which have been found to reflect vagal modulation of the SA node and correlate strongly with the high frequency (HF) power band (Pagani et al., 1986).

The frequency domain indices represent power density of HRV and provide information on the distribution of power as a frequency band; formed of both the high frequency band and the low frequency band. The HF (above 15Hz) frequency reflects respiratory mediated HRV, while LF (0.04 to 0.15Hz) is modulated by both the sympathetic and parasympathetic nervous systems (Stein and Kleiger, 1999). In addition to HF and LF, frequency domain measures also include very low frequency (VLF) and ultra-low frequency (ULF), although the underlying physiological mechanisms involved are less distinguished than HF and LF (Task Force, 1996).

The Current Body of Knowledge

Measurement of HRV

There are a considerable amount of reliability and reproducibility studies of HRV in adults, although these have not been conclusive, as determined by a review by Sandercock et al. (2005). Freed et al. (1994), Sinnreich et al. (1998), and Marks and Lightfoot (1999) have all found HRV is a moderately reliable measurement from stable ECG recorded under controlled, resting conditions. Within individuals, resting measures of HRV have been found to be reliable including; RMSSD ($r = 0.20–0.98$), pNN50 ($r =0.43–0.97$) HF ($r = 0.48–0.96$), LF ($r = 0.60–0.97$), and TP ($r = 0.52–0.97$) (Hohnloser et al., 1992; Pitzalis et al., 1996; Melanson, 2000). However, Sandercock et al. (2005) concluded that further research was required to accurately assess the reliability of HRV. Furthermore, LF was reproducible under all three conditions of rest, tilt and controlled respiration, total power was reproducible at rest and HF only during controlled respiration. Therefore, the reproducibility of the frequency domain parameters depends on the analysed condition (Pitzalis et al., 1996).

However, in relation to children there have been very few such studies looking at reproducibility (test-retest reliability) of HRV. This is important in terms of interpretation of research as reliable results for adults may not generalise in younger individuals (Dietrich et al., 2010) due to the age-dependent differences in autonomic functioning (Tanaka et al., 1998). One of the first to precisely investigate the reliability of HRV measures at rest in children was Winsley et al. (2003) in which a sample of 12 children, ages 11-12 years old had HRV assessed for a period of 5 minutes in a supine position, with breathing controlled at 12 breaths/minute. The outcome of this study was to suggest that HRV measures at rest in children are unreliable. However, this study has limitations in its sample size of only 12 children and using just one age range of 11-12 years old. Furthermore, controlling the breathing rate for children may have lead to the lack of reliability of the measures taken. This is because it may have led to excess anxiety as the children attempted to maintain the required 12 breaths/minute, thus affecting the resting heart rate of the children. The authors of this study concluded that more research was required in this area to which led Dietrich et al. (2010) to conduct a study on 57 children ranging from the ages of 10-13 years. HRV was measured by ECG in both the supine and standing position for a period of 5 minutes, and found to be moderate-to-high in terms of reproducibility according to the magnitude of relative and absolute reliability. The authors of this study conclude that relative reliability of short term measurements of HRV in the time and frequency domains may be considered satisfactory in the supine and standing positions in children, thus implicating a significant capacity to detect real differences between children (Dietrich et al., 2010).

Although the use of the electrocardiogram (ECG) is the 'gold standard' for measuring HRV, there are limitations both in terms of measurement/ analysis and in field based studies looking at exercise/ physical activity as the equipment is not easily portable. The limitations in terms of measurement and analysis of HRV from the ECG come from the requirement to apply algorithms to locate the peak of R waves, and R-R intervals, which could lead to errors due to drift, and biologic and electromagnetic interference (Bolanos, Nazeran, and Haltiwanger, 2006). The limitations of the ECG in the analysis of HRV outside of the laboratory and especially in the physical training conditions led to the development of wireless heart rate monitors allowing for the exposure of R-R intervals to be detected. Several studies have therefore investigated the validity and reliability of such heart rate monitors in analysing HRV (mainly the Polar S810), all of which have concluded that specifically the Polar S810 heart rate monitor was a valid and reliable measure of R-R intervals and subsequent HRV analysis in the supine position for adults (Gamelin, Berthoin, and Bosquet 2006; Nunan et al., 2009). Additionally, a study of children aged 9.6±0.9 years found that the Polar S810 was a valid measure of R-R intervals in the supine position, although this study only consisted of 12 children (Gamelin et al., 2008).

Age, Gender and Ethnic Differences in HRV

Age and gender significantly affect heart rate and various components of HRV in the supine position and in response to standing (Fagard, Pardaens, and Staessen, 1999). The increase in HRV and respectively the decrease in heart rate through childhood have been related to the growth of cardiac mass and stroke volume (Kmit and Rubleva, 2001). Measures of HRV (M, SDNN, RMSSD, TF, VLF and HF) in children aged 6-16 years old increase with age in a wavelike way changing from year to year, although it is believed that HR control is stabilised between 15-16 years old as no differences were observed (Galev, Igisheva, and Kazin 2002). This is supported by research that has found that overall HRV measures increased with age and were not influenced by gender, and also indices of parasympathetic function increased up to the age of 10, again gender-unrelated (Silvetti, Drago, and Ragonese, 2001). HRV parameters are known to decrease with an associated increase in age (Bonnemeier et al., 2003). The effect of aging on HRV is linear up to the age of 60 years; thereafter the age-related decrease in HRV stabilizes (Koskinen et al., 2009).

Several studies have investigated gender differences in the measures of HRV, with the evidence somewhat divisive with certain studies suggesting that females have a higher HRV than in males (Evans et al., 2001; Koskinen et al., 2009). However, other researchers have found the opposite, suggesting that males have a higher HRV than females (Umetani et al., 1998; Bonnemeier et al., 2003). There is also evidence to suggest that there is no gender difference in HRV (Sloan et al., 2008). Bonnemeier et al. (2003) however, stated that the significant Gender differences decrease with age. Furthermore, studies in the adult population have also investigated whether gender differences in HRV are observable in children. Research on this issue is equivocal with certain studies suggesting that there is an absence of HRV differences related to gender (Reed et al., 2006; Krishnan et al., 2009), and other suggesting differences between boys and girls in HRV parameters are observable from 12 years of age for some parameters (SDNN, RMSSD and HF) and as early as 9 years of age in parameter M (Galev, Igisheva, and Kazin, 2002). However, it has been found that measures of HRV are significantly higher in boys than in girls irrespective of age (in the range of 1-20 years) (Silvetti, Drago, and Ragonese 2001). The mechanisms underlying age-related gender differences in HRV are undistinguished, but it has been suggested there are lower levels of parasympathetic activity in young females, which declines (above the age of 30) compared to more stable levels of sympathetic activity (Umetani et al., 1998).

Another variable that may have an effect on HRV in individuals is race or ethnicity. Firstly, Liao et al. (1995) reported that African Americans had a lower LF, higher HF, and a larger HF/LF ratio than Caucasians. These findings have been substantiated by further research, suggesting that both in adults and adolescents, African American individuals have lower measures of HRV although mainly measured in the frequency domain (Guzzetti et al., 2000; Faulkner, Hathaway, and Tolley, 2003; Zion et al., 2003). This has been suggested to be due to parasympathetic activity decreasing progressively with age only in Caucasians and not in African Americans, with African Americans having a lower parasympathetic activity comparable to similar aged Caucasian populations. This is reflected by HF and LF measures of HRV (Choi et al., 2006). However, there is evidence to suggest that African Americans have higher resting HRV than European Americans (Wang et al., 2005; Li et al., 2009). While most research has focused on the comparison between African Americans with Caucasians, Reed et al. (2006) were the first to examine differences between Asian and Caucasian children within a Canadian community following suggestions that there may be differences between Asian and Caucasian individuals. Their results suggested that Asian children had a higher HF: LF ratio than Caucasian children of the same age. However, although not significant, Caucasian children registered higher time domain measures (SDNN, RMSSD) in the supine position than Asian children.

Weight Status and HRV

Childhood obesity is a major epidemic concerning the health and wellbeing of children, with the acute effects of obesity on children being an increase in the likelihood of developing an impaired glucose tolerance, hypertension and fatty liver disease (Rudolph, 2004). Furthermore, the greatest health problems occur when children move into adulthood with obesity-related illnesses such as diabetes, cancers, gall bladder disease, endocrine disorders and osteoarthritis (Lobstein et al., 2004). Previous data suggests that the sympathetic nervous system (SNS) is important in the regulation of an individual's energy balance, and altered SNS activity may affect the amount of fat mass in humans (Acheson et al., 1988; Spiegelman and Flier, 2001). The effect of increased Body Mass Index (BMI) on the cardiovascular system is a reduced HRV caused by a withdrawal of the parasympathetic tone and/or the increase in sympathetic modulation, attributed to the decreased adreno-receptor responsiveness, vagal withdrawal and/or increased sympathetic activity (Ramaeker et al., 1998; Fraley et al., 2005; Schmid et al., 2010). Changes in weight status in either direction have also been associated with changes in HRV (Hirsch et al., 1991; Poirier et al., 2003).

Studies of autonomic activity and HRV in obese children have produced conflicting results. Some studies have found that obese children exhibit higher sympathetic activity and a reduction of parasympathetic activity with a withdrawal of vagal activity in comparison to normal weight children (Karason et al., 1999; Sekine et al., 2001). This is reflected in HRV measures, with lower RMSSD, SDRR and HF and an increased LF:HF ratio (Martini et al., 2001; Rabbai et al., 2003). However, more recent studies have concluded that obese children have both a reduced sympathetic and parasympathetic tone (Nagai et al., 2003; Vanderlei et al., 2010). Furthermore, there is research to suggest there is no change in sympathetic activity but a reduction/hypoactivity of the parasympathetic tone linked to RMSSD and LF (Yakinci et al., 2000; Kim et al., 2005). In addition, Rabbia et al. (2003) found that children who were obese for a period of less than 4 years had significantly increased sympathetic activity, but children who had been obese for more than 4 years had HRV values no different to healthy individuals, suggesting that the period of obesity may be an important variable to consider when evaluating obesity and HRV.

Physical Activity and HRV in Adults and Children

It is now a widespread belief that the most people in the developed world are not meeting current guidelines for physical activity (PA) attributed to the increase in pleasurable sedentary activities such as T.V. and especially for children video games (Buchhiet et al., 2007). The decrease in habitual physical activity has been suggested as a causality of increases in cardiovascular risk (Kohl, 2001), and low habitual PA has been found to lead to a decrease in HRV (Buchheit et al., 2007; Dietrich et al., 2008; Blom et al., 2009). In turn regular physical activity has beneficial effects on the autonomic control of the heart accompanied with an increase in HRV (Dietrich et al., 2008) and is a predictor of LF, HF and SDNN (Blom et al., 2009). Regular PA is partially associated with increased vagal modulation, linked to increased HF power (Hull et al., 1994) and moderate-to-high PA results in higher parasympathetic indices/ outflow (Melanson, 2000; Bucheit et al., 2004). Most of the research into habitual PA and the relationship with HRV has focussed around the adult population, thus very little data exists for children on habitual PA on both cardiorespiratory and health indexes, although it is said that identified cardiovascular risk factors may be found in early childhood or adolescence (Buchhiet et al., 2007), thus provide an interesting and important area of research.

Intervention Studies to Increase HRV

Regular PA/exercise has been associated with an increased HRV (Jurca et al., 2004; Dietrich et al., 2008), and as such forms a basis for many intervention studies looking to increase HRV in certain populations. It is well documented that long-term endurance training has a beneficial effect on cardiac modulation of the heart with increases in HRV, parasympathetic activity, and a decrease in the sympathetic activity of the heart at rest (Shi et al., 2005; Gregoire et al., 1996; Chen and Dicarlo, 1998). Training intervention studies however are inconsistent in that studies in middle-aged participants have shown an increase in parasympathetic tone after aerobic training (Melanson and Freedson, 2001; Amano et al., 2001; Jurca et al., 2004), whilst other studies show no improvement/effect on HRV following training (Boutcher and Stein, 1995). Although it is suggested that moderate to high intensity physical activity or exercise has a greater effect on vagal related indexes of HRV (Buchheit et al., 2005; Buchheit et al., 2007). However, in a recent review, it is suggested that exercise therapy may improve HRV in myocardial infarction, and chronic heart failure patients from resulting increased vagal tone and decreased sympathetic activity (Routledge et al., 2010).

Several studies have examined the effect of different exercise intensities on children, however again the research is inconsistent. Following a 13 week endurance training program (3×1 h week^{-1}; intensity > 80% HR_{max}), it was found that endurance training has a positive effect on nocturnal global HRV without changes in parasympathetic or sympathetic activity (Mandigout et al., 2002). Negai et al. (2004) followed this study with a 12 month school-based exercise program (20mins/day, 5days/ week, 130-140bpm) in 300 children aged 6-11years. Results suggested that moderate exercise training has a positive effect on cardiac ANS activity in children with initially low HRV. Conversely, a 7 week high intensity intermittent training program in 52 children aged 9 years, found that there was no significant effect on the autonomic control of the heart, measured by HRV, despite improvements in aerobic fitness (Gamelin et al., 2009), which may suggest that moderate exercise intensities may be more beneficial in increasing HRV in children. Although it may be the training load (intensity, duration and frequency of training) that may account for the different effects on HRV (Gamelin et al., 2009).

Self-Assessed PA Studies

One of the first studies to look at habitual PA and the HRV in adults was by Melanson (2000), with an aim of assessing day-to-day resting HRV, whether habitual PA affects reliability of measures and whether HRV is related to self-reported habitual PA levels. The study consisted of 37 male subjects aged between 25-49, each asked to complete a modified Aerobics Centre Longitudinal study of PA questionnaire reporting the number of sessions and minutes per week spent in purposeful exercise. After which participants were categorised into low, moderate, or high PA. HRV was recorded in the supine position for 15 minutes using an ECG allowing for time and frequency domain indices measured to be recorded. The findings of this study suggest that HRV measures were highly reproducible, and that time and frequency domain measures (HF and total power) were greater in active individuals compared to sedentary individuals, but that HRV does not appear to increase with increasing levels of physical activity.

However, this study has several limitations that may have affected the above results. The study included highly trained endurance athletes in the high PA category, which is not representative of the normal population, and also endurance training has been shown to increase HRV (Levy et al., 1998; Stein et al., 1999). Furthermore, the use of an ECG has limitations as discussed earlier in analysis of HRV (Bolanos, Nazeran, and Haltiwanger, 2006). Further studies have been conducted looking at self-reported PA and HRV both in adults and in adolescents using various questionnaires, either measuring the amount of times per session or week that an individual is sweating or hard breathing. However, theses studies seem to be inconclusive with authors claiming that either there is a significant relationship between self-reported PA and HRV (Dietrich et al., 2008; Blom et al., 2009), whilst other authors claim to have found the opposite with no significant interaction between self-reported PA and HRV measures (Sandercock et al., 2008)

The use of self-report as a means to assess PA has been questioned (Shephard, 2003). The use of self-report questionnaires was found to have limited reliability and validity as a measure of PA, and as such may be argued is a major limitation within these studies (Shephard, 2003). Furthermore, some studies have used the occurrence of sweat per day/session as a measure of PA which has also been suggested as being limited in the ability to distinguish between inactive subjects in epidemiological studies (Washburn et al., 1990). Limitations of self-reported PA in children involve errors from human cognitive processes, the definition of the desired variables, inadequate length of assessment and failure to account for weekdays, weekend and seasonal variations (Baronowski, 1988; Cale, 1994), although self-reported questionnaires are still a valid and reliable measure of PA in children (Argiropoulou et al., 2004).

A common feature within the literature around the use of self-reported PA is that authors tend to confuse or inter-change between physical activity and physical exercise. However, these terms are independent as physical activity is defined as any body movement produced by skeletal muscle that results in energy expenditure above rest, whereas physical exercise is a specific type of PA for the sole purpose of improving fitness (Trost, 2001). Researchers from ACSM found that the definition of moderate physical exercise such as "'moderate intensity' is a pace at which you break a sweat, have a slight increase in heart rate, but are still able to talk," were not sufficient in helping women understand the intensity required to meet the ACSM recommendations (ACSM, 2006) further causing a possible limitation of self-report methods as the population may have different understandings of what intensity PA they had done.

Objective Measures of PA

With self-report studies having limitations in the accurate assessment of PA (Washburn et al., 1990; Shephard, 2003), objective measures should be considered in future studies of PA and HRV as they provide a valid and reliable measure (Trost, 2001; Duncan, Schofield, and Duncan, 2007). Methods of measuring PA in both adults and children include the use of accelerometers or daily step count from pedometers. The use of pedometers has become a popular monitoring tool due to their low cost and feasibility (Cardon, and Bourdeaudhuij, 2007) and have been to found be reliable and valid measures of PA in adolescents and children (Rowe et al., 2004; Tudor-Locke et al., 2004; Eisenmann and Wickel, 2005).

Additionally accelerometers have been found to be a reliable measure of PA, specifically the TriTrac (Professional Products, Inc., Madison, WI) in both young adults (Nichols et al., 1999) and in children (Coleman et al., 1997).

However, a search of relevant databases and search engines revealed that currently no studies have researched the relationship between pedometer measured PA and HRV in either adults or children, although a relationship between a low daily step count and coronary heart disease risk factors has been found in adolescent girls (Schofield et al., 2009). Conversely accelerometers have been used as an objective measure to examine the effect of habitual on HRV. Some studies have combined self-report methods with accelerometers in middle aged men (aged 61±4years) (Buchheit et al., 2005) and in 12 year-old children (Buchheit et al., 2007). In the case of the latter, it has been suggested that regular moderate activities are adequate to influence physical fitness but higher vagal related HRV indexes were found in those that took part in moderate to very high intensity PA. Furthermore, Gutin et al. (2005) found favourable HRV profiles were significantly associated with higher amounts of moderate-vigorous physical activity.

Conclusion and Future Directions

The current body of literature based on habitual PA and HRV has limitations in its use of self-reported PA with the use of questionnaires, with little research assessing PA and HRV using other objective tools such as accelerometers or pedometers. Furthermore, although there have been several studies linking PA with HRV in adults and adolescents, there are very few studies with pediatric populations. The extant literature base also contains confusion in the terms physical activity and physical exercise which may explain why the literature is equivocal.

The limitations identified earlier in this chapter provide areas for further research, specifically the need to examine the relationship between objective measures of PA (pedometers/ accelerometers) and HRV in adults/adolescents and children. Furthermore, as research examining gender and ethnic differences is inconsistent, future research is needed to determine whether these variables do actually impact upon HRV measures, so that it can be said that both intervention and PA studies reporting that improved HRV has occurred is truly independent of age, gender and ethnic influences.

References

Acheson, K.J. Ravussin, E. Schoeller, D.A. Christin, L. Bourquin, L. Baertschi, P. Danforth, E., and Jequier, E. (1988). 'Two-week stimulation or blockade of the sympathetic nervous system in man: Influence on body weight, body composition, and twenty four-hour energy expenditure'. *Metabolism,* 37 (1), 91-98.

ACSM (2006). 'What is "Moderate Intensity" physical activity? New study suggests better to show than tell' *American College of Sports Medicine* .

Amano, M. Kanda, T. UE, H., and Moritani, T. (2001). 'Exercise training and autonomic nervous activity in obese individuals' *Medicine and Science in Sports and Exercise,* 33 (8), 1287-1291.

Aubert, A.E, Beckers, F., and Ramaekers, D. (2001). 'Short-term heart rate variability in young athletes' *Journal of Cardiology,* 37 (Suppl. 1), 85–88.

Argiropoulou, E. Michalopoulou, M. Aggeloussis, N., and Avgerinos, A. (2004). 'Validity and reliability of physical activity measures in Greek high school age children' *Journal of Sports Science and Medicine,* 3, 147-159.

Baronowski, T. (1988). 'Validity and reliability of self-reported measures of physical activity: an information-processing perspective' *Research Quarterly for Exercise and Sport,* 59, 314-327.

Berntson, G.G. Norman, G.J. Hawkley, L.C. Cacioppo, J.T. (1997). 'Cardiac autonomic balance versus cardiac regulatory capacity.' *Psychophysiology,* 45, 643-652.

Bigger, J, T., Fleiss, J, L. Steinman, Rolnitzy, L, M., Kleigner, R, E., and Rottman, J, N. (2007). 'Frequency domain measures of heart period variability and mortality after myocardial infarction.' *Circulation,* 85, 164 –167.

Blom, E., Olsson, E., Serlachius, E., Ericson, M., and Martin, I., (2009). 'Heart rate variability is related to self-report physical activity in a healthy adolescent population' *European Journal of Applied Physiology,* 106, 877-883.

Bolonas, M. Nazeran, H., and Haltiwanger, E. (2006). 'Comparison of heart rate variability signal features derived from electrocardiography and photoplethymography in healthy individuals' *IEEE Engineering in medicine and biology society conference proceedings,* 1, 4289.

Bonnemeier, H. Wiegand, U. Brandes, A. Kluge, N. Katus, H. Richardt, G., and Potratz, J. (2003). 'Circadian profile of cardiac autonomic nervous modulation in healthy subjects: Differing effects of aging and gender on heart rate variability' *Journal of Cardiovascular Electrophysiology,* 14, (8) 791-799.

Boutcher, S., and Stein, P. (1995). 'Association between heart rate variability and training response in sedentary middle-aged men' *European Journal of Applied Physiology and Occupational Physiology,* 70, 75–80.

Buchheit, M. Simon, C. Piquard, F. Ehrhart, J., and Brandenberger, G. (2004). 'Effects of increased training load on vagal-related indexes of heart rate variability: A novel sleep approach' *American Journal of Physiology: Heart and Circulatory Physiology* ,287, 2813-2818.

Buchheit, M. Simon, C. Charloux, A. Doutreleau, S. Piquard, F., and Brandenberger, G. (2005). 'Heart rate variability and intensity of habitual physical activity in middle-aged persons' *Medicine and Science in Sports and Exercise,* 37 (9), 1530-1534.

Buchheit, M. Platat, C. Oujaa, M., and Simon, C. (2007). 'Habitual physical activity, physical fitness and heart rate variability in preadolescents' *International Journal of Sports Medicine,* 28, 204-210.

Cale, L. (1994). 'Self-reported measures of children's physical activity: Recommendations for future development and a new alternative measure' *Health Education Journal,* 53, 439-453.

Cardon, G, and De Bourdeauhuij, I. (2007). 'Comparison of pedometer and accelerometer measures of physical activity in preschool children' *Pediatric Exercise Science,* 19, 205-214.

Chen, C., and Dicarlo, S. (1998). 'Endurance exercise training-induced resting bradycardia: A brief review' *Sports Medicine, Training, and Rehabilitation,* 8 (1), 37.

Choi, JB. Hong, S. Nelesen, R. Bardwell, W. Natarajan, L. Schubert, C., and Dimsdale, J. (2006). 'Age and ethnicity differences in short-term heart-rate variability' *Psychosomatic Medicine,* 68, 421-426.

Coleman, K. Saelens, B. Wiedrich-Smith, M. Finn, J., and Epstein, L. (1997). 'Relationship between TriTrac-R3D vectors, heart rate, and self-report in obese children' *Medicine and Science in Sport and Exercise,* 29 (11), 1535-1542.

Dietrich, D. F. Ackermann-Liebrich, U. Schindler, C. Bartelemy, J. C. Brandli, O. Gold, D. R. Knopfli, B. Probst-Hensch, N.M. Roche, F. Tschopp, JM. Von Eckardstein, A., and Gaspoz, J. M. (2008). 'Effect of physical activity on heart rate variability in normal, overweight, and obese subjects: Results from the SAPALDIA study' *European Journal of Applied Physiology,* 104, 557-565.

Dietrich, A. Rosmalen, J. Althaus, M. Van Roon, A. Mulder, L. Minderaa, R. Oldehinkel, A. and Riese, H. (2010). 'Reproducibility of heart rate variability and baroreflex sensitivity measurements in children' *Biological Psychology,* 85, 71-78.

Duncan, S. Schofield, G., and Duncan, E. (2007). 'Step count recommendations for children based on body fat' *Preventative Medicine,* 44, 42-44.

Evans, J. Ziegler, M. Patwardhan, A. Ott, B. Kim, C. Leonelli, F., and Knapp, C. (2001). 'Gender differences in autonomic cardiovascular regulation: spectral, hormonal, and hemodynamic indexes' *Journal of Applied Physiology,* 91, 2611-2618.

Eisenmann, J., and Wickel, E. (2005). 'Moving on land: an explanation of pedometer counts in children' *European Journal of Applied Physiology,* 93 (4), 440-446.

Fagard, R. Pardaens, K., and Staessen, J. (1999). 'Influence of demographic, anthropometric and lifestyle characteristics on heart rate and its variability in the population' *Journal of Hypertension,* 17 (11), 1589-99.

Faulkner, M. Hathaway, D., and Tolley, B. (2006). 'Cardiovascular autonomic function in healthy adolescents' *Heart and Lung: The Journal of Acute and Critical Care,* 32 (1), 10-22.

Fraley, M. Birchem, J. Senkottaiya, N., and Alpert, M. (2005). 'Obesity and the electrocardiogram' *Obesity Reviews,* 6 (4), 275.

Galev, A. Igisheva, L., and Kazin, E. (2002). 'Heart rate variability in healthy six-to sixteen-year-old children' *Human Physiology,* 28 (4), 428-432.

Gamelin, F.X. Berthoin, S., and Bosquet, L. (2006). 'Validity of the Polar S180 heart rate monitor to measure R-R intervals at rest' *Medicine and Science in Sports and Exercise,* 38 (5), 887-893.

Gamelin, F.X. Baquet, G. Berthoin, S., and Bosquet, L. (2008). 'Validity of the Polar S180 to measure R-R intervals in children' *International Journal of Sports Medicine,* 29 (2), 134-138.

Gamelin, F.X. Baquet, G. Berthoin, S. Thevenet, D. Nourry, C. Nottin, S., and Bosquet, L. (2009). 'Effect of high intensity intermittent training on heart rate variability in prepubescent children' *European Journal of Applied Physiology,* 105, 731-738.

Goldberger,J, G., Challapalli, S., Tung, R., Parker, M, A., and Kadish, A, H. (2001). 'Relationship of heart rate variability to parasympathetic effect.' *Circulation,* 1977-1983.

Gregoire, J. Tuck, S. Yamamoto, Y., and Hughson, R. (1996). 'Heart rate variability at rest and exercise: Influence of age, gender and physical training' *Canadian Journal of Applied Physiology,* 21, 455-470.

Guzzetti, S. Mayet, J. Shahi, M. Mezzetti, S. Foale, R. Sever, P. Poulter, N. Porta, A. Mallaini, A., and Thom, S. (2000). 'Absence of sympathetic overactivity in Afro-Caribbean hypertensive subjects studied by heart rate variability' *Journal of Human Hypertension,* 14 (5), 337.

Hirsch, J. Leibel, RL. Mackintosh, R., and Aguirre, A. (1991). 'Heart rate variability as a measure of autonomic function during weight change in humans' *American Journal of Physiology,* 261 (6 pt 2), R1418-1423.

Hohnloser, S. Klingenheben, T. Zabel, M. Schroder, F., and Just, H. (1992). 'Intraindividual reproducibility of heart rate variability' *PACE,* 15 (Part II) ,2211-2214.

Hull, S. Vanoli, E. Adamson, P. Verrier, R. Foreman, R., and Schwartz, P. (1994). 'Exercise training confers anticipatory protection from sudden death during acute myocardial ischemia' *Circulation,* 89 (2), 548-552.

Jurca, R. Church, T. Morss, G. Jordan, A., and Earnest, C. (2004). 'Eight weeks of moderate-intensity exercise training increases heart rate variability in sedentary postmenopausal women' *American Heart Journal,* 147 (5), e8-e15.

Karason, K. Molgaard, H. Wikstrand, J., and Sjostrom, L. (1999). 'Heart rate variability in obesity and the effect of weight loss' *American Journal of Cardiology,* 83, 1242-1247.

Kim, J. Park, YG. Cho, KH. Hong, MH. Han, HC. Choi, YS., and Yoon, D. (2005). 'Heart rate variability and obesity indices: Emphasis on the response to noise and standing' *The Journal of the American Board of Family Practice,* 18, 97-103.

Kleiger, R. Miller, P. Bigger, T., and Moss, A. (1987). 'Decreased heart rate variability and its association with increased mortality after acute infarction' *The American Journal of Cardiology,* 59 (4), 256-262.

Kmit, G., and Rubleva, L. (2001). 'Age-related features of morphological and functional development of myocardium in children of five to nine years' *Human Physiology,* 27 (5), 556-560.

Kohl, H.W. (2001). 'Physical activity and cardiovascular disease: Evidence for a dose response' *Medicine and Science in Sports and Exercise,* 33, S472-483.

Lobstein T, Baur L, and Uauy R (2004). 'Obesity in children and young people: A crisis in public health' *Obesity Reviews,* Vol.5 (suppl. 1), pp 4-85.

Kosiknen, T. Kahonen, M. Jula, A. Laitinen, T. Keltikangas-Jarvinen, L. Viikari, J. Valimaki, I., and Raitakari, O. (2009). 'Short-term heart rate variability in healthy young adults: The Cardiovascular risk in young Finns study' *Autonomic Neuroscience: Basic and Clinical,* 145, 81-88.

Krishnan, B. Jeffery, A. Metcalf, B. Hosking, J. Voss, L. Wilkin, T., and Flanagan, D. (2009). 'Gender differences in the relationship between heart rate control and adiposity in young children: A cross-sectional study (Early Bird 33)' *Pediatric Diabetes,* 10, 127-134.

Leicht, A, S., Sinclair, W, H., and Spinks, W, L. (2008). 'Effect of exercise mode on heart rate variability during steady state exercise.' *European Journal Applied Physiology,* 102, 195-204.

Li, Z. Sneider, H. Su, S. Ding, X. Thayer, F. Treiber, F., and Wang, X. (2009). 'A longitudinal study in youth of heart rate variability at rest and in response to stress' *International Journal of Psychophysiology,* 73, 212-217.

Liao, D. Barnes, R. Chambless, L. Simpson, R. Sorlie, P., and Heiss G. (1995). 'Age, Race, and sex differences in autonomic cardiac function measured by spectral analysis of heart rate variability- The ARIC study' *American Journal of Cardiology,* 76 (1), 906-912.

Mandigout, S. Melin, A. Fauchier, L. N'Guyen, L. Courtiex, D., and Obert, P. (2002). 'Physical training increases heart rate variability in healthy prepubertal children' *European Journal of Clinical Investigation,* 32, 479-187.

Martin, G. Magid, N. Myers, G. Barnett, P. Schaad, J. Weiss, J. Lesch, M., and Singer D (1987). 'Heart rate variability and sudden death secondary to coronary artery disease during ambulatory electrocardiographic monitoring' *The American Journal of Cardiology,* 60 (1), 86-89.

Martini, G. Riva, P. Rabbia, F. Molini, V. Ferrero, GB. Cerutti, F. Cerra, R., and Veglio, F. (2001). 'Heart rate variability in childhood obesity' *Clinical Autonomic Research,* 11 (2), 87-91.

Melanson, E. (2000). 'Resting heart rate variability in men varying in habitual physical activity' *Medicine and Science in Sports and Exercise,* 32 (11), 1984-1901.

Melanson, E., and Freedson, P. (2001). 'The effect of endurance training on heart rare variability in sedentary adult males' *European Journal of Applied Physiology,* 85 (5), 442-449.

Nagai, N. Matsumoto, T. Kita, H., and Moritani, T. (2003). 'Autonomic nervous system activity and the state and development of obesity in Japanese school children' *Obesity Research,* 11 (1), 25-32.

Nagai, N. Hamada, T. Kimura, T., and Moritani, T. (2004). 'Moderate physical exercise increases cardiac autonomic nervous system activity in children with low heart rate variability' *Child's Nervous System,* 20 (4), 209-214.

Nichols, J. Morgan, C. Sarkin, J. Sallis, J., and Calfas, K. (1999). 'Validity, reliability, and calibration of the Tritrac accelerometer as a measure of physical activity' *Medicine and Science in Sport and Exercise,* 31 (6), 908-912.

Nunan, D. Donovan, G. Jakovljevic, D. Hodges, L. Sandercock, G., and Brodie, D. (2009). 'Validity and reliability of short-term Heart-Rate Variability from Polar S810' *Medicine and Science in Sports and Exercise,* 41 (1), 243-8.

Pagani, M., Lombardi, F., Guzzeti, S., Rimoldi, O., Fulan, R., Pizzinelli, P., Sandrone, G., Malfatto, G., Dell'Orto, S., and Piccaluga, E. (1986). 'Power spectral analysis of heart rate and arterial pressure variabilities as a marker of sympatho-vagal interaction in man and conscious dog.' *Circulation Research,* 59, 178-193.

Pitzalis, M. Mastropasqua, F. Massari, F. Forleo, C. Di Maggio, M. Passantino, A. Colombo, R. Di Biase, M., and Rizzon, P. (1996). 'Short-and long-term reproducibility of time and frequency domain heart rate variability measurements in normal subjects' *Cardiovascular Research,* 32, 226-233.

Poirier, P. Hernandez, TL. Weil, KM. Shepard, TJ, and Eckel, RH. (2003). 'Impact of diet-induced weight loss on the cardiac autonomic nervous system in severe obesity' *Obesity Research,* 11 (9,) 1040-1047.

Rabbia, F. Silke, B. Conterno, A. Grosso, T. De Vito, B. Rabbone, I. Chianduss, L., and Veglio, F. (2003). 'Assessment of cardiac modulation during adolescent obesity' *Obesity Research,* 11 (4), 541-548.

Ramaekers, D. Ector, H. Aubert, AE. Rubens, A., and Van de Werf, F. (1998). 'Heart rate variability and heart rate in healthy volunteers. Is the female autonomic nervous system cardioprotective?' *European Heart Journal,* 19 (9), 1334-1341.

Reed, K., Warburton, D., Whitney, C., and McKay, H., (2006). 'Differences in heart rate variability between Asian and Caucasian children living in the same Canadian community' *Applied Physiology, Nutrition and Metabolism,* 31 (3), 277.

Rudolph, M. (2004). 'The obese child' *Archives of Disease in Childhood- Education and Practice,* 89 pp ep57-67.

Routledge, F. Campbell, T. McFetridge-Durdle, J., and Bacon, S. (2010). 'Improvements in heart rate variability with exercise therapy' *Canadian Journal of Cardiology* 26 (6) 303-312.

Rowe, D. Mahar, M. Raedeke, T., and Lore, J. (2004). 'Measuring physical activity children with pedometers: Reliability, reactivity, and replacement of missing data' *Pediatric Exercise Science,* 16 (4), 343-354.

Sandercock, G.R., Bromley, P.D., Brodie, D.A., (2005). 'The reliability of short-term measurements of heart rate variability' *International Journal of Cardiology,* 103, 238-247.

Schofield, G. Schofield, L. Hinckson, E., and Mummery, K. (2009). 'Daily step count and selected coronary heart disease risk factors in adolescent girls' *Journal of Science and Medicine in Sport,* 12, 148-155.

Schmid, K. Schonlebe, J. Drexler, H., and Mueck-Weymann, M. (2010). 'Associations between overweight, variability in heart rate, and well-being in the young men' *Cardiology of the Young,* 20, 54-59.

Sekine, M. Izumi, I. Yagagami, T., and Kagamimori, S. (2001). 'Obesity and cardiac nerve activity in healthy children: Results of the toyama birth cohort study' *Environmental Health and Preventive Medicine,* 6 (3), 149-153.

Shephard, R. (2003). 'Limitations to the measurement of habitual physical activity by questionnaires' *British Journal of Sports Medicine,* 37, 197-206.

Shi, X. Stevens, G. Foresman, B. Stern, S, and Raven, P. (1995). 'Autonomic nervous system control of the heart: Endurance exercise training' *Medicine and Science in Sports and Exercise,* 27, 1406-1413.

Silvetti, M. Drago, F., and Ragonese, P. (2001). 'Heart rate variability in healthy children and adolescents is partially related to age and gender' *International Journal of Cardiology,* 81, 169-174.

Sinnreich, R. Kark, J. Fiedlander, Y. Sapoznikov, D., and Luria M. (1998). 'Five minute recordings of heart rate variability for population studies: Repeatability and age-sex characteristics' *Heart,* 80, 156-162.

Sloan, R. Huang, MH. McCreath, H. Sidney, S. Lui, K. Williams, D., and Seeman, T. (2008). 'Cardiac autonomic control and the effects of age, race, and sex: The CARDIA study' *Autonomic Neuroscience: Basic and Clinical,* 139, 78-85.

Spiegelman, B., and Flier, J. (2001). 'Obesity and the regulation of energy balance' *Cell,* 104, 531-543.

Stein,P, K., and Kleiger, R, E. (1999). 'Insights from the study of heart rate variability' *Annual Review Medicine,* 50, 249-261.

Tanaka, H. Hyllienmark, L. Thulesius, O. Brisma, T. Ludvigsson, J. Ericson, M.O. Lindblad, L.E., and Tamai, H. (1998). 'Autonomic function in children with type 1 diabetes mellitus' *Diabetic Medicine,* 15, 402-411.

Task Force of the European Society of Cardiology and the North American Society of Pacing Electrophysiology European Heart journal (1996). 'Heart rate variability' *European Heart Journal,* 12, 354-381.

Tudor-Locke, C. Williams, J. Reis, J., and Pluto, D. (2004). 'Utility of pedometers for assessing physical activity: Construct validity' *Journal of Sports Medicine,* 34 (5), 281-291.

Trost, S. (2007). 'State of the Art Reviews: Measurement of physical activity in children and adolescents' *American Journal of Lifestyle Medicine,* 1, 299.

Umetani, K. Singer, D. McCraty, R., and Atkinson, M. (1998). 'Twenty-four hour time domain heart rate variability and heart rate: Relations to age and gender over nine decades' *Journal for American College of Cardiology,* 31, 593-601.

Vanderlei, L. Pastre, C. Junior, I., and Godoy, M. (2010). 'Fractal correlation of heart rate variability in obese children' *Autonomic Neuroscience: Basic and Clinical,* 155, 125-129.

Wang, X. Thayer, J. Treiber, F., and Snieder, H. (2005). 'Ethnic differences and Heritability of heart rate variability in African-and European American youth' *The American Journal of Cardiology,* 96 (8), 1166-1172.

Washburn, R. Goldfield, S. Smith, K., and McKinlay, J. (1990). 'The validity of self-reported exercise-induced sweating as a measure of physical activity' *American Journal of Epidemiology,* 132 (1), 107-113.

Winsley, R.J. Armstrong, N. Bywater, K., and Fawkner, S.G. (2003). 'Reliability of heart rate variability measures at rest and during light exercise in children' *British Journal of Sports Medicine,* 37 (6), 550.

Yakinci, C. Mungen, B. Karabiber, H. Tayfun, M., and Evereklioglu, C. (2000). 'Autonomic nervous system functions in obese children' *Brain and Development,* 22, 151-153.

Yutaka, A,J., Saul,P., Albreicht,L., Hartley, H., Leonard, S,L., Cohen, R,J., and Colucci, W.S. (1989). 'Modulation of cardiac autonomic activity during and immediately after exercise.' *American Journal of Physiology,* 256, H132–H136.

Zion, A. Bond, V. Adams, R. Williams, D. Fullilove, R. Sloan, R. Bartels, M. Downey, J., and De Meersman, R. (2003). 'Low arterial compliance in young African-American males' *American Journal of Physiology in Heart and Circulatory Physiology,* 285, 457-462.

In: Reviews in Pediatric Exercise Science
Editor: Michael Duncan, pp. 161-180
ISBN: 978-1-61470-978-7

Chapter XI

Thermoregulation in Children and Adolescents

Michael J. Price
Coventry University, UK.

Introduction

The ability to undertake prolonged exercise in the heat has long been of interest to physiologists. Of the many limiting factors to exercise performance, body temperature responses in both cool and hot conditions in particular have been the subject of considerable interest. Research in this area has examined the underlying concepts of heat balance within the body with wide ranging applications from marathon running (Pugh et al., 1967) and other athletic performances (Marsh and Sleivert, 1999; Myler et al., 1989) to the effects of protective clothing on vocational and military operations (Giesbrecht et al., 2007, Cheung and McLellan, 1998; House et al., 1997). More recent research has focussed upon methods to improve the ability to work in the heat such as cooling techniques (Marino, 2000), cool fluid (Lee et al., 2007) and 'slushie' ingestion (Ross et al., 2010) and populations with thermal dysfunction (Price, 2006).

Of the populations traditionally considered to be at risk of increased heat injury, research examining thermoregulation in children has received considerable interest (Falk and Dotan, 2011; Naughton and Carlson, 2008; Rowland 2008). Previous research studies have generally reported differences in thermoregulatory responses between children and adults as a result of the greater body surface area (BSA) to body mass ratio in children when compared to adults, maturational difference in exercise economy and lower sweat rates in children when compared to adults, with children thus relying more on dry heat exchange for heat dissipation (Falk and Dotan, 2011; Rowland, 2008; Shibasaki et al., 1997). These differences also imply that children absorb more heat from the environment as well as demonstrating a reduced heat loss potential which may compromise heat tolerance while exercising in thermally stressful environments (Rivera-Brown et al., 2006).

In a recent review Rowland (2008) revisited the area of thermoregulation in children during exercise in the heat. It was noted that previous literature had not used appropriate child-adult comparisons, failed to match subjects by relative exercise intensity or had involved extremes of ambient temperature. With such factors in mind it was concluded that the current literature failed to indicate differences in thermoregulatory responses between adults and children. Furthermore, it was noted that there was no convincing evidence that children were at any greater risk than adults of exercising in the heat, a view that was similarly taken by Naughton and Carlson (2008). The current review will consider the comments of Rowland (2008) in considering thermoregulatory responses from an absolute and relative exercise intensity perspective as well as considering heat injury and prevention in the paediatric population, exercise performance in the heat and thermal factors at exhaustion in children, thermoregulatory aspects of specific clinical subgroups within the paediatric population and future research directions. Where possible, existing data from studies of adult thermoregulation will be briefly reviewed in order to provide context from which the associated responses from the paediatric literature can be compared.

Heat Injury and Prevention in the Paediatric Population

Marshall (2011) presented a recent article on heat injury in youth sport. The author presented three main factors contributing to heat injury in the child and adolescent populations namely; physiological factors, exposure to heat and factors relating to social and/or behavioural contexts. The physiological reasons, as noted above, have recently been challenged (Rowland, 2008) bringing a new perspective to research design in this area, some of which will be considered in this review. In discussing the factor of children's exposure to heat Marshall noted that seventeen times more high school aged American football players were exposed to the heat during August pre season practices when compared to collegiate football players (i.e. 1.1 million vs. 65, 000, respectively) significantly increasing children's exposure time to the environment. In addition, it was noted that many children in the United States are involved in summer sports camps which would increase the potential for greater exposure to warmer environmental conditions. In light of this, an important point to consider is that some states in America have three to seven times greater risk of heat death than the United States as a whole (Centre for Disease Control and Prevention, 2005). Consequently, regional differences in heat risk and injury may be expected.

From a social and behavioural context, Marshall (2011) noted that the primary heat injury prevention strategies still remain the same as those expected for adults such as frequent rests and hydration breaks. In summarising recommendations from a range of key heat injury prevention sources the following factors were considered of key importance for heat injury prevention in children; heat acclimation, knowledge of temperature and humidity in reducing or modifying activity when these are high, frequent rest and hydration strategies, educating health care providers on heat illness and having an emergency plan, being prepared to rapidly reduce core temperature and wearing only one layer of lightweight and light coloured clothing.

Exertional Heat Injury

Nelson et al. (2011) examined the extent of exertional heat related injuries reporting to emergency departments in the United States between 1997 – 2006. Although high core temperature can present with exertional heat injuries, this particular form of heat injury does not necessarily require a large environmental load in order to occur. Patients under 19 years of age represented the largest population affected by exertional heat injury with 75% of cases resulting from performing sport or exercise and 11% from yard work. This age group also represented the population with the largest number of exertional heat related injuries from sport and exercise activities. In contrast, the older groups (40 – 59 years and 60+ years) experienced more exertional heat injuries from yard work. Consequently, sports activities pose a specific risk, especially in children and adolescents. As the data critiqued by Rowland (2008) did not necessarily show differences between children and adults in terms of their thermoregulatory responses, it is reasonable to suggest that the important factors for children in preventing heat injury may be those relating more to heat exposure duration and social and behavioural challenges. With an awareness of increasing childhood obesity and the knowledge that obese children acclimate at a slower rate than lean children (Dougherty et al., 2009), social and behavioural aspects may be considered just as important as physiological ones. This may be of particular importance where an increase in physical activity in younger populations is consistently encouraged.

Heat Stroke Deaths

Deaths from heat stroke have been examined in relation to specific locations where high summer temperatures exist such as; Japan (Nakai et al., 1999; Honda et al., 1995), Singapore (Tham et al., 1989), South Australia (Green et al., 2001) and the United States, (Centre for Disease control and Prevention, 2005; Guard and Gallagher, 2005), although not all have focussed on children. From such location specific studies the relationship between mortality and environmental conditions has been examined (Honda et al., 1991, Nakai et al., 1999). For example, Tham et al. (1989) noted that of 27 exertional heat injury cases 25 were in patients less than 30 years of age. Honda et al. (1995) noted that in children between 0 – 4 years mortality was not environmental temperature dependent whereas in children between 5 and 14 years old death rates were greater when environmental temperatures were greater than 33°C, possibly as a result of increased outdoor activities and increased heat exposure. Similarly, Nakai et al. (1999) observed that heat related deaths were most likely on days where peak temperature was greater than 38°C however, 50% of these occurred in children of four years and under. There are also data available regarding heat related deaths in children as a result of being trapped in parked cars (Guard and Gallagher, 2005) highlighting the social and behavioural aspects of heat illness noted by Marshall (2010), particularly in those of a very young age.

An important point to note here is that many countries, not usually experiencing long periods of warmer environmental temperature, can still be exposed to relatively rapid and unexpected changes in environmental conditions. Such ‘heat waves’ do not give the opportunity for natural and progressive heat acclimation to occur. More sudden environmental stresses in cooler countries may therefore be just as crucial as for those countries with habitually warm environmental conditions. Research design focussing on both one off heat exposures and more prolonged but increasing environmental temperatures should be considered, as well as studies relating to native and visiting populations.

Absolute and Relative Exercise Intensities

Rowland (2008) noted that previous child-adult thermoregulatory comparisons had not considered exercise at similar relative exercise intensities, i.e. at similar percentages of maximal oxygen uptake (VO_{2max}). When comparing thermoregulatory responses across groups demonstrating different levels of VO_{2max} the relative exercise intensity is indeed an important factor in research design and explanation of the data. For example, trained and untrained adults elicit different VO_{2max} values (Gant et al., 2004) as do participants undertaking different exercise modes such as arm cranking and cycle ergometry (Young et al., 1987; Sawka et al., 1984) and persons with different levels of spinal cord injury resulting in different amounts of recruitable muscle mass (Price and Campbell, 2003; Hopman et al., 1993). Thus, when exercising at fixed absolute exercise intensities, such as a given treadmill speed or ergometer power output, those individuals with greater functional capacities will find the exercise less stressful. Therefore, when considering physiological responses across groups with different functional capacities relative workloads are often used in research designs.

Absolute and Relative Exercise Intensities in Adults

The importance of absolute and relative exercise intensities on thermoregulatory responses to exercise was first noted by Saltin and Hermansen (1966). Here, core temperature responses during 60 minutes of cycle ergometry at 25, 50 and 75% VO_{2max} in participants with a range of fitness levels were compared. Two further participants differing in VO_{2max} but with the same body surface area (~$1.9m^2$) exercising at 52%VO_{2max} were also examined. Core temperature estimates for both rectal and oesophageal temperature were much more closely related to the relative exercise intensity (%VO_{2max}) than the absolute intensity (absolute oxygen consumption). Such responses have since been confirmed for a larger group of participants during cycle ergometry (Greenhaff, 1989) and for treadmill running using a cross sectional design of trained and untrained runners (Gant et al., 2004). Furthermore, able-bodied upper body trained athletes and athletes with low level spinal cord injuries have also been shown to demonstrate the same increase in core temperature at the same relative intensity during prolonged arm crank ergometry in cool conditions even though absolute metabolic rates differed significantly (Price and Campbell, 1999, 1997). Differences in heat production and heat loss between populations should therefore be considered in such instances. This is of particular important for child-adult comparisons in light of the potential difference in sweating and dry heat exchange responses and absolute VO_{2max} values.

Absolute and Relative Exercise Intensities in Children

Figure 1 summarizes the data from Saltin and Hermansen (1966), Greenhaff (1989) and Gant et al. (2004) for the reported increases in rectal temperature in relation to relative exercise intensity (Price, 2009). It was the aim of this section of the review to present a similar plot for child and adult core temperature data in the literature in order to demonstrate whether fundamental thermoregulatory differences exist between these populations. However, sufficient data for increases in core temperature during exercise in cool conditions over a range of intensities for the paediatric population is lacking. Recent studies have predominantly considered environmental temperatures of between 31 – 41°C (Dougherty et al., 2009; Rivera-Brown et al., 2008, 2006; Rowland et al., 2008; Inbar et al., 2004) confirming the comments of Rowland (2008) when noting that many studies have examined extremes of environmental temperature rather than cooler environments. If data from studies of children undertaking exercise in cooler environments (19°C; Rowland et al., 2008) are considered it can be seen that increase in core temperature (0.5°C) does not fit the expected core temperature increase noted for adult data. Affecting factors could include the use of rectal temperature as a core estimate and exercise duration. The latter possibly being affected by the associated thermal lag of rectal temperature measures. Future research is therefore required in order to establish whether fundamental differences exist in thermoregulation between adults and children.

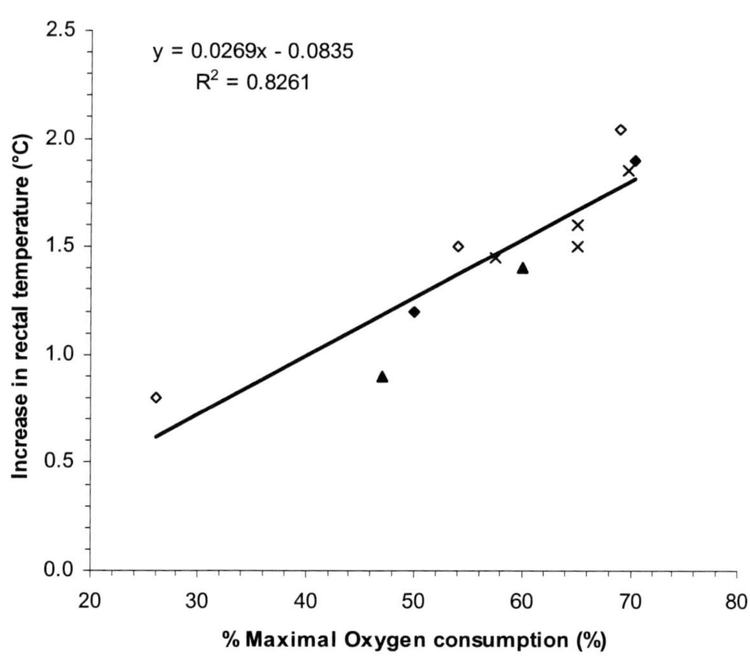

Figure 1. Increase in rectal temperature against relative exercise intensity (% $\dot{V}$ O_{2max}) during cycle ergometry and treadmill running. Data plotted from Saltin and Hermansen (1966) (empty diamond), Greenhaff (1989) (filled diamond), Sawka et al (1984) (filled triangle) and Gant et al., 2004) (cross). With permission.

Studies comparing child and adult groups that have matched participants for VO_{2max} may help to overcome differences in metabolic rate and heat production. However, where this is done for VO_{2max} values relative to body weight (i.e. $ml.kg^{-1}.min^{-1}$) the absolute VO_{2max} values ($l.min^{-1}$) will still be significantly larger for the adult groups simply as a function of body mass. For example, Rowland et al. (2008) examined body temperature responses in boys and men with similar relative VO_{2max} (42 and 40 $ml.kg^{-1}.min^{-1}$, respectively). Due to the difference in body mass (47 vs. 82 kg, respectively) absolute VO_{2max} values would approximate to 2.08 and 3.28 $l.min^{-1}$, respectively. Consequently the heat production potential for the adults at a given percentage of the maximal oxygen consumption is greater than for the groups of boys. If core temperatures between the two groups are similar at the end of exercise in the heat (e.g. Rivera-Brown et al., 2008, 2006; Rowland et al., 2008) this implies that the children produce less heat, but are unable to dissipate heat as effectively and is in agreement with the traditional view of maturational differences in sweating responses. Of course, matching child and adolescent groups for absolute VO_{2max} is not possible unless large differences in aerobic capacity are warranted. However future research considering body temperature responses in relation to absolute and metabolic rates should be considered.

Environmental Temperature and Exercise Performance

Exercise performance is significantly affected by environmental temperature (Drust et al., 2005; Parkin et al., 1999; Galloway and Maughan, 1997; Tatterson et al, 2000). For example, Galloway and Maughan (1997) demonstrated the effects of four different environmental temperatures on performance at a relative exercise intensity of $70\%VO_{2max}$ to exhaustion in eight healthy males. Optimal performance was observed at 11°C (Figure 2). Indeed, literature relating to the effects of environmental temperature on endurance performance generally considers temperatures of between 3-11°C to be optimal (Nimmo, 2004). From Figure 2 it can be seen that the 'warmer' environmental temperatures, and those most likely experienced by the general population, occur on the right hand side of optimal where there is a steep decrease in performance as environmental temperature increases.

Studies of exercise performance in a range of environmental conditions for children are lacking however, a small number of studies have reported such data. Recently, Rowland et al (2008) examined the performance of boys (11.7 years) and men (31.8 years) at $65\%VO_{2peak}$ until exhaustion in 19 and 31°C conditions. Both groups were matched for relative VO_{2max} (44 and 40 $ml.kg^{-1}.min^{-1}$, respectively). The results showed that both groups performed equally well in both cool and hot conditions; 41.4 and 42.9 minutes in cool conditions and 29.3 and 30.5 minutes in hot conditions, respectively. These times represent a reduction in performance of ~29% for both groups. When compared to the performance data in Figure 2 there was a decrease in performance of ~36% between the 21 and 31°C conditions. It should be noted though that the performance times were shorter than for Galloway and Maughan's participants who demonstrated a moderate training status (VO_{2max} 4.01 l.min-1, ~57 $ml.kg^{-1}.min^{-1}$). Furthermore, the boys and men studied by Rowland et al. exercised at a slightly lower relative exercise intensity, performing for a shorter durations of time which also suggests a lower training status.

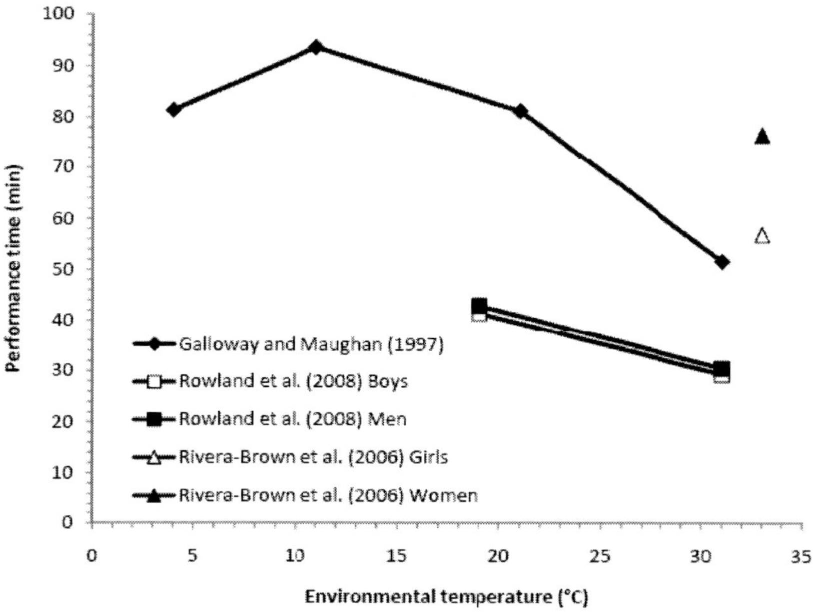

Figure 2. Performance times for continuous exercise in a range of environmental conditions for children and adults. Main figure redrawn from data of Galloway and Maughan, (1997) (filled diamonds).

Two of the many factors which may affect exercise performance in hot conditions are the training status of participants and the degree of heat acclimation (Cheung and McLellan, 1998). In accommodating these factors, Rivera-Brown et al., (2006) examined the exercise performance of girls (11.3 years) and women (26.8 years) in hot conditions. All participants were born and raised in a tropical climate undertaking 110 – 120 min of exercise per day, 4-5 times each week for at least six months and were therefore acclimated to exercise in hot conditions. The relative VO_{2max} values for the girls and women were similar to those in the study by Rowland et al. (2008) (46 and 43 $ml.kg^{-1}.min^{-1}$, respectively) allowing easier comparison of the performance data. The exercise intensity was set to 60% peak oxygen uptake with participants exercising to exhaustion. The exercise trials were undertaken on a cycle ergometer outdoors with an ambient dry bulb temperature of 33°C and wet bulb temperature of 28°C. The girls managed an exercise performance time of 56.9 min which was 25% shorter, but not significantly different, to that for the women (76.5 min). The lack of significance may be due to the considerable range of performance times observed. If, like the data of Rowland et al. (2008), we compare the performance trials to that for men at $70\%VO_{2max}$ to exhaustion we can see that the performance times in the heat for the women and girls were longer. It is possible that this is due to both the lower exercise intensity undertaken and the trained and heat acclimated status of the female participants.

Core Temperature at Exhaustion

A high core temperature (eosphageal temperature of 40.0°C, rectal temperature of ~39.5°C) has been implicated as a contributing limiting factor to endurance exercise, most likely acting on the central nervous system in a protective manner to reduce muscular activity and heat production (Hargreaves, 2008; Neilsen and Nybo 2003; Nybo and Nielsen, 2001). Rectal temperatures at exhaustion from exercise in the heat have been shown to reach ~40°C with athletes fatiguing at the same core temperature but after different durations of performance (Nybo and Neilsen, 2001). Furthermore, rectal temperatures of 41°C have also been shown in marathon runners competing in cool conditions (Pugh et al., 1969).

It is possible that the training status of participants may also determine the level of core temperature reached at fatigue. For example, the athletes studied by Nybo and Neilsen (2001) elicited VO_{2max} values of 65 $ml.kg^{-1}.min^{-1}$, fatiguing at rectal temperature of 39.5°C. Similarly, Cheung and McLellan (1998) reported core temperature values at fatigue of 39.2°C for participants with VO_{2max} values of ~60 $ml.kg.^{-1}min^{-1}$. Rectal temperature values at fatigue following exercise in the heat in less well trained groups (VO_{2max} ~53 and 46 $ml.kg^{-1}.min^{-1}$) have been reported to be 38.7 – 38.8 °C (Sabiosky et al., 2003; Cheung and McLellan, 1998). However, data from the study of Galloway and Maughan (1997) noted end rectal temperature of 40.1°C in participants with moderate levels of aerobic fitness (57 $ml.kg^{-1}min^{-1}$). These participants also undertook performance trials in other ambient temperatures terminating exercise at core temperatures proportional to the environmental temperature. Even though there were differences in the protocols used in the aforementioned studies there does, on the whole, appear to be a relationship between rectal temperature at exhaustion during exercise in the heat and aerobic fitness. With this in mind rectal temperature values reported at exhaustion in children can be compared along with possible reasons for exercise termination.

Rowland et al. (2008) observed similar rectal temperature values for boys (37.9°C) and men (38.2°C) exercising to exhaustion at 65%VO_{2peak} in 19 and 31°C conditions. During exercise in cool conditions final rectal temperatures for both groups were 38.1°C. Although not exercising to exhaustion, rectal temperature values for heat acclimated and trained boys during 4 × 20 minute exercise bouts with 25 minutes between bouts in 33°C heat were reported as ~38.0°C (Rivera-Brown et al., 2008). Following cycle ergometry at ~60% VO_{2peak} to exhaustion in 33°C conditions rectal temperatures for heat acclimated and trained girls (38.2°C) and women (38.4°C) were also similar (Rivera-Brown et al., 2006). However, the range of end core temperatures observed was between 37.8 – 38.9° for the girls and 38.0 to 39.3°C for the women. There was also a similarly wide range of performance times for the women when compared to the girls (76.4 min vs. 64.1 min). Unfortunately no analysis of the relationship between rectal temperature and performance was undertaken. Such an approach may have been revealing as it may be expected that those exposed to the heat for longer would have the greater potential for increased heat gain (Nielsen, 1996).

The reason reported by the girls and women for stopping exercise in the study of Rivera-Brown et al. (2006) was that participants 'felt it was too hot'. Three of the five girls who stated this exercised for less than 50 minutes (Rivera-Brown, et al., 2006). Indeed the rating of thermal perception during exercise was significantly warmer for the girls being rated as 'very hot' when compared to a rating of 'hot' for the women. Of the six participants stating that the exercise felt too hot five were girls and only one was in the adult group. The authors suggested that the girls greater thermal strain may have acted as a protective mechanism, preventing themselves from being overexerted (Rivera-Brown et al., 2006). In comparison, Cheung and McLellan (1998) reported that highly fit adult males who were stopped due to reaching the rectal temperature safety cut off point (39.3°C) stated that they could have continued exercise whereas males in the moderate fitness group ceased exercising due to volitional exhaustion rather than thermal factors, even though some coincidently reached the thermal cut off point. Future studies should consider both reasons for fatigue and motivational factors during exercise and thermal stress. Such studies would complement the existing literature on exertional heat injury. Rivera-Brown et al. (2006) noted that the mode of exercise may also have been a limitation to performance. Where modes of exercise have a local fatigue component, such as cycle ergometry or arm crank ergometry in none specifically trained or untrained populations, this may be the main factor terminating exercise performance. Indeed, training studies of such exercise modes demonstrate a reduction of the local fatigue component (Volianitis et al., 2004; Magel et al., 1978). Whether this would correlate with changes in reasons for exercise termination should be examined further in children and athletes.

To conclude, values for rectal temperatures reported at the end of exercise performance trials in hot conditions appear to represent the expected range of core temperatures for lesser trained adult males. However, data is lacking for endurance trained boys and girls during mode specific performance trials in hot conditions. Data is also lacking for adult male-female comparisons in terms of heat tolerance and the affect of training status to which comparison of child data can be made.

Clinical and Practical Applications

Studies of adults with thermal dysfunction or clinical populations have considered a range of groups including multiple sclerosis patients (Reynolds et al., 2011), vascular dysregulation (Gompper et al., 2010), spinal cord injury (Hopman et al., 1993; Price and Campbell, 2003) and ectodermal dysplasia (Totel, 1974). The literature for clinical aspects of children's thermoregulation has focussed upon side effects of drug treatments (Ben-Zeev et al., 2003; Nieto-Barrera et al., 2002; Arcas et al., 2001), children with burns (McEntire et al., 2010, 2009, 2006; Micak et al., 1993) and children with cerebral palsy (Maltais et al., 2004a, 2004b). Recent more applied studies have examined the thermal responses of children during water based activities whilst wearing wet suits (Wakabayashi et al., 2007) and 'stinger suits' (Sinclair et al., 2009). These aspects will be discussed in the following sections.

Drug Treatment and Sweat Gland Dysfunction

One area of thermal dysfunction that has been more recently reported in the literature for the paediatric population is hypohidrosis as a side effect of the drug Topiramate (TPM). TPM is an anti-epileptic drug which is usually well tolerated in children (Arcas et al., 2001). However, there are a number of reports of children demonstrating side effects. The studies described below are important for the exercise professional in contact with children who may be on such medication and exercising in warm environments a well as for the families of these children. However, it goes without saying that a physician's advice should always be sought prior to undertaking exercise when any medication or treatment is being taken.

The first study to report observations of thermal dysfunction with TPM treatment noted three cases of reduced sweating in children who were either newly prescribed with TPM treatment or who developed a sweating decrease whilst on TPM treatment (Arcas et al., 2001). All sweating dysfunction occurred two to three months after reaching their target dose. The three cases consisted of; a 17 month old boy presenting with daily hyperthermia up to 38.5°C which disappeared after bathing; a 9 year old boy presenting with daily hyperthermia and fatigue with symptoms which also disappearing after bathing and; a 16 year old boy presenting an inability to produce sweat during moderate physical exercise. Interestingly, the latter case did not show any symptoms during exercise in water. The dorsal foot sweat rates measured via iontophoresis in 22-24°C conditions for the first two cases were 188 and 180 sweat glands per cm^2. Once TPM treatment was discontinued (10 days and 5 weeks, respectively) sweat gland activity returned to expected norm levels of 328 and 392 sweat glands per cm^2. The authors concluded that awareness of such side effects could avoid 'inappropriate investigations or treatments'.

In observing febrile episodes relating to environmental temperature and physical activity in a 6 year 2 month old boy, Ben-Zeev et al., (2003) reported a reduction in sweat rate to 5% that expected for age matched controls. This led the authors to further examine the experiences of thirteen other patients using TPM (aged 1 to 37 years). Of these patients, nine demonstrated a reduced sweat quantity of 0.089 g per 30 minutes compared to that of 0.21 g per 30 minutes for matched controls. Of these, eight were children below 16 years old but only three had symptoms related to heat intolerance. In relation to TPM and heat intolerance, a previous study by Nieto-Barrera et al., (2002) observed the responses of children (average age of 7 years 8 months) on TPM treatment in the summer months with ambient temperature of up to 37°C. The authors observed red faces and tiredness which worsened on effort, the signs of which reduced on discontinuation of the treatment and in cooler environments. Since the above studies of children and TPM treatment related hypohidrosis, the incidence of hypohidrosis has also been reported in adults (Markowitz et al., 2010; de Carolis et al., 2003).

The underlying mechanism for the observed reductions in sweating responses are generally noted to be due to inhibition of carbonic anhydrase (Arcas et al., 2001) or the co-enzymes of carbonic anhydrase localised in eccrine sweat glands (Cerminara et al., 2006). In addition to the iontophoretic analysis usually reported electrophysiological methods have also been considered. Margari et al. (2008) undertook an electrophysiological analysis of two children demonstrating TPM related hypohidrosis. The data revealed normal function of beta and delta sensory fibres to the sweat glands but absent sympathetic skin responses, these responses though returned to normal after treatment was discontinued. These results supported previous suggestions of a transient carbonic anhydrase block at the level of the sweat gland without involvement of the peripheral nervous system.

Burns

One of the classic reports of thermal dysfunction in adults considered the loss of evaporative cooling in a participant due to a large area of healed burns scar tissue and subsequent loss of sweating capacity (Totel, 1974). Burn scar tissue reduces the available surface area for sweating and could result in reduced tolerance to exercise and thermal stress

(Micak et al., 1993). Data reported for the adult patient with burn scar tissue covering 56% of the BSA demonstrated core temperature at rest in warm conditions could be maintained, albeit at a greater level of core temperature, with greater sweat gland output when compared to an able-bodied individual (Totel, 1974).

Although subsequent data for body temperature regulation during exercise in adults with burns is lacking a case study report of responses to heat acclimation has been considered (Wingo et al., 2008), as well as body temperature regulation at relatively low levels of exercise and heat stress (Austin et al., 2003). The former of these studies demonstrated an increased heat tolerance after seven days acclimation with associated increases in sweat sensitivity in uninjured skin and reductions in heart rate and both rating of perceived exertion (18 to 14) and thermal sensation (7.5 to 6.5) on day seven compared to day one. The latter study of adults observed that moderate levels of exercise intensity (75W) for one hour in the heat (30°C, 60% relative humidity) in two groups of burns patients (33% vs. 78% BSA affected) did not show any heat intolerance. Similar rectal temperature responses to those of unburned participants were observed. More recent data has focussed upon thermal responses of skin grafts (Crandall and Davis, 2010; Davis et al., 2009; 2007a; 2007b) Studies concerning thermal responses of children with burns scar tissue are similarly sparse, although a number of key studies have been undertaken. These are described below.

Micak et al., (1993) examined the thermoregulatory responses of thirty-two children with a mean time since injury of 2.3 years and mean burns surface area of 44% BSA. During an incremental exercise test in a temperature controlled environment the children all reached the same level of endurance capacity regardless of burn surface area and without any excessive rise in core temperature. Since these preliminary findings little was reported in the literature until a series of studies by McEntire et al. (2010, 2009, 2006). The first of these studies examined children with mean burn area of greater than 40% BSA or without burns during exercise at 75% peak aerobic power for 20 minutes at room temperature (McEntire et al., 2006). Differences were observed during the later stages of exercise between burned and non burned skin in those children with burns. However, no differences were observed between tympanic temperature or unburned skin between the two groups of children. Consequently the authors concluded that there was no thermoregulatory impairment under the conditions tested.

When considering 30 minutes of treadmill exercise at 75W but in warm conditions McEntire et al., (2010) observed only three out of ten children with burns were able to complete the exercise test. However, only one of these reached a core temperature of greater than 39°C. In comparison, all the children without burns managed to complete the exercise test. Although the burned children demonstrated warmer core temperature in the first 12 minutes of exercise hyperthermia was not typically observed. A more extreme case of a boy with 99% BSA burn area exercising under the same test conditions (31°C, 40% relative humidity) completed just 12 minutes of the 30 minute test. The early termination of exercise though was not due to exertional hyperthermia, as the increase in core temperature was ~0.7°C, but rather the low level of fitness and heat intolerance (McEntire et al., 2009).

Cerebral Palsy

As with the other clinical populations noted above little research is available regarding body temperature regulation in children, and adults, with cerebral palsy (CP). This particular population exhibits a wide range of conditions which can be graded into a range of functional movement classifications (Palisano et al., 1997). With respect to body temperature regulation, children with CP have varying degrees of antagonistic limb muscle co-activation resulting in inefficient movement patterns and increased metabolic rate when compared to children without CP (Unnithan et al., 1996a, 1996b) which may affect body temperature regulation due to increased heat production.

One condition which is associated with CP is that of cold extremities, a factor which is reported more in those who are non ambulatory than those able to walk (Svedberg et al., 2008). A range of approaches have been reported in order to offset this aspect of CP including acupuncture (Svedberg et al., 2001a, 2001b) and low temperature sauna bathing (~60°C; Iiyama et al., 2008). The former observed that acupuncture may improve skin temperature in some of the children tested whereas the sauna increased core temperature by 1.0°C with an accompanying increase in skin blood flow and blood flow velocity. The latter study however was under taken in a CP group with an age range from 19 to 53 years rather than children.

Zurek et al. (2008) examined the skin temperature responses in the lower limbs in a group of children with spastic CP (6 – 16 years old) during simulated hippotherapy (therapeutic horse riding). Hippotherapy is an activity often undertaken by children with CP. It was hypothesized that the rhythmic lower leg motion may stimulate blood flow in the lower limbs which are usually subject to large temperature variability. In those children with unilateral palsy the mean healthy leg skin temperature at rest was 32.0°C compared to the paralysed leg at 30.5°C. Cooler lower body skin temperatures have previously been observed in persons with spinal cord injury as a result of reduced metabolic rate and blood flow (Price and Campbell, 1997, Price and Goosey-Tolfrey, 2008). During exercise there were similar decreases in leg skin temperature (1.3 – 1.5 °C) to approximately 30.5 and 29.2°C in the healthy and paralysed legs, respectively. In those children with diplegia, both legs were approximately 31°C at rest and again decreased by similar amounts during exercise (~0.6 – 0.8°C). The authors noted that this response was likely due to continuous vasoconstriction during exercise and decreased blood flow, the opposite of what was hypothesized. The protocol thus did not help in offsetting the cold extremities associated with the disability by increasing blood flow. However, Zurek et al., (2008) did note that the decrease in skin temperature should not exclude the use of long term use of hippotherapy in terms of psychological and physical benefits.

It is possible that simply sitting on the saddle and the action of the child's body mass could have caused occlusion of the lower limb arterial supply to varying degrees. This process could also have resulted in reduced blood flow and consequently decreased skin temperatures rather than active vascoconstriction. In a previous study Barnett and Ablarde, (1995) examined active hyperaemia of the skin overlying the ischial tuberosities after being seated on a hard surface for 5, 10 and 15 minutes. The group tested consisted of able-bodied and spinal cord injured participants as well as one with CP. All six participants were noted to demonstrate an increase in blood flow after the seating period indicative of hyperaemia. Furthermore, all participants demonstrated a relationship between the interface pressures of seating and the vascular responses. It is likely therefore, that skin temperature after hippotherapy could well have increased once the child was out of the saddle, the degree of which may be affected by the level of paralysis in CP children.

Two studies have examined the thermoregulatory responses of children with CP to durations and intensities of exercise representative of physical activity patterns for this particular group (Maltais et al., 2004a, 2004b). Both studies examined children with CP individually matched by age, biological maturity and body size. The exercise protocol involved 3 × 10 minute bouts of exercise with 10 minute recovery between them in 35°C, 45-50% relative humidity conditions. One study examined arm crank exercise at an intensity eliciting 120 – 130 beats.min^{-1} (Maltais et al., 2004a) whereas the other examined treadmill walking at an intensity of 140 – 150 beat.min^{-1} (Maltais et al., 2004b). These intensities were determined for each CP participant and compared to a carefully matched pair exercising at the same absolute intensity. During arm exercise in the heat there were no differences in metabolic rate (~0.5 l.min^{-1} oxygen consumption) or heat production, sweat losses and little increase in rectal temperature in either group. The change in skin temperature however was ~0.6°C lower for the CP children. The lack of difference between groups was suggested to reflect the relatively mild motor impairment in the upper limbs of the CP group and the 10 minutes exercise bouts not being of sufficient duration to elicit changes in core temperature. The latter may also have been a function of the CP groups' inability to exercise for a longer duration. The authors concluded that mild to moderate CP did not affect thermal or physiological responses under the conditions examined.

In contrast to upper body exercise in the heat when tested during treadmill exercise in hot conditions children with CP demonstrated greater oxygen consumption (~0.86 vs. ~0.60 litres.min^{-1}, respectively) and heart rate (~37 beats.min^{-1} difference between groups) than the control group as well as earlier and greater increases in rectal temperature (38.0 vs. 37.6°C) and skin temperature during exercise when compared to the control group. Although there were warmer core temperatures in the CP group there were no differences in sweat rates suggesting a greater reliance on dry heat exchange in this group. This was also reflected in the greater heart rate values for the CP group representing a greater proportion of cardiac output being delivered to the skin as well as the working muscles. The authors suggested future work should consider comparisons of groups representing different severities of CP.

In summary, the specific groups of children considered from more clinical populations have often demonstrated an inability to exercise in hot condition due to factors relating to fitness rather than hyperthermia. Thus, studies examining the physiological responses of these groups to aerobic training programmes are required, not just from a thermoregulatory perspective but also from functional capacity, physical activity and exercise tolerance perspectives. In addition, hydrotherapy or water therapy is often used with clinical populations and involves water temperatures of ~39°C (Gass et al. 2001). If both fitness and thermal tolerances of the groups involved can be improved this may have subsequently enhance the effectiveness or duration of various clinical procedures.

Thermoregulatory Effects of Swim Suits

Considering the application to leisure time activities, surprisingly little research has been reported regarding thermoregulation during swimming in children. Two recent studies have considered the use of thermal wet suits (Wakabayashi et al., 2007) and protective lifesaving suits in this population (Sinclair et al., 2008). Wakabayashi et al. (2006) determined the thermoregulatory responses of prepubescent children to 30 minutes of exercise at an intensity of 130 – 140 beats.min^{-1} in water of 23°C while wearing either a normal swim suit (NSS) or a neoprene based thermal swim suit (TSS). On immersion in water there was a reduced rate of skin temperature cooling while wearing the TSS with values stabilising around 28°C after 10 minutes when compared to 25°C for the NSS. Rectal temperature was also greater during exercise in the TSS trial (37.4 – 37.5°C) when compared to the NSS trial (37.1 – 37.2°C). The relationship between the children's percentage body fat and change in rectal temperature and change in body temperature was positively related for the NSS trial. However, during the TSS trial there was no relationship observed as rectal temperature was maintained. The TSS was able to maintain a warmer body temperature than the NSS which may be advantageous for children with lower body fat percentages.

In an applied field based study Sinclair et al. (2008) examined the thermal responses of junior lifesavers with and without a mandatory 'stinger suit' (SS). These suits are used to protect from marine stinger species in the waters around the north Australian coastline. The suits cover the whole body with exception of the head, hands and feet and could potentially result in greater thermal strain during beach activities in the high ambient temperatures. The exercise protocol used involved beach and water activities typical of junior surf lifesavers, undertaken in field conditions of ~27°C and 80% relative humidity. When wearing the SS core temperature increased from baseline (37.8°C) when compared to a decrease for the normal swim suit (NSS; 37.6°C) whereas skin temperatures were lower than baseline after both beach and water activities. Male core temperatures were greater than the female values for the beach activities. There were no differences in sweat rates between suits. The study concluded that the protective suits elicited increased thermoregulatory strain during exercise in warm and humid environment.

Conclusions and Future Work

In conclusion, a number of authors consider children and adults to elicit similar thermoregulatory responses. If future research supports this then it is more likely that social and behavioural aspects of thermoregulation are predominantly responsible for heat injuries. Children appear to have a protective mechanism to cease exercise in order prevent overheating, occurring at a similar core temperature to that of lesser trained adults. This is important practically as children may be exposed to environmental stress for longer than adults as a result of self selected physical activities and/or more structured leisure time activities. In more clinical populations, such as children with burns, exercise tolerance appears to be related to fitness rather than hyperthermia.

There is large scope for future work within the area of thermoregulation in children, and indeed adults, from both fundamental and applied directions. Investigations of absolute and relative exercise intensities will provide data examining whether underlying differences in body temperature regulation exist between children and adults. Although some studies have considered body temperature regulation in applied settings there is a need for examining responses to real world scenarios. Although thermal and fluid balance factors have been examined in competitive boys tennis (Bergeron et al., 1997) such scenarios are generally lacking in the current literature (Rowland, 2008). With the increased drive for greater physical activity in the children due to increases in childhood obesity studies of body temperature regulation from a health perspective are also required. Examining changes in thermal responses and exercise tolerance may aid some children to exercise for longer or at greater intensities. Consequently, the results of increased heat exposure duration whilst undertaking suitable activity patterns should also be considered. Future research should also focus upon research designs applied to thermoregulatory differences as a result of training status (i.e. sedentary children to child athletes) such as the pre acclimation observed with endurance training in adults (Schvartz et al., 1974) and optimal heat acclimation models for all fitness levels. Knowledge regarding the relationship between core temperature and fatigue in groups of differing fitness may also be expanded upon from such studies. Finally, research into water based activities will yield important leisure time and clinical applications.

References

Arcas J, Ferrer T, Roche MC, Martínez-Bermejo A, López-Martín V. (2001). Hypohidrosis related to the administration of topiramate to children. *Epilepsia*, 42(10):1363-5.

Austin KG, Hansbrough JF, Dore C, Noordenbos J, Buono MJ. (2003). Thermoregulation in burn patients during exercise. *Journal of Burn Care and Rehabilitation*, 24(1),9-14.

Barnett RI, Ablarde JA. (1995). Skin vascular reaction to short durations of normal seating. *Archives of Physical Medicine and Rehabilitation*, 76(6), 533-40.

Ben-Zeev B, Watemberg N, Augarten A, Brand N, Yahav Y, Efrati O, Topper L, Blatt I. (2003). Oligohydrosis and hyperthermia: pilot study of a novel topiramate adverse effect. *Journal of Child Neurology*,. 18(4), 254-7.

Bergeron MF, Maresh CM, Armstrong LE, Signorile JF, Castellani JW, Kenefick RW, LaGasse KE, Riebe DA. (1995). Fluid-electrolyte balance associated with tennis match play in a hot environment. *International Journal of Sport Nutrition*, 5(3), 180-93.

Cerminara C, Seri S, Bombardieri R, Pinci M, Curatolo P. (2006). Hypohidrosis during topiramate treatment: a rare and reversible side effect. *Pediatric Neurology*, 34(5), 392-4.

Centers for Disease Control and Prevention (CDC). (2005). Heat-related mortality--Arizona, 1993-2002, and United States, 1979-2002. *MMWR Morbidity and Mortality Weekly Reports,* 54(25), 628-30.

Cheung, S.S. and McLellan, T.M. (1998). Heat acclimation, aerobic fitness, and hydration effects on tolerance during uncompensable heat stress. *Journal of Applied Physiology,* 84, 1731-9.

Crandall CG, Davis SL. (2010). Cutaneous vascular and sudomotor responses in human skin grafts. *Journal of Applied Physiology*, 109(5), 1524-30.

Davis SL, Shibasaki M, Low DA, Cui J, Keller DM, Wingo JE, Purdue GF, Hunt JL, Arnoldo BD, Kowalske KJ, Crandall CG. (2009). Sustained impairments in cutaneous vasodilation and sweating in grafted skin following long-term recovery. *Journal of Burn Care Research*, 30(4), 675-85.

Davis SL, Shibasaki M, Low DA, Cui J, Keller DM, Purdue GF, Hunt JL, Arnoldo BD, Kowalske KJ, Crandall CG. (2007a). Skin grafting impairs postsynaptic cutaneous vasodilator and sweating responses. *Journal of Burn Care Research*, 28(3), 435-41.

Davis SL, Shibasaki M, Low DA, Cui J, Keller DM, Purdue GF, Hunt JL, Arnoldo TB, Kowalske KJ, Crandall CG. (2007b). Impaired cutaneous vasodilation and sweating in grafted skin during whole-body heating. *Journal of Burn Care Research*, 28(3), 427-34.

de Carolis P, Magnifico F, Pierangeli G, Rinaldi R, Galeotti M, Cevoli S, Cortelli P. (2003). Transient hypohidrosis induced by topiramate. *Epilepsia*, 44(7), 974-6.

Drust B, Rasmussen P, Mohr M, Nielsen B, Nybo L. (2005). Elevations in core and muscle temperature impairs repeated sprint performance. *Acta Physiologica Scandinavia*, 183(2), 181-90.

Dougherty KA, Chow M, Kenney WL. (2009). Responses of lean and obese boys to repeated summer exercise in the heat bouts. *Medicine and Science in Sports and Exercise*, 41(2), 279-89.

Falk B, Dotan R. (2008). Children's thermoregulation during exercise in the heat: a revisit. *Applied Physiology Nutrition and Metabolism*, 33(2), 420-7.

Galloway, S.D., Maughan, R.J. (1997). Effects of ambient temperature on the capacity to perform prolonged cycle exercise in man. *Medicine and Science in Sports and Exercise,* 29(9), 1240-9.

Gant N, Williams C, King J, Hodge BJ. (2004). Thermoregulatory responses to exercise: relative versus absolute intensity. *Journal of Sports Sciences,* 22(11-12), 1083-90.

Gass EM, Gass GC. (2001). Thermoregulatory responses to repeated warm water immersion in subjects who are paraplegic. *Spinal Cord.* 39(3),149-55.

Greenhaff PL. (1989). Cardiovascular fitness and thermoregulation during prolonged exercise in man. *British Journal of Sports Medicine*, 23(2), 109-14.

Gompper B, Bromundt V, Orgül S, Flammer J, Kräuchi K. (2010). Phase relationship between skin temperature and sleep-wake rhythms in women with vascular dysregulation and controls under real-life conditions. *Chronobiology International*, 27(9-10), 1778-96.

Giesbrecht, G.G., Jamieson, C. and Cahill, F. (2007). Cooling hyperthermic firefighters by immersing forearms and hands in 10 degrees C and 20 degrees C water. *Aviation Space and Environmental Medicine,* 78, 561-7.

Green H, Gilbert J, James R, Byard RW. (2001). An analysis of factors contributing to a series of deaths caused by exposure to high environmental temperatures. *American Journal of Forensic Medicine and Pathology*, 22(2), 196-9.

Guard A, Gallagher SS. (2005). Heat related deaths to young children in parked cars: an analysis of 171 fatalities in the United States, 1995-2002. *Injury Prevention*, 11(1), 33-7.

Hargreaves M. (2008). Physiological limits to exercise performance in the heat. *Journal of Science and Medicine in Sport*, 11(1),66-71.

Honda Y, Ono M, Sasaki A, Uchiyama I. (1995). Relationship between daily high temperature and mortality in Kyushu, Japan. *Japanese Journal of Public Health*, 42(4), 260-8.

Hopman MT, Oeseburg B, Binkhorst RA. (1993). Cardiovascular responses in persons with paraplegia to prolonged arm exercise and thermal stress. *Medicine and Science in Sports and Exercise*, 25(5), 577-83.

House, J.R., Holmes, C., Allsopp, A.J. (1997). Prevention of heat strain by immersing the hands and forearms in water. *Journal of the Royal Naval Medical Service*. 83:26-30.

Iiyama J, Matsushita K, Tanaka N, Kawahira K. (2008). Effects of single low-temperature sauna bathing in patients with severe motor and intellectual disabilities. *International Journal of Biometeorology*, 52(6), 431-7.

Inbar O, Morris N, Epstein Y, Gass G. (2004). Comparison of thermoregulatory responses to exercise in dry heat among prepubertal boys, young adults and older males. *Experimental Physiology*, 89(6), 691-700.

Lee JK, Maughan RJ, Shirreffs SM. (2009). Cold drink ingestion improves exercise endurance capacity in the heat. *Medicine and Science in Sports and Exercise*, 40(9), 1637-44.

Magel JR, McArdle WD, Toner M, Delio DJ. (1978). Metabolic and cardiovascular adjustment to arm training. *Journal of Applied Physiology*, 45(1), 75-9.

Maltais D, Wilk B, Unnithan V, Bar-Or O. (2004b). Responses of children with cerebral palsy to treadmill walking exercise in the heat. *Medicine and Science in Sports and Exercise*, 36(10), 1674-81.

Maltais D, Unnithan V, Wilk B, Bar-Or O. (2004a). Responses of children with cerebral palsy to arm-crank exercise in the heat. *Medicine and Science in Sports and Exercise*, 36(2), 191-7.

Margari L, Ventura P, Buttiglione M, Presicci A, Lucarelli E, Sardaro M, Di Fruscolo O, de Tommaso M. (2008). Electrophysiological study in 2 children with transient hypohidrosis induced by topiramate. *Clinical Neuropharmacology*, 31(6), 339-46.

Marino, F.E. (2002). Methods, advantages, and limitations of body cooling for exercise performance. *British Journal of Sports Medicine*, 26, 89-94.

Markowitz SY, Robbins MS, Cascella C, Sheikh HU, Grosberg BM. (2010). Reversible hypohidrosis with topiramate therapy for chronic migraine. *Headache*, 50(4), 672-4.

Marsh, D. and Sleivert, G. (1999). G. Effect of precooling on high intensity cycling performance. *British Journal of Sports Medicine*, 33, 393-7.

Marshall S. W. Heat injury in youth sport. (2010). *British Journal of Sports Medicine*, 44(1), 8-12.

McEntire SJ, Chinkes DL, Herndon DN, Suman OE. (2010). Temperature responses in severely burned children during exercise in a hot environment. *Journal of Burn Care Research*, 31(4), 624-30.

McEntire SJ, Lee JO, Herndon DN, Suman OE. (2009). Absence of exertional hyperthermia in a 17-year-old boy with severe burns. *Journal of Burn Care Research*, 30(4), 752-5.

McEntire SJ, Herndon DN, Sanford AP, Suman OE. (2006). Thermoregulation during exercise in severely burned children. *Pediatric Rehabilitation*, 9(1), 57-64.

Micak RP, Desai MH, Robinson E, McCauley RL, Robson MC, Herndon DN. (1993). Temperature changes during exercise stress testing in children with burns. The *Journal of Burn Care and Rehabilitation,* 14(4), 427-30.

Myler, G., Hahn, A.G and Tumilty, D.McA. (1989). The effects of preliminary skin cooling on performance of rowers in hot condition. *Excel*, 6, 17-21.

Nakai S, Itoh T, Morimoto T. (1999). Deaths from heat-stroke in Japan: 1968-1994. *International Journal of Biometeorology*, 43(3), 124-7.

Naughton GA, Carlson JS. (2008). Reducing the risk of heat-related decrements to physical activity in young people. *Journal of Science and Medicine in Sport*, 11(1), 58-65.

Nielsen B. (1996). Olympics in Atlanta: a fight against physics. *Medicine and Science in Sports and Exercise,* 28(6), 665-8.

Nielsen B, Nybo L. (2003). Cerebral changes during exercise in the heat. *Sports Medicine,* 33(1), 1-11.

Nelson NG, Collins CL, Comstock RD, McKenzie LB. (2011). Exertional heat-related injuries treated in emergency departments in the U.S., 1997-2006. *American Journal of Preventive Medicine*, 40(1), 54-60.

Nieto-Barrera M, Nieto-Jiménez M, Candau R, Ruiz del Portal L. (2002). Anhidrosis and hyperthermia associated with treatment with topiramate. *Revista de Neurologia,* 34(2), 114-6.

Nimmo M. (2004). Exercise in the cold. *Journal of Sports Sciences*, 22(10), 898-915.

Nybo, L. and Nielsen, B. (2001). Hyperthermia and central fatigue during prolonged exercise in humans. *Journal of Applied Physiology*, 91, 1055-60.

Parkin JM, Carey MF, Zhao S, Febbraio MA. (1999). Effect of ambient temperature on human skeletal muscle metabolism during fatiguing submaximal exercise. *Journal of Applied Physiology*, 86(3), 902-8.

Palisano R, Rosenbaum P, Walter S, Russell D, Wood E, Galuppi B. (1997). Development and reliability of a system to classify gross motor function in children with cerebral palsy. *Developmental Medicine and Child Neurology*, 39(4), 214-23.

Price, M.J. (2009). 'The effects of absolute exercise intensity on core temperature responses of athletes with a spinal cord injury. In '*Body Temperature Regulation'*, Austin B. Cisneros and Bryan L. Goins (eds) Nova Biomedical Books Inc, New York., 227-241.

Price, M.J. (2006). Thermoregulation during Exercise in Individuals with Spinal Cord Injuries. *Sports Medicine*, 36(10), 863-879.

Price MJ, Campbell IG. (2003) Effects of spinal cord lesion level upon thermoregulation during exercise in the heat. *Medicine and Science in Sports and Exercise*, 35(7), 1100 – 1107.

Price MJ, Campbell IG. (1999). Thermoregulatory responses of able-bodied, paraplegic and a tetraplegic athlete at rest, during prolonged upper body exercise and during passive recovery. *Spinal Cord,* 37, 772-779.

Price MJ, Campbell IG. (1997). Thermoregulatory responses of able-bodied and paraplegic athletes to prolonged upper body exercise. *European Journal of Applied Physiology*, 76, 552-560.

Price MJ, Goosey-Tolfrey VL, (2008). Heat Flow of the paraplegic and Able-bodied lower limb during resting heat exposure. *Journal of Thermal Biology*, 33, 255-260.

Pugh LG, Corbett JL, Johnson RH. (1967). Rectal temperatures, weight losses, and sweat rates in marathon running. *Journal of Applied Physiology*, 23(3), 347-52.

Reynolds LF, Short CA, Westwood DA, Cheung SS. (2011). Head pre-cooling improves symptoms of heat-sensitive multiple sclerosis patients. *Canadian Journal of Neurological Science*, 38(1), 106-11.

Rivera-Brown AM, Ramírez-Marrero FA, Wilk B, Bar-Or O. (2008). Voluntary drinking and hydration in trained, heat-acclimatized girls exercising in a hot and humid climate. *European Journal of Applied Physiology*, 103(1), 109-16.

Rivera-Brown AM, Rowland TW, Ramírez-Marrero FA, Santacana G, Vann A. (2006). Exercise tolerance in a hot and humid climate in heat-acclimatized girls and women. *International Journal of Sports Medicine*, 27(12), 943-50.

Ross, M.L., Garvican, L.A,, Jeacocke, N.A., Laursen, P.B., Abbiss, C.R., Martin, D.T., Burke, L.M. 2010. Novel Pre-Cooling Strategy Enhances Time Trial Cycling In the Heat. *Medicine and Science in Sports and Exercise*. [Epub ahead of print].

Rowland T. (2008). Thermoregulation during exercise in the heat in children: old concepts revisited. *Journal of Applied Physiology*, 105(2), 718-24.

Rowland T, Hagenbuch S, Pober D, Garrison A. (2008). Exercise tolerance and thermoregulatory responses during cycling in boys and men. *Medicine and Science in Sports and Exercise*, 40(2), 282-7.

Saboisky, J., Marino, F.E., Kay, D. and Cannon, J. (2003). Exercise heat stress does not reduce central activation to non-exercised human skeletal muscle. *Experimental Physiology,* 88, 783-90.

Saltin B, Hermansen L. (1966). Esophageal, rectal, and muscle temperature during exercise. *Journal of Applied Physiology*. 21(6), 1757-62.

Sawka MN, Pimental NA, Pandolf KB. (1984). Thermoregulatory responses to upper body exercise. *European Journal of Applied Physiology and Occupational Physiology*, 52(2), 230-4.

Schvartz E, Magazanik A, Glick Z. (1974). Thermal responses during training in a temperature climate. *Journal of Applied Physiology*, 36(5), 572-576.

Shibasaki M, Inoue Y, Kondo N, Iwata A. (1997). Thermoregulatory responses of prepubertal boys and young men during moderate exercise. *European Journal of Applied Physiology and Occupational Physiology*, 75(3), 212-8.

Sinclair WH, Crowe MJ, Spinks WL, Leicht AS. (2008). Thermoregulatory responses of junior lifesavers wearing protective clothing. *Journal of Science and Medicine in Sport,* 11(6), 542-8.

Svedberg LE, Englund E, Malker H, Stener-Victorin E. (2008). Parental perception of cold extremities and other accompanying symptoms in children with cerebral palsy. *European Journal of Pediatric Neurology*, 12(2), 89-96.

Svedberg LE, Nordahl UE, Lundeberg TC. (2001a). Effects of acupuncture on skin temperature in children with neurological disorders and cold feet: an exploratory study. *Complementary Therapies in Medicine*, 9(2), 89-97.

Svedberg L, Nordahl G, Lundeberg T. (2001b). Effects of acupuncture on skin temperature in children with neurological disorders and cold feet. *Developmental Medicine and Child Neurology*, 43(5), 358-60.

Tatterson AJ, Hahn AG, Martin DT, Febbraio MA. (2000). Effects of heat stress on physiological responses and exercise performance in elite cyclists. *Journal of Science and Medicine in Sport*, 3(2), 186-93.

Tham MK, Cheng J, Fock KM. (1989). Heat stroke: a clinical review of 27 cases. *Singapore Medical Journal*, 30(2), 137-40.

Totel GL. (1974). Physiological responses to heat of resting man with impaired sweating capacity. *Journal of Applied Physiology*, 37(3), 346-52.

Unnithan VB, Dowling JJ, Frost G, Volpe Ayub B, Bar-Or O. (1996a). Cocontraction and phasic activity during GAIT in children with cerebral palsy. *Electromyography and Clinical Neurophysiology*, 36(8), 487-94.

Unnithan VB, Dowling JJ, Frost G, Bar-Or O. (1996b). Role of cocontraction in the O_2 cost of walking in children with cerebral palsy. *Medicine and Science in Sports and Exercise*, 28(12), 1498-504.

Volianitis S, Yoshiga CC, Nissen P, Secher NH. (2004). Effect of fitness on arm vascular and metabolic responses to upper body exercise. *American Journal of Heart and Circulatory Physiology*, 286(5), H1736-41.

Wakabayashi H, Kaneda K, Okura M, Nomura T. (2007). Insulation and body temperature of prepubescent children wearing a thermal swimsuit during moderate-intensity water exercise. *Journal of Physiological and Anthropology*, 26(2), 179-83.

Wingo JE, Low DA, Keller DM, Davis SL, Kowalske KJ, Purdue GF, Hunt JL, Crandall CG. (2008). Heat acclimation of an adult female with a large surface area of grafted skin. *Journal of Burn Care Research*, 29(5),848-51.

Young AJ, Sawka MN, Epstein Y, Decristofano B, Pandolf KB. (1987). Cooling different body surfaces during upper and lower body exercise. *Journal of Applied Physiology*. 63(3), 1218-23.

Zurek G, Dudek K, Pirogowicz I, Dziuba A, Pokorski M. (2008). Influence of mechanical hippotherapy on skin temperature responses in lower limbs in children with cerebral palsy. *Journal of Physiology and Phamacology*, 59 Suppl 6, 819-24.

In: Reviews in Pediatric Exercise Science
Editor: Michael Duncan, pp. 181-199
ISBN: 978-1-61470-978-7

Chapter XII

Injuries in Sport among Children and Adolescents

Sheila Leddington Wright and Andrew King
Coventry University, UK.

Introduction

Sporting injuries occur among children and adolescents just as among adults, but there are important differences in the rate of incidence, the nature of the injuries, and the recovery afterwards. This chapter will examine the evidence as it currently stands in relation to the incidence of different types of sporting injuries in young people, noting the lack of authoritative evidence for the UK. It will divide injuries into the acute and traumatic on the one hand – contusions, bruises, sprains, lacerations and fractures – and the overuse injuries on the other. Traumatic acute injuries have a definite onset and occur after large tensile, load or impact forces cause tissue failure or breakdown. In contrast, overuse injuries result from repetitive low loading, and often have no specific onset. Skeletally immature athletes are different from their adult counterparts mainly because of the different physiology and biomechanics in immature bone. These differences mean different points of weakness compared to those in the adult musculoskeletal system. Common overuse injuries in children include osteochondroses such as Osgood-Schlatter's syndrome, anterior knee problems, and bony problems such as fractures of the lumbar spine or spondylolisthesis. Although the literature is sparse, the chapter will review any evidence on the effectiveness of rehabilitation and prevention strategies in relation to these injuries. Some short case studies will illustrate how young athletes often react to injury and present to coaches, parents, and medical and sports injury professionals. The chapter will conclude with some points regarding assessment, and the roles of coaches and parents in detecting and preventing injuries, noting that it is necessary to take measures to confirm the presence or absence of less common pathologies that would need further investigation. Any pain in a young athlete that lasts more than a few weeks requires detailed assessment, investigation and analysis.

For the purposes of research and surveillance studies it is easiest to define young people in terms of age (for example under 18, or under 16), but it is more appropriate to define young people in terms of their physiological development. Adolescents before puberty have characteristic physiology that differs from that of adults, whereas under-18s who have completed puberty tend to incur injuries similar to those of adult sportsmen and women (Hawkins, and Metheny, 2001). Children may be defined as under-10s, but again it might be better to define them in terms of their development, as in the state of their bony growth, and epiphyseal distinction. For example, in this field of paediatric injuries Haywood and Boyce (1996) define children as 'all individuals prior to the age of skeletal maturity', although this could include some males up to the age of 25!

Relevant Physiology

The necessity for longitudinal bone growth during human development, and for growth in response to the stresses of exercise and weight-bearing, requires that at birth long bones bear little resemblance to the adult skeleton. During gestation the bones are initially cartilaginous, and at birth the long bones are only beginning to ossify at the shaft (diaphysis). At each end there are one or more cartilaginous centres (the epiphysis or epiphyses) which then also start to ossify. Until maturation of the skeleton, longitudinal growth is provided by the epiphyseal end plates lying between the primary and secondary centres of ossification. The developing growth cartilage at the end plates is weaker than bone, and less able to resist forces, so that the epiphyses at the sites of muscular attachment are particularly prone to microtrauma (Martini and Nath, 2009). 'The same strain that might cause tendon, ligament, capsule, or bone damage in an adult is likely to cause epiphyseal or apophyseal damage in a child.' (Haywood and Boyce, 1996) The end plates only disappear when the epiphysis fuses to the shaft at the end of adolescence (usually in the late teens or early twenties). On average girls mature physiologically two years earlier than boys, although there is wide variation in the ages at which different bones and different individuals completely ossify. The adolescent growth spurt is usually greatest between 11 and 13 years in girls, and 13 and 15 years in boys. Girls tend to reach their maturity in height at about 15, while males continue to grow, often until the mid-20s (Hawkins and Metheny, 2001). Bone growth continues throughout childhood and adolescence, with the pelvis and wrist enlarging until the age of 25 (Martini and Nath, 2009).

Biomechanically the variance in the timing of limb growth – in both length and mass – means that there are differences in the limb moments of inertia in each individual. This in turn results in a variety of body and limb performances, which again alters in each sport and even in particular manoeuvres such as tackles (Hawkins and Metheny, 2001). The changes in length and tissue strength in response to stress can lead to marked increases in the stresses on bone and the attachments to bone. The stresses of bone growth can also be manifest in some pathologies associated with growth, such as the development of a spinal scoliosis or Scheuermann's syndrome. The gender differences in the growth spurt, and advances in its timing over the last century, indicate that there are both nutritional and hormonal influences on body and bony changes (Martini and Nath, 2009), as well as the effects of exercise and prolonged posture.

Simultaneously soft tissues such as muscle, ligaments, and joint capsules adapt in response to the stretch put on them by the lengthening skeleton, and to the increased muscular demands necessary to move the longer and heavier limb levers. At times the growth spurt in the skeleton requires a remarkable lengthening of the musculo-tendinous component, which may result in areas of tightness. This tightness is thought to be a critical factor in overuse injuries (Hawkins and Metheny, 2001). As bones grow in length and mass, muscular adaptation does not always keep pace, and muscles may have to work at nearer their current maximum force to achieve the same functional movements (Hawkins and Metheny 2001). Muscle mass increases at varying rates along with weight from birth through adolescence. The rate of muscle mass increase in boys peaks at puberty. Girls do not experience this same peak in the rate of muscle mass increase. The total muscle mass peaks in girls between 16 and 20 years, and in boys between 18 and 25 (Martini and Nath, 2009).

The modern phenomena of obesity and type 2 diabetes in adolescence can also impact on the incidence of recreational and sporting injuries, although their effects are difficult to quantify, and are not so obvious in the sporting population. Some obese individuals starting sport have particular musculo-skeletal patterns which can predispose them to injury. For example, the combination of flat feet, valgus knees and weak hip extensors and abductors, combined with the weight overload, can create excessive stresses at the knee, leading to anterior knee pain and pathology (McConnell, 1996). However, this is a growing area of interest, since it is important to encourage participation in sport and exercise in young people particularly with a view to preventing obesity and type 2 diabetes (Hardman and Stensel, 2009).

The physiological responses of the immature athlete to the stresses and strains of exercise are in many ways similar to those of the adult. However, microtrauma that in the adult results in ligament damage or tendinopathies, in the skeletally immature tends to involve the epiphyses of the bone. This can have effects on length, width, rotation, and shape, impacting in turn on joint alignment. In most young athletes conditions are self-limiting, in part as a result of the faster rate of healing in childhood, but in some individuals the conditions may cause "substantial lifelong disability" (Ecklund and Jaramillo, 2002).

Incidence and Prevalence

What injuries occur among young athletes, and how often, are questions fraught with difficulty. The incidence of different kinds of sporting injuries among young people forms a subject with its own challenges of definition and measurement. Evidence on incidence is sporadic, and certainly not systematic. A recent review of the literature by Caine *et al.* (2006) remarked on the lack of standardised epidemiological data, and the difficulties in making comparisons between studies. Goldberg's study (2007) identified the problems in surveillance studies as follows: defining 'sports injury', classifying the injuries reported, and the methods of data collection. Definitions of 'child', 'youth', 'adolescent', and 'young athlete' vary from study to study. In addition the ways of measuring the incidence (numbers of injuries per match hours, per hours of training and competition, per exposures as in the number of competitions or training sessions, or simply per year) and the risk of incurring an injury (per hour of exposure including training, per hour of competition, or per year) vary between studies, and are sometimes not specified. Methods for carrying out incidence surveillance studies have not been agreed (Goldberg *et al.,* 2007).

Whilst there is research from a range of countries around the world, the variations in popularity of different sports around the world makes generalisation from individual studies quite difficult. For example, the literature relating to American high school sporting injuries is dominated by American football, wrestling, basketball and ice-hockey (e.g. Hutchinson and Nasser, 2000, Centers for Disease Control and Prevention, 2006). Indeed the census of sports-related injuries in US high school athletes only looked at nine sports: baseball, football and wrestling for boys, softball and volleyball for girls, and basketball and soccer for both boys and girls (Centers for Disease Control and Prevention, 2006). By contrast the European literature is dominated by soccer. A recent study of sports injuries causing fractures among adolescents presenting at a hospital in Scotland (Wood *et al.,* 2010) listed football (soccer), rugby and skiing as the sports responsible for two thirds of the total number. A Swiss study identified the main culprits for knee injuries as ice hockey, handball, soccer, downhill skiing and basketball (de Loes *et al.,* 2000). On the other hand, the prominence of ice hockey, handball and skiing would probably not be repeated in England and Wales.

There is some analysis in the literature of the types, and anatomical locations, of injuries that occur most frequently – ankle and knee being most common (e.g. Frisch *et al.* 2009). Other evidence relates to when injuries take place – in training or competition, at school or at organised sports clubs, early or late season, or, more specifically, for example, in the tackle or on landing.

The following generalisations are supported by the literature:

- risk of sports injury is smaller in the lower age groups (<10 years), no doubt due to the lower mass, lower speeds of collisions, and lower hours of organised participation (for relevant biomechanics see Hawkins and Metheny, 2001);
- risk of sports injury increases with age, in some sports reaching a peak at approximately 14-16 years (Froholdt *et al.*, 2009, Sundblad *et al.*, 2005, le Gall *et al.*, 2006, Haseler, 2010);
- as participants get older, injuries are more likely to occur in matches and competitions during contact sports, e.g. in the tackle (Cloke, 2009), whereas younger participants incur relatively more injuries in training (le Gall *et al.*, 2006);
- girls have a higher risk than boys of incurring injury as calculated from injuries incurred per hour of exposure (McNoe *et al.*, 2010, Messina *et al.*, 1999, Parkkari *et al.*, 2008, de Loes *et al.*, 2000), although boys more commonly need to seek medical advice with severe injuries;
- anatomically, the most frequent injuries occur at the ankle (see case study 1), and the knee (Cloke, 2009, Messina *et al.*, 1999, Haywood and Boyce, 1996, Frisch *et al.*, 2009, Purnell *et al.*, 2010);
- particular sports show their own incidence patterns: for example, in gymnastics common injuries are ankle and knee problems associated with landings, especially in floor routines (Caine *et al.*, 2003, Purnell *et al.*, 2010, Kirialanis *et al.*, 2002);
- in rugby there are relatively more shoulder injuries related to tackling (Haseler 2010, Junge *et al.*, 2004);

- ice hockey had a particular pattern of facial and eye injuries associated with stick use (reduced by mandatory use of full face shields) (Benson and Meeuwisse, 2005);
- taekwondo has a pattern of foot and toe injuries (Pieter, 2005);
- the sports with the highest rates of injury per 1000 hours of exposure in an international review of the literature are ice-hockey, rugby, and soccer among boys, and soccer, basketball and gymnastics among girls (Caine *et al.*, 2006);
- other sports which feature, when rates are calculated in terms of the numbers of injury per competition or training session, are cross-country running and baseball among boys, and cross-country running and softball among girls (Caine *et al.*, 2006, Plisky *et al.*, 2007);
- there is limited evidence that some injuries are more common in early season, presumably before athletes are conditioned in strength, speed or flexibility to cope with the strains of a new season, or alternatively as a result of the new levels of workload being placed on the body (le Gall *et al.*, 2006, Garraway and Macleod, 1995)

Traumatic Injuries

Traumatic and acute injuries are easier to record and to investigate retrospectively through Hospital Casualty records, visits to the school sick bay, or accident reports, whereas the insidious overuse injuries are often under-represented in such records. So, although some studies focus entirely on acute injuries, other information suggests that overuse injuries are nearly half of the total (Caine *et al.,* 2006). For example the investigation of nine sports in US high schools in the school year 2005-6 relied on injuries coming to the notice of certified athletic trainers at certain representative high schools, with the consequence that traumatic injuries are almost certainly over-represented in the results (Centers for Disease Control and Prevention, 2006). Sprains, strains and contusions as a group were almost two thirds of the injuries, and together with fractures made up 75% of the total. Of the rest there were a significant group of concussion injuries (higher in competition than in practice), mainly in American football.

The priority in the young athlete is to ensure that there are no severe injuries that require attention, such as fractures, epiphyseal complications or joint damage. For example an effusion of the knee joint may be the result of soft tissue damage, but it may also obscure a disruption of an epiphyseal plate (which could cause abnormal bone growth) (Salter and Harris, 1963), or a torn cruciate ligament. Shoulder dislocations should be appropriately investigated and relocated by a professional with the requisite level of training, since there may be tears to the glenoid labrum, which may be missed or even exacerbated during relocations by unqualified staff (Deitch *et al.,* 2003). There is therefore a need for vigilance among coaches, trainers, teachers and first aid staff. They should communicate effectively with parents about any injury or concerns about overload so as to enable effective early management such as x-ray or MRI screening.

Concussion requires careful consideration in the young athlete, since the growing central nervous system is particularly sensitive to trauma. Athletes below the age of 10 present with different symptoms from those in the adult, and recovery may be slower. Physiologically the response to cerebral swelling differs from that in the adult. The revised Sport Concussion Assessment Tool, or SCAT2, has been recommended as a mechanism to identify and monitor different grades of injury (SCAT2) The consensus statement on concussion in sport recommended that children should not return to sport practice until 'completely symptom free' (McCrory *et al.,* 2009).

Soft tissue lesions such as bruises and contact injuries rarely present to therapists or local General Practitioners, since the young athlete will recover from such injuries remarkably quickly. One complication may be the 186aximize186ion of a haematoma within a large muscle group. Good management is essential to avoid complications such as myositis ossificans (Best 1995, Jackson, 1973), which may take from 6 to 12 months to resolve (Thomas, 2009). Effective treatment depends on an appreciation of the cause of injury and the requirements for return to play. Initial treatment strategies for sprains and contusions are similar to those for adult injuries, with the proviso that healing is often quicker in the younger sports person. The PRICE strategy (protection, rest, ice, compression, elevation) is generally the first response after assessment (ACPSM, 2010, Betts, 2006). The aims of treatment are to decrease pain, 186aximize the healing process and restore normal function. Good management is required in the rehabilitation stage to ensure that progressive loading is maintained and integrated during the return to sport (case study 1). Every person and their injury is individual, and although a rough estimate can be made for a time to return to sport based on the soft tissue healing framework (e.g. Watson, 2011), such estimates will have to take into account the many factors involved, such as the severity of the injury, area of injury, individual healing rates, general health and age of the child, their lifestyle, and their outlook.

Case Study 1. Netball Player with Ankle Pain

History

15 year-old girl who plays goal attack presents complaining of lateral ankle pain preventing her returning to netball. She has an England schools trial in 3 weeks and is very anxious.

2 weeks ago in a match she turned her ankle in a game. There was no immediate swelling and she was able to continue by swapping position with the goal shooter which meant less running around. It was sore to walk at the end of the match, worsening as the ankle became swollen. She walked home with friends and spent the evening watching television.

Previous History

No previous ankle injuries
Plays netball at school every lunch break and for a club at the week-end
Has recently had a growth spurt

Aggravating Activities

Unable to run. Aches at the end of the school day.
Easing activities
Rest and bandage

General

Lives with parents who are both working

On Examination

Height 1.71 metres; Weight 62 kg; BMI 21.5
Swelling posterior ankle joint. Not hot to touch.
Active ROM equal right and left ankles
Resisted ROM equal right and left
Passive overpressure of inversion painful
Inversion stress test positive
Tender on palpation of Anterior Talo-Fibular Ligament
Balance equal with eyes open, less stable with eyes closed
Tight gastrocnemius and hamstring (bilaterally)
Stands with slight inversion the calcaneum, bilaterally.

Provisional Diagnosis

Anterior Talo-Fibular Ligament strain

Management and Treatment

Part of the problem for this young girl is the early management of the soft tissue injury. She had felt pressure to continue the game because she was a good shooter and the reserve was not a shooter. She also reports feelings of not wishing to let the team down as it was "not that painful at the time". The teacher did not examine the ankle during the game or afterwards. After injury of the ligament, the bleeding from the disruption would continue as the foot continued to be used. If she had stopped and applied ice this would have minimised bleeding. Walking home and sitting in the evening would slow the healing process as venous stasis would occur with inactivity and the leg being in a dependent position. To maximise healing she should have been encouraged to stop playing and apply ice in elevation for 10 minutes (PRICE). Being taken home in a car would have been preferable, as would resting the limb in elevation with ice applied every 2 hours for pain relief plus paracetamol. Gentle ankle exercise could have been commenced at that point. As the injury resolved through the healing stages, gradual progressive loading would have been encouraged with return to normal activity as soon as possible.

When she presented to therapy services this young netballer had thus inadvertently made the injury worse by her actions. Healing was not maximised by allowing venous stasis to occur.

Better management, initially with use of PRICE and advice on progressive graded loading, enabled this girl to attend the trial for England Schools netball. As a precaution she wore kinesiology tape as she returned to training although she had a full pain-free range of movement with good balance and muscle strength.

During her rehabilitation she was advised to maintain cardiovascular fitness with cycling, then to progress to jogging, then to run in straight lines.

General stability and conditioning was recommended, as she had experienced a growth spurt and it was possible that she had not adapted to her new height in terms of muscle control and proprioception.

Outcome and Progression

Following the initial consultation the client reported that she was much happier and understood management in the future for any similar situations. She was keen to perform better than before her injury, so in the early stages she was encouraged to shoot from a standing position.

Prognosis

Encouraging improved balance and proprioception with general strength and conditioning may ensure she is less vulnerable to lateral ligament strains. Although she was able to play and be asymptomatic, it is important for the future that her general conditioning matches her skills.

Overuse Injuries

Overuse injuries occur as a result of repetitive low loading of particular tissues. While they rarely appear during free play activities (Micheli and Fehlandt, 1992), they are on the increase as a result of children participating in organised sport. It was seen above that overuse injuries may make up nearly a half of all injuries to skeletally immature athletes (Hawkins and Metheny, 2001). In addition the very nature of these injuries may mean that these injuries cause a disproportionately high loss of time away from the sport, as well as a high risk of reinjury if not well-managed and rehabilitated. Factors contributing to overuse injuries can be divided into intrinsic and extrinsic.

Factors intrinsic to the skeletally immature athlete include the physiology of immature bone, changes in size and weight during growth, increased biomechanical stresses due to anatomical malalignment, the increased stresses associated with obesity, and psychological factors such as maturity and self-esteem. Malalignment can be due to a range of causes, such as altered foot mechanics, increased Q angle (i.e. the angle between axes of the thigh and the lower leg) and other skeletal problems such as hypermobility, genu valgus and genu valgum (summary in Hawkins and Metheny, 2001). In addition, particular pathologies of bone growth, such as Perthes' disease at the hip, Freiberg's disease of the metatarsals, scoliosis and Scheuermann's syndrome in the back, produce their own symptoms, but also cause changes in biomechanical stresses elsewhere in the neuromusculo-skeletal system. These in turn can increase the risk of overuse injury. The increased risks associated with these biomechanical intrinsic stressors mean that athletes, coaches and parents should monitor carefully when there are changes in extrinsic factors.

The extrinsic factors are changes external to the athlete, for example in training intensity, duration or frequency resulting in an increase in the loading that the neuromusculo-skeletal tissues have to bear. Alternatively extrinsic factors may be changes in equipment such as shoes or rackets, a change in role within a team, poor technique, uneven or troublesome playing surfaces, or even peer pressure. In cases where athletes are known after screening to have an intrinsic condition which results in greater risk of strain, management of training intensity and of training alterations becomes much more important. In addition such athletes need to pay closer attention to possible preventative strategies such as joint protectors, foot orthotics, or careful choice of footwear.

Sports with multiple repetitions of similar movement patterns are perhaps more liable to cause overuse injuries, such as distance running, tennis, swimming, baseball (pitching), cricket (bowling), and gymnastics (e.g. Plisky *et al.,* 2007). However, some of these sports are lacking detailed research on injuries in the younger athlete.

Overuse injuries in the young athlete tend to affect the maturing skeleton for the physiological reasons discussed above. Chief among these are the osteochondroses, such as Osgood-Schlatter's disease and Sinding-Larsen-Johannson disease at the patellar tendon of the knee, and Sever's disease at the Achilles tendon insertion at the ankle. Cross-country runners are particularly prone to medial tibial stress syndrome ('shin splints'), as well as other complaints of the knee and ankle, featuring high in sports with a high incidence of injuries (Rauh *et al.,* 2000, Plisky *et al.,* 2007).

Osteochondroses and Inflammation at Tendinous Apophyses

Osteochondrosis is an injury characterisitic of adolescents. It is thought to be due to overuse (Micheli and Fehlandt, 1992, Adirim and Cheng, 2003), but with a multifactorial pathogenesis. Osteochondrosis or apophysitis is irritation at the insertion of a tendon into the developing cartilaginous bone (apophysis). The common sites of apophysitis are the attachment of the patellar tendon to the tibial tuberosity (Osgood-Schlatter's disease), the insertion of the Achilles tendon and fascia to the calcaneum (Sever's disease), and the common flexor origin at the medial epicondyle of the elbow (Adirim and Cheng, 2003).

One of the most common orthopaedic conditions of the skeletally immature athlete under the age of 16 is Osgood-Schlatter's syndrome, a traction apophysitis of the tibial tuberosity, where the patellar tendon applies huge forces to its developing point of attachment to the tibia (see case study 2). Symptoms include pain and tenderness over the tibial tuberosity that is exacerbated by exercise, particularly on jumping, or ascending or descending hills or stairs. Although the cause remains unclear, repetitive trauma in sport is considered an important factor (Gholve *et al.,* 2007). The common ages reported for this condition are between 12-15 in boys and 8-12 in girls, with occurrence being greater in boys. This age of incidence probably relates to bony development as opposed to chronological growth. Osgood-Schlatter's syndrome is a clinical diagnosis, derived from an assessment of the history, signs and symptoms. Plain x-rays of the knee are recommended to exclude other pathologies such as infection or tumours (Gholve *et al.,* 2007), and they can sometimes identify a detached particle of bone. Other authors remark that x-ray is not usually required unless there is severe anterior knee pain with more swelling than expected, which may indicate a bony tumour (Bruckner and Khan, 2001).

There are no prospective randomised controlled trials evaluating the efficacy of treatment, so reviews have used retrospective studies (Bloom, 2004). Standard treatment is behaviour modification (generally by limiting activity), ice, protective padding and may include anti-inflammatory medication. The question arises in particular cases whether the best activity limitation means complete rest with immobilisation, or complete abstention from sport, or change to a different activity, or just a marked reduction in training. There are no prospective studies looking at such variations in dosage of rest, so the therapist, coach, trainer or parent needs to assess objectively the degree of irritation and pain reported by the athlete (and the readiness of the athlete to be honest in this regard). Ross and Villard (2003) recommend a conditioning program once the acute symptoms have resolved. There are few published reports describing the effects of Osgood-Schlatter's on disability levels of athletes beyond adolescence but one study indicates that subjects with a history of the syndrome score higher on functional disability scores later on in life (Ross and Villard 2003). Osgood-Schlatter's syndrome is self limiting in 90% of patients (Gholve *et al.,* 2007) resolving over a period of 12-18 months (Haywood and Boyce, 1996). In severe cases surgery can be used to excise detached ossicles, or fragments of bone or cartilage, and the case reports report a much quicker return to activity than in conservatively-treated cases (e.g. summary in Bloom, 2004). This raises the question of whether more of the recalcitrant cases would do better with surgery than the current conservative approach, or whether only those that are mechanically dysfunctional with positive signs on x-ray are suitable for such action.

The principles of rest, advice and good management apply to the other osteochondroses too. For Sever's disease at the heel, there is also the option of viscoelastic heel inserts to absorb shock exerted on the tendon (White, 2006), while orthotics can change the ankle joint angle and the tension exerted on the tendon and its apophysis. Some authors also recommend use of ketoprofen gel (White, 2006). In the young athlete with an osteochondrosis a progressive conditioning programme incorporating strength training, stretching and flexibility, and development of balance skills and coordination is recommended as symptoms recede (Haywood and Boyce, 1996). The nature of the condition may preclude the strengthening part of the programme before the flexibility and balance components. For the athlete (and parent, therapist, teacher or coach) the flexibility and balance components then become a focus for maintaining fun and interest, whilst normal participation in their chosen sport is not possible.

Case Study 2: Footballer with Knee Pain

History

14 year-old left-footed footballer who complains of left knee pain increasing over the past few months.

Intense ache during playing and for a few hours afterwards

Slow onset over past few months

Plays mid-field for his school team, and also in the local football academy

Has been attending more intense training sessions recently, and been practising kicking on his own.

Previous History

No previous knee injuries

Plays football every day with friends, and has played since he could walk

Has recently had a growth spurt

Aggravating Activities

Pain worse on running, jumping, squatting and kneeling, and sometimes on going up and down stairs

Easing Activities

Rest. Has tried ice pack which sometimes helps

General

One older brother who also plays football; lives with parents

On Examination

Height 1.79 metres; Weight 53Kg; BMI 16.5

Mild swelling at the proximal end of the tibial tuberosity

Tender on palpation of the tibial tuberosity

Full pain-free active and passive range of movement

Balance on right foot better than on left

Muscle strength: inner range left quadriceps slightly weaker than the right; poor hamstring control bilaterally

Tight hamstrings, iliopsoas and quadriceps

Stands with slight pronation of both feet

Provisional Diagnosis

Osgood-Schlatter's syndrome

Management and Treatment

Post-activity management – ice if painful.

Advice on reducing activity level, aiming to keep the level just below symptom production. This will change over time, so at times there will be some discomfort when testing the level of activity.

Gentle passive stretching of iliopsoas, quadriceps, hamstrings and gastrocnemius to increase length

Strengthening exercise: eccentric exercises for quadriceps to strengthen the muscle

Maintain cardiovascular fitness

General stability and conditioning

Education on activity modification/avoidance of aggravating activities.

Explain diagnosis and treatment plan and prognosis to client and his parents

30 minute sessions weekly for 2-3 weeks to ensure that the client is happy with self management; then monthly maintenance as necessary

Review after each session to continue treatment or refer as appropriate.

Outcome and Progression

Following the initial consultation the client reported that he reduced training that evening and that there was a slight decrease in symptoms during training and afterwards – he used the ice as instructed and noted the time and intensity of the training session.

Although the symptoms were managed better, following the third visit at the parents' insistence the boy consulted his General Practitioner who arranged an X-ray which confirmed the diagnosis.

Prognosis

He may continue to experience symptoms since activity does not affect the healing process of the condition. Osgood-Schlatter's will tend to resolve itself over a period of 6 months to 2 years when tibial tuberosity ossifies and fuses to the tibia.

Assessment, and the Role of the Coach or Parent after Injury to the Skeletally Immature Athlete

While traumatic injuries present their own challenges of first aid, diagnosis and treatment, the presence of an injury is at least obvious. With insidious overuse injuries there is a more gradual onset, and reporting is much more variable. Aching rather than frank pain is often the first symptom to alert the athlete, and then the coach or parent, to a potential problem. Other dysfunctions which may ring alarm bells are limping, locking (e.g. of the knee), loss of balance (around the ankle), or just a change in demeanour and the athlete's reluctance to participate in sports where previously they were very enthusiastic. It is vital to prevent a frustrating cycle of pain, rest, return of symptoms on return to sport, followed by repetition of the same stages with increasing frustration and irritation. Parents sometimes think that their child's vague slow-onset mild pain must be "growing pains" (Foster, Boyd and Jandial 2008). An active sporting child is usually irritable with the aches and pain, but goes away still very keen to continue sport. As the pain occurs more frequently and sometimes more intensely the parents worry more and the child becomes agitated, irritable or annoyed. The parents consult the General Practitioner (GP), but often by the time of the appointment there is little or nothing to see other than some tenderness around the area. The joint concerned moves freely, pain is not elicited and no other symptoms are found. The GP is understandably reluctant to investigate further and the child is told to "rest". The young athlete rests and when the ache is gone tries to return to sport but is frustrated when the pain returns. At this point a cycle emerges of seeing the GP, resting, and experiencing pain and frustration. An unknown number of children drop out of sport at this stage.

Careful attention to the history, combined with a detailed holistic understanding of the athlete's behaviour, facilitates an accurate analysis of the problem, and any potential underlying factors. The athlete's mental and emotional maturity is an important consideration when investigating the history. While under-10s may be honest in answering direct questions, they may not see the relevance of signs and symptoms not specifically mentioned, such as waking in the night, or feeling stiff in the morning. On the other hand, older adolescent athletes may be more incomplete or canny in their answers, ready to give a particular slant if they anticipate an undesirable verdict, for example being forced to rest and miss an important competition. An increase in training frequency, intensity, or overall duration can all have implications for overload. Pain during training and competition might reflect a direct mechanical relationship between the injury and the activity. However, pain on waking, symptoms of stiffness in the morning and after periods of inactivity, difficulty getting up from the floor, and warm joints, are all signs suggestive of inflammatory disease, either of joints or muscles. It is important that such symptoms are investigated further by medically trained professionals. Pain of insidious onset and/or the presence of night pain require careful assessment and testing in order to exclude potential serious pathology. The following have been listed as important indications for concern, requiring referral for further investigation:

- 'Systemic upset…
- [Indications of] sepsis or malignancy, [such as] fever, malaise, anorexia, weight loss, raised inflammatory markers, bone pain, persistent or worsening night pain;

- Abnormal growth (e.g. height and weight);
- Abnormal developmental milestones, e.g. delay in achieving major milestones, or regression from those milestones already achieved;
- Impaired functional ability (ask about play, sport, schoolwork, 'clumsiness');
- Limping (persistent or intermittent);
- Morning symptoms (other than tiredness after disturbed sleep);
- Widespread pain (such as upper limbs and back);
- School absenteeism'

(Foster *et al.,* 2008b)

Since overuse injuries are a particular area of concern in young athletes, there is a need for proactive steps to minimise incidence. A good guideline is the 10% rule, which states that no single element of training intensity, duration or frequency should be increased by more than 10% in any one week (Dalton, 1992). Young athletes are susceptible to pressure and high expectations from coaches, parents, peers, and themselves. It is therefore essential that all adults involved are aware of the possibilities for abuse, and in this connection parents, coaches and carers would be well advised to consider and observe any attitudes, behaviour and developments that may possibly indicate neglect or abuse. A set of standards for protecting children in sport has been produced in the UK by the NSPCC and the Child Protection in Sport Unit (Child Protection in Sport Unit, 2006).

Prevention of Sporting Injuries in Young Athletes

Prevention is, of course, much better than cure. In this regard coaches must monitor the growth of their charges, since growth spurts are an important predictor for overuse injuries. Pre-season conditioning and on-going flexibility training (especially for boys who have a tendency to lose flexibility between 8 and 13 years) are important weapons in the war against overuse injury (Hawkins and Metheny, 2001).

Intelligent coaches will be able to identify the presence of conditions and factors which predispose to injury. For example, hypermobility syndrome is not uncommon, and can be an important factor increasing the risk of traumatic injury in sports such as netball (Smith 2005). A Danish study found that in 12-13 year old school children hypermobility was present in about a tenth the sample, and of these half had injuries which prevented them currently participating in sport (Gyldenkerne *et al.,* 2007). An Australian questionnaire study with 200 under-16 netball players found that there was a significantly higher incidence of injuries (most commonly in the ankle, knee and fingers) among those with a higher Beighton score for joint hypermobility (Smith, 2005). A new assessment tool for people with benign hypermobility was published in 2000, the revised Brighton score (Grahame *et al.,* 2000), which should be incorporated into examination of such athletes (Russek 2000).

Prevention of injuries can cover a whole range of strategies, but MacKay and colleagues collect them under the three E's of Engineering, Education and Enforcement (MacKay *et al.,* 2004). For example, there is sometimes a need to pay careful attention to the condition of the playing surface, since many injuries are lower extremity problems associated with slipping and change of direction. In tennis, the overuse injuries like patellar tendon problems and tennis elbow are less of a problem in the younger athlete than ankle injuries (Bylak and Hutchinson, 1998). The authors of a New Zealand study into injuries in young tennis players felt that attention to the court surface, and introducing new surfaces gradually, were as important in injury prevention as the gradual introduction of new skills and gradual increase in intensity of practice (Bylak and Hutchinson, 1998). Interventions related to intrinsic factors may be just as critical. An important well-structured prospective study from Norway has provided fairly convincing evidence that a structured series of exercises as a warm-up before handball training and competitions can significantly reduce the number of severe ankle and knee ligament injuries in young sporting females (Olsen *et al.,* 2005). However, the intervention was multi-faceted, so it was not clear whether the benefits came from learning good techniques of ankle and knee stabilisation particularly on landing, from improved proprioception and joint awareness, from strengthening (especially in eccentric hamstring strength), or from the specific warm-up effects (Olsen *et al.,* 2005).

Educating athletes, coaches and parents in how to prevent and manage injuries in various sporting activities presents a considerable challenge. New research on the critical interventions in conditioning, whether in stretching, strengthening, improving endurance or coordination, may be difficult for the individual coach to access and then apply appropriately, however motivated he or she might be to prevent traumatic or overuse injuries in their charges. Where there is good evidence it is incumbent on the relevant sport's governing body to adopt findings and disseminate them via regulation and enforcement, in order to prevent unnecessary injuries.

Enforcement can come in a variety of guises, but an example would be the enforcement in rugby of the IRB rules on scrums for the under-19 age-group, such as reducing the distance which a more powerful scrum is allowed to push backwards less powerful opponents, and the banning of intentional wheeling of scrums. These rules were introduced to reduce the risk of serious spinal injuries during scrummaging (IRB, 2008). In Judo the junior age-group participants are not allowed to use arm or shoulder locks, or chokes, that are permissible in adult contests (UMA 2010).

Conclusions

Sporting injuries in the younger athlete can be very straight-forward with remarkably quick healing times, but, on the other hand, some overuse injuries can be very troublesome and long-lasting. With both traumatic and overuse injuries there is the potential to miss serious underlying conditions. In the case of traumatic injuries, good assessment and treatment can ensure that hidden complications are brought to light quickly. Good initial management and treatment (ACPSM 2010) will maximise healing rates, and minimise the scar tissue that sometimes becomes a factor in muscular injuries several years later. In the case of the overuse injuries with insidious onset there is often a much more complicated multi-factorial picture, and the treatment is similarly less straight forward. The young athlete can often be too quick to return to the provoking activities, and risks entering a frustrating cycle of irritation and pain, enforced rest, followed by reinjury on return to sport. With athletes in this predicament there is an important role for coaches and parents to motivate their charges, but also to be imaginative in formulating entertaining and effective conditioning programmes which will maintain interest during advisable reduction in participation in the preferred sport, and also help to prevent recurrence. At the same time, intelligent analysis of the factors that caused the increased stresses should lead coaches and therapists to alter intrinsic factors, for example by the use to shoe orthotic supports or by a stretching programme, so altering the biomechanical forces throughout the lower limb. Above all, the young athlete complaining of pain should be listened to carefully, and where the pain lasts for more than a few weeks, it is vital that further detailed investigation and analysis should be undertaken to exclude any serious underlying cause of the problem.

References

ACPSM (2006) *PRICE Guidelines: Guidelines for the management of soft tissue (musculoskeletal) injury with Protection, Rest, Ice, Compression, Elevation (PRICE) in the first 72 hours*. Association of Chartered Physiotherapists in Sport. (A new edition was compiled in 2010, but is not yet published.)

Adirim, T., and Cheng, T. (2003). Overview of Injuries in the Young Athlete. *Sports Medicine, 33(1),* 75-81.

Baumgarten, T.E. Andrews, J.R., and Satterwhite, Y.E. (1998). The Arthroscopic Classification and Treatment of Osteochondritis Dissecans of the Capitellum *American Journal of Sports Medicine 26(4):* 520-523

Benson, B., and Meeuwisse, W. (2005). Ice-hockey injuries. In, Caine, D., and Maffulli, N. (eds) *Epidemiology of Pediatric Sports Injuries. Team Sports. Medical Sports Science 49*, 31-61

Best, T.M. (1995). Muscle-tendon injuries in young athletes. *Clinics in Sports medicine 14(3),* 669-686.

Betts,T. (2006). 'Physiotherapy – General principles', in Narvani, A., Thomas, P., and Lynn, B., (Eds.), *Key Topics in Sports Medicine.* London: Routledge.

Bloom, J. (2004). What is the best treatment for Osgood-Schlatter disease? *Journal of Family Practice, 53(2),* 153-4.

Bruckner, P., and Khan, K. (2001). *Clinical Sports Medicine*. 2nd Edition. Sydney: McGraw Hill.

Bylak, J., and Hutchinson, M. (1998). Common sports injuries in young tennis players *Sports Medicine, 26(2),* 119-132.

Caine, D., Knutzen, K., Howe, W., Keeler, L., Sheppard, L., Henrichs, D., Fast, J. (2003). A three-year epidemiological study of injuries affecting young female gymnasts. *Physical Therapy in Sport, 4(1),* 10-23.

Caine, D., Caine, C., and Maffulli, N. (2006a). Incidence and Distribution of Pediatric Sport-Related Injuries. *Clinical Journal of Sport Medicine, 16(6),* 500-513.

Caine D., DiFiori J., and Maffulli N. (2006b) Physeal injuries in children's and youth sports: reasons for concern? *British Journal of Sports Medicine, 40,* 749-760.

Centers for Disease Control and Prevention (2006). Sports-related injuries among high school athletes – United States, 2005-6 school year. *Morbidity and Mortality Weekly Report, 55(38),* 1037-1040.

Child Protection in Sport Unit (2006). *Standards for Safeguarding and Protecting Children in Sport.* 2nd edition. Retrieved from http://www.nspcc.org.uk/Inform/cpsu/resources/publications/StandardsForSafeguarding_wda61582.html

Cloke, D. (2009). The epidemiology of ankle injuries occurring in English Football Association academies. *British Journal of Sports Medicine, 43(14),* 1119-1125.

Dalton, S. (1992). Overuse injuries in adolescent athletes. *Sports Medicine, 13(1),* 58-70.

De Loes, M., Dahlstedt, L.J., and Thomee, R. (2000). A 7-year study on risks and costs of knee injuries in male and female youth participants in 12 sports. *Scandinavian Journal of Medicine and Science in Sports, 10(2),* 90-97.

Deitch, J., Mehlman, C.T., Foad, S.L., Obbehat, A., Mallory, M. (2003). Traumatic anterior shoulder dislocation in adolescents. *American Journal of Sports Medicine 31(5),* 758-363.

Ecklund, K. and Jaramillo, D. (2002). Patterns of Premature Physeal Arrest: MR Imaging of 111 Children *American Journal of Roentgenology, 178(4),* 967-972.

Foster, H., and Jandial, S. (2008a). pGALS – A screening examination of the musculo-skeletal system in school-aged children. *Reports on the Rheumatic Diseases Series 5(15),* 1-7. Arthritis Research Campaign.

Foster, H. E., Boyd, D., and Jandial, S. (2008b). 'Growing pains' A practical guide for primary care. *Reports on the Rheumatic Diseases Series 6(1),* 1-6. Arthritis Research Campaign.

Frisch, A., Seil, R., Urhausen, A., Croisier, J. L., Lair, M. L., Theisen, D. (2009). Analysis of sex-specific injury patterns and risk factors in young high-level athletes. *Scandinavian Journal of Medicine and Science in Sports, 19(6),* 834-841.

Froholdt, A., Olsen, O.E., Bahr, R. (2009). Low Risk of Injuries Among Children Playing Organized Soccer: A Prospective Cohort Study. *American Journal of Sports Medicine 37(6),* 1155-1160.

Garraway, M., and Macleod, D. (1995). Epidemiology of rugby football injuries. *Lancet 345,* 1485-1487.

Gholve, P.A., Scher, D.M., Khakharia, S., Widmann, R.F., Green, D.W. (2007). Osgood-Schlatter Syndrome. *Current Opinion in Pediatrics, 19(1),* 44-50.

Goldberg, A. S., Moroz, L., Smith, A., Ganley, T. (2007). Injury surveillance in young athletes. *Sports Medicine, 37(3),* 265-278.

Grahame, R., Bird, H.A., Child, A. (2000). The revised (Brighton 1998) criteria for the diagnosis of benign joint hypermobility syndrome (BJHS). *Journal of Rheumatology, 27(7),* 1777-9.

Gyldenkerne, B., Iversen, K., Roegind, H., Fastrup, D., Hall, K., Remvig, L. (2007). Prevalence of general hypermobility in 12-13-year-old school children and impact of an intervention against injury and pain incidence. *Advances in Physiotherapy, 9(1),* 10-15.

Hardman, A., and Stensel, D.J. (2009). *Physical Activity and Health. The evidence explained.* Routledge: London 2nd edition chapters 2 and 10.

Haseler, C. (2010). The epidemiology of injuries in English youth community rugby union. *British Journal of Sports Medicine, 44(15),* 1093-1099.

Hawkins, D., and Metheny, J. (2001). Overuse injuries in youth sports: biomechanical considerations. *Medicine and Science in Sports and Exercise, 33(10),* 1701–1707.

Haywood, H., and Boyce, W. (1996). Knee overuse injuries in the skeletally immature athlete. *Physiotherapy Canada, 48 (3):* 190-196.

IRB (International Rugby Board) (2008) *U19 variations* [to the Laws of the Game of Rugby Football]. Retrieved from, http://guide.rugbyrugby.com/Rugby%20Sections/ Beginners% 20Guide/2008-IRB-U19-Law-Variations.pdf.

Jackson, D.W., Feagin, J.A. (1973). Quadriceps contusions in young athletes. Relation of severity of injury to treatment and prognosis *Journal of Bone and Joint Surgery (Am.) 55(1),* 95-105.

Junge, A., Cheung, K., Edwards, T., Dvorak, J. (2004). Injuries in youth amateur soccer and rugby players – a comparison of incidence and characteristics *British Journal of Sports Medicine 38(2),* 168-172.

Kirialanis, P., Malliou, P., Beneka, A., Gourgoulis, V., Giofstidou, A., Godolias, G. (2002). Injuries in artistic gymnastic elite adolescent male and female athletes. *Journal of Back and Musculoskeletal Rehabilitation 16(4)*: 145-151.

Le Gall, F., Carling, C., Reilly, T., Vadewalle, H., Church, J., Rochcongar, P. (2006). Incidence of injuries in elite French youth soccer players: a 10-season study. *American Journal of Sports Medicine, 34(6),* 928-938.

McConnell, J. (1996). Management of patello-femoral problems. *Manual Therapy, 1:* 60-66.

McCrory, P., Meeuwisse, W., Johnston, K., Dvorak, J., Aubry, M., Molloy, M., Cantu, R. (2009). Consensus statement on concussion in sport, 3rd International Conference on Concussion in Sport, held in Zurich, November 2008. *Clinical Journal of Sport Medicine, 19,* 185-200.

Mackay, M., Scanlan, A., Olsen, L., Reid, D., Clark, M., McKim, K., Raina, P. (2004). Looking for the evidence: a systematic review of prevention strategies addressing sport and recreational injury among children and youth. *Journal of Science and Medicine in Sport, 7 (1),* 58-73.

McNoe, B. M., Chalmers, D. J. (2010). Injury in Community-Level Soccer. *American Journal of Sports Medicine, 38(12),* 2542-2551.

Messina, D.F., Farney, W.C., DeLee, J.C. (1999). The Incidence of injury in Texas high school basketball: a prospective study among male and female athletes. *American Journal of Sports Medicine, 27(3),* 294-299.

Micheli, L.J., and Fehlandt, A.F. (1992). Overuse injuries to tendons and apophyses in children and adolescents. *Clinics in Sports Medicine, 11(4),* 713-26.

Olsen, O., Myklebust, G., Engebretsen, L., Holme, I., Bahr, R. (2005). Exercises to prevent lower limb injuries in youth sports: cluster randomised trial. *British Medical Journal, 330,* 449-452.

Parkkari, J., Pasanen, K., Mattila, V. M., Kannus, P., Rimpelä, A. (2008). The risk for a cruciate ligament injury of the knee in adolescents and young adults: a population-based cohort study of 46 500 people with a 9 year follow-up. *British Journal of Sports Medicine, 42(6*), 422-426.

Pieter, W. (2005). Martial Arts Injuries. In, Caine, D., and Maffulli, N. (Eds) *Epidemiology of Pediatric Sports Injuries. Individual Sports. Medicine and Sport Science 48,* 59-73.

Plisky, M., Rauh, M., Heiderscheit, B., Underwood, F., Tank, R. (2007). Medial tibial stress syndrome in high school cross-country runners: incidence and risk factors. *Journal of Orthopaedic and Sports Physical Therapy, 37(2),* 40-47.

Purnell, M., Shirley, D., Nicholson, L., Adams, R. (2010). Acrobatic gymnastics injury: Occurrence, site and training risk factors. *Physical Therapy in Sport, 11(2):* 40-46.

Rauh, M.J., Margherita, A.J., Rice, S.G., Koepsell, T.D., Rivara, F.P. (2000). High school cross country running injuries: a longitudinal study. *Clinical Journal of Sport Medicine, 10,* 110-116.

Ross, M., and Villard, D. (2003). Disability levels of college-aged men with a history of Osgood-Schlatter disease. *Journal of Strength and Conditioning Research, 17(4),* 659-663.

Russek, L. (2000). Examination and Treatment of a Patient with Hypermobility Syndrome. *Physical Therapy, 80(4)*, 386-398.

Salter, R., and Harris, W.R. (1963). Injuries involving the epiphyseal plate. *Journal of Bone and Joint Surgery, 45,* 587-622.

Smith, R., Damodaran, A., Swaminathan, S., Campbell, R., Barnsley, L. (2005). Hypermobility and sports injuries in junior netball players. *British Journal of Sports Medicine, 39(9),* 628-631.

SCAT2 (2008). *Sport Concussion Assessment Tool 2.* Retrieved from, http://links.lww.com/JSM/A11.

Sundblad, G., Saartok, T., Engstrom, L-M., Restrom, P. (2005). Injuries during physical activity in school children. *Scandinavian Journal of Medicine and Science in Sports, 15(5),* 313-323.

Thomas, P. (2006). Paediatrics - Sports Medicine. In, Narvani, A.A., Thomas, P., and Lynn, B. (Eds.) *Key Topics in Sports Medicine.* London: Routledge.

UMA (2010). *Judo Ne Waza Rules and Regulations.* Retrieved from, http://www.umauk.co.uk/UMA_Event_Rules,%20Regulations_Divisions_and_Brackets_in_PDF_Format/UMA_Judo_Ne-Waza_Rules.pdf.

Verhagen, E. (2009). A prospective cohort study on physical activity and sports-related injuries in 10–12-year-old children. *British Journal of Sports Medicine, 43(13),* 1031-1035.

Verhagen, E. A., Chin A.P., Marijke, J.M., van Mechelen, W., Collard, D.C.M. (2008). Acute physical activity and sports injuries in children. *Applied Physiology, Nutrition and Metabolism, 33(2),* 393-400.

Watson, T. (2011). *Tissue Repair.* Retrieved from, http://www.electrotherapy. org/ modalities/tissuerepair.htm

White, R.L. (2006). Ketoprofen gel as an adjunct to physical therapist management of a child with Sever's disease. *Physical Therapy, 86(3),* 424-433 .

Wojciechowski, M. (2007). Working with kids: physical therapy and the pediatric athlete. *Physical Therapy Magazine,* March 2007, 52-58.

Wood, A., Robertson, G., Rennie, L., Caesar, B., Court-Brown, C. (2010). The epidemiology of sports-related fractures in adolescents. *Injury, 41(8),* 834-838.

In: Reviews in Pediatric Exercise Science
Editor: Michael Duncan, pp. 201-215
ISBN: 978-1-61470-978-7

Chapter XIII

Sprinting and Plyometric Ability in Youths: The Effect of Natural Development and Training

***Michael G. Hughes*[1]*, Rhodri Lloyd*[2] *and Robert Meyers*[1]**
[1] University of Wales Institute Cardiff, Cardiff, UK.
[2] University of Gloucestershire, UK.

Introduction

It is established that children and adolescents, defined here as individuals up to the age of 18 years (Faigenbaum et al., 2009), often perform activity in bursts of high intensity exercise interspersed with rest (Ratel, Bedu, Hennegrave, Doré, and Duché, 2004). Such intermittent activity is also characteristic of many sports (Glaister, 2005) and is likely to be crucial to competitive success in racket sports, court sports and field sports (Doré et al., 2005). Additionally, underlying components of high-intensity exercise performance such as strength, speed and stretch-shortening cycle characteristics are developed in childhood and become crucial determinants of exercise capacities in adulthood. The development of plyometric ability, sprint speed and strength tends to occur naturally as infants develop into adults but these aspects of physical performance are also increased by physical training. The purpose of this chapter is to discuss the development of aspects of explosiveness in children and adolescents (i.e., youths). The development of strength in this way has been reviewed elsewhere (Faigenbaum et al., 2009) so the focus here is to review the effects of maturation, development and training on sprinting and plyometric ability in youths.

Sprinting in Youths

Introduction to Sprinting

Forward locomotion in humans may be categorized into walking, running and sprinting. Each of these categories of locomotion represents the optimal movement strategy through progressively increasing movement velocities. Walking may be distinguished from other forms of forward locomotion by periods of double support (both feet in contact with the ground) during the stance phase of the gait cycle (Novacheck, 1998). The progressive increase in velocity experienced through running and sprinting results in periods of 'double-float', where both feet are simultaneously in the air. A distinction between running and sprinting may be made through both the increase in velocity between the two forms of locomotion, and the nature of foot strike during ground contact. Typically when sprinting, an athlete will use a forefoot strike with the ground, in contrast to the rearfoot strike usually seen in running (Hasegawa, Yamauchi, and Kraemer, 2007).

Sprint activity is often regarded as a key element of performance in many sporting tasks (Rimmer and Sleivert, 2000; Taylor, 2003), with bouts of sprint activity often influencing the success of game specific tasks. Children and adults may show a similar prevalence of sprint performance in sports (Castagna, D'Ottavio, and Abt, 2003) and sprinting is frequently used by children during playground games and activities (Faigenbaum et al., 2009).

Despite the relative importance of sprinting, there is much inconsistency in the results of biomechanical evaluations of sprint running (Nesser, Latin, Berg, and Prentice, 1996), however, the foundation of sprinting speed lies in the interaction of stride length (SL) and stride frequency (SF) (Weyand, Sternlight, Bellizzi, and Wright, 2000; Hunter, Marshall, and McNair, 2004). It is also common to see the terms step length and step frequency (Hunter et al., 2004) used in the description of sprint performance, and whilst these represent similar variables it is important to clarify that a 'stride' is considered as occurring between ground-contacts with the same foot, while the 'step' refers to the strikes of opposite feet.

In adult populations there are well-established hierarchical models for sprinting performance (Hay, 1993) that have been the driving force in the research on sprinting and speed training to date. These hierarchical models suggest that step length is influenced by both the distance achieved during flight and distance achieved during the ground contact. The flight distance may be derived from the angle and velocity at take-off, which in turn are influenced by the application of ground reaction forces in the vertical and horizontal planes. The step distance may be considered a product of lower limb placement at touchdown and take-off from ground contact. The step rate may be influenced by the time spent during contact and during flight, with the main focus of the flight phase being the repositioning of the lower limbs for subsequent ground contact. The relative contributions of the determinants of step length and step frequency to the different phases of sprinting (Hunter et al., 2004) are still unknown, and therefore uncertainty exists on the key to optimal sprint performance.

In adult populations, faster sprinters have been shown to apply greater support forces during ground contact, leading to the attainment of higher speeds through elevated SL and SF in conjunction with reduced ground contact periods (CT) (Weyand et al., 2000). However other research highlighting the importance of improvements in only SL, only SF or both SL and SF concurrently can be found in equal measure (Hunter et al., 2004).

The volume of work exploring the development of sprint characteristics in paediatric populations is somewhat limited. However, Schepens, Willems, and Cavagna (1996) have reported similar SF and CT with children and adults, and therefore the increases in maximum speed observed with developing age were attributed to increased SL. It should be noted that these data were expressed in terms of chronological age and no consideration for maturation was made. When data from cross-sectional studies are expressed using a maturation offset relative to peak height velocity (PHV) (Mirwald, Baxter-Jones, Bailey, and Beunen, 2002) it has been suggested that longer CT, slower SF and greater SL are observed in boys pre-PHV compared to more mature boys, resulting in no significant improvement in speed between three years and one year prior to PHV (Meyers, Oliver, Hughes, Stembridge, and Cronin, 2010). These data also suggest that improvements in speed were evident around the time of PHV but only once both CT and SF stabilized, which could suggest a learning period is required for children to adapt to growth related changes before improvements in maximum speed become evident.

Natural Development of Sprinting in Youths

There has been considerable research into the natural development of speed throughout childhood and adolescence (Malina, Bouchard, and Bar-Or, 2004). However, the wide variation in experimental design has led to significant variation in the data reported (Viru et al., 1999). The majority of research has been cross sectional in nature. These cross-sectional studies have indicated that in 3-7 year olds, improvements in maximal running speed in both sexes are largely linear with advancing age (Morris, Williams, Atwater and Wilmore, 1982), however it has also been suggested that improvements may be greater between the ages of 5-8 years old, after which the improvement may be less (Malina et al., 2004). In an analysis of eight cross-sectional articles, Viru et al. (1999) also reported accelerated development in speed between the ages of 7-11 years in boys and 6-9 years in girls. In contrast, where longitudinal studies are reviewed the equivalent period for both boys and girls is suggested to be between 5-9 years of age (Viru et al., 1999). Despite the disparity in age ranges reported by different study designs, a period of accelerated development between 5-9 years years of age for girls and 5-11 years of age for boys may be termed the "pre-adolescent spurt" in motor performance (Malina et al., 2004).

Preceding and throughout the pre-adolescent spurt, similar improvements in speed are reported for boys and girls. In most cases the data suggest boys have a slightly better performance than girls (Papaiakovou et al., 2009), although most of the girls fall within one standard deviation of the boys' results (Malina et al., 2004). It has been suggested that the improvements in speed during this period are largely due to maturation of the neuromuscular system (Borms, 1986), which may include reduced co-contraction (Frost, Dowling, Dyson, and Bar-Or, 1997; Lambertz, Mora, Grosset, and Perot, 2003), improved reflex muscle activity (Grosset, Mora, Lambertz, and Perot, 2007) and improved muscle activation (Ozmun, Mikesky, and Surburg,1994). Such developments of the neuromuscular system in turn result in improved co-ordination and technique (Borms, 1986; Viru et al.,1999) which may facilitate more effective transfer of support forces during sprinting activity.

A second "adolescent spurt" in performance (Malina et al., 2004) has been reported between ages 12-15 years old for boys and 10-12 years for girls (Viru et al., 1999; Borms,

1986). Data suggest that the adolescent spurt in performance occurs at the same time as, or just in advance of PHV (Philippaerts et al., 2006; Beunen, and Malina, 1988) in both boys and girls and may also be associated with developing sexual maturity (Malina et al., 2004). In boys it has been suggested that greatest improvements in sprint speed coincide with developing sexual maturation equivalent to approximately 1.5 years prior to PHV (Volver and Viru, 1997; Viru et al., 1999), whereas in girls it may correspond to approximately 1 year prior to PHV (Szczesny and Coudert, 1993; Viru et al., 1999). After the adolescent spurt, sprint performance in girls often reaches a plateau, whilst conversely boys' speed continues to improve (Malina et al., 2004).

The difference in the timing of the adolescent spurt in performance between boys and girls seems to support that maturation is associated with improvements in sprint speed (Ford et al., 2011). In boys the mechanisms associated with improvements in speed during the adolescent spurt are thought to be related to increases in body size (Borms, 1986), the 10-fold increase in testosterone (Viru et al., 1999) and large increases in muscle mass (Malina, 1969). The influence of circulating androgen levels and the onset of the biological changes associated with female adolescence (Malina et al., 2004) may also help to explain the deviation in performance level of between the sexes around the age of 15 years.

Other factors have also been proposed as possible mechanisms for the development of speed throughout childhood. Physical increases in the surface area of the muscle–tendon junction from childhood into adulthood (Ovalle, 1987) and changes in the visco-elastic properties of the musculotendinous unit (Kubo, Kanehisa, and Fukunaga, 2003) seen throughout childhood may favour improved sprint performance. Increased musculotendinous stiffness with advancing age (Lin, Brown, and Walsh,1997; Lambertz et al., 2003) and the potential transformation of slow to fast twitch motor units (Van Praagh and Doré, 2002) may also be considered as potential contributing factors to improved sprint performance throughout childhood and adolescence. Adolescent boys have also been reported to have increased anaerobic enzyme activity and increased serum lactate levels following exercise compared to pre-adolescent boys (Naughton, Farpour-Lambert, Carlson, Bradney, and van Praagh, 2000), suggesting that increased anaerobic metabolic capacity may also play a role in improved anaerobic performance throughout adolescence.

In summary, the development of speed throughout childhood and adolescence is well reported, with evidence for pre-adolescent and adolescent periods of accelerated adaptation. The mechanisms associated with improvements in speed performance are multi-faceted with a complex interaction of neuromuscular, hormonal, metabolic and structural changes assisting in improved performance. At this stage there is insufficient evidence to identify whether the changes in performance are predominantly influenced by progressing chronological age or maturation and future longitudinal studies should look to advance the understanding of this area.

Plyometric Activity in Youths

Introduction to Plyometric Activity

Plyometric training is a common exercise mode used to develop explosive muscular power (Potach and Chu, 2008), and is becoming increasingly implemented within youth-based training programmes (Faigenbaum et al., 2009). Plyometric training is normally associated with drills such as jumping, hopping and skipping, but could also include forms of running and sprinting. Plyometric activity requires the effective utilization of the stretch-shortening cycle (SSC), which is characterized by an initial eccentric stretching of the muscle, a short isometric phase, and a subsequent powerful concentric action (Potach and Chu, 2008). This naturally occurring sequence of muscular contractions underpins most forms of human locomotion (Nicol, Avela and Komi, 2006). According to Komi (2000), a human action must satisfy certain criteria in order to be deemed a SSC, those being: (1) preactivation of the muscle before ground contact occurs; (2) a brief and rapid eccentric phase; and (3) an immediate transition between the stretch and shortening actions. In addition to these criteria, based on a ground contact time threshold of 250 ms, the SSC has been categorized into slow (> 250 ms) and fast (< 250 ms) actions (Schmidtbleicher, 1992).

It has previously been reported that a SSC action produces a more powerful force output than a concentric contraction in isolation (Cavagna, Dusman and Margaria, 1968), and a number of mechanisms have been proposed to explain this phenomenon. Storage and reutilization of elastic energy (Komi and Bosco, 1978; Cavagna et al., 1968), contributions from stretch reflexes (Komi and Gollhofer, 1997), and neural potentiation of the contractile machinery (Walshe, Wilson, and Ettema, 1998) have all been suggested as theories underpinning fast-SSC movements. Conversely, the increased ground contact times associated with slow-SSC movements have been deemed to enable an increased time for cross-bridge formation (Bobbert, Gerritsen, Litjens and van Soest, 1996; Van Ingen Schenau, Bobbert and de Haan, 1997). Therefore, it can be concluded that the most suitable mechanisms to explain the performance benefits emanating from the SSC are dependent on the demands of the plyometric task (Lloyd, Oliver, Hughes and Williams, 2011a).

Task-specificity is an important factor to consider when examining the developmental literature surrounding plyometric ability in children and adolescents, as variations in testing methods may confound our overall understanding. Previous research has measured jump heights from squat and countermovement jumps, and the percentage difference between the two (attributed to pre-stretch) has been used to quantify SSC performance in youths (Gerodimos et al., 2008; Harrison and Gaffney, 2001; Isaacs, 1998). However, such methods fail to produce movements indicative of true SSC function, primarily owing to a lack of preactivation, and the absence of a rebound (Lloyd et al., 2011a; Komi and Gollhofer, 1997). More recently, researchers have used alternative protocols, such as drop jumps (Lazaridis et al., 2010), maximal hopping (Lloyd, Oliver, Hughes and Williams, 2009) and sub-maximal hopping (Lloyd, Oliver, Hughes and Williams, 2011b) to assess SSC function. These testing protocols enable the calculation of leg stiffness and reactive strength index, measures that more closely resemble true SSC behaviour (Lloyd et al., 2009). Leg stiffness represents the ratio between peak centre of mass displacement and peak ground reaction force, which typically occur at the midpoint of the stance phase when rebounding from the ground (McMahon and Cheng, 1990). Whereas reactive strength index assesses SSC function by measuring the ratio between the height jumped and the time spent in contact with the ground developing the forces needed to execute the jump (McClymont, 2005).

Natural Development of Plyometric Activity in Youths

Previous research has shown that plyometric performance, as measured by a range of field-based tests of SSC function, improves with age (Lloyd et al., 2011b). Specifically, the research of Lloyd and colleagues demonstrated that as children become older, they utilize a greater degree of lower limb stiffness when hopping bilaterally, however the development was non-linear throughout childhood (Lloyd et al., 2011b). Significance testing revealed similar patterns of non-linear development for reactive strength index, and squat and countermovement jump height (Lloyd et al., 2011b). Additional research examining developmental issues in paediatric plyometric performance identified an age effect, stating that irrespective of the type of jump performed (squat jump, countermovement jump, or countermovement jump with arm swing), jump height increased consistently between children, adolescents and adults (Gerodimos et al., 2008). The research also stated that children's countermovement jump performance was more variable, and that this variability reduced with age. This suggests that a child's plyometric ability is likely to develop naturally with experience, as they improve their motor coordination. This notion is supported by earlier work which suggested that less mature perceptual systems, slower response times, and a reduced coordinative ability, were causes of greater variation in jump performance and vertical jump take-off velocities (Harrison and Gaffney, 2001).

Preactivation refers to the feedforward neural control strategy experienced by the extensor musculature during the preparatory phase of human movement, under both self-initiated and mechanically-induced perturbation movement conditions (Horita, Komi, Nicol and Kyrolainen, 2002; Hortobágyi and DeVita, 2000). It has previously been reported that increased levels of preactivation are associated with concomitant increases in leg stiffness (Kubo et al., 2007; Kubo, Kanehisa, and Fukunaga, 2001), with greater stiffness producing a more explosive plyometric action. Previous research has shown that when performing 20 cm drop jumps, men jumped higher and displayed greater levels of preactivation than prepubescent boys (Lazaridis et al., 2010). Similarly, it has been shown that as frequency is increased during bilateral hopping, men produce greater relative leg stiffness, shorter ground contact times, and make greater use of feedforward and reflex muscle activity than boys (Oliver and Smith, 2010). Elsewhere in the literature, authors have reported that during vertical jump performance, post-pubescent subjects displayed greater pre-landing co-contraction ratios, whilst pre-pubescent subjects recorded greater co-contraction during the impact phase (Croce, Russell, Swartz and Decoster, 2004). It was suggested that the younger cohort displayed more reflexive activation patterns during ground contact, whereas the older participants displayed greater levels of preactivation. These studies suggest that with age, children experience naturally occurring developments in preparatory muscle activity, enabling a more efficient rebound during ground contact.

Muscular co-contraction is defined as activation of both the agonist and antagonist muscle groups crossing the same joint (Winter, 2005). Despite co-contraction serving as a protective mechanism to provide joint stability and prevent injury, thus explaining the reason why young children appear to have higher co-contraction ratios, for plyometric performance, increased co-contraction is deemed detrimental to performance. This is due to the increased antagonist activation resulting in a reduced agonist force output and overall net joint moment (Winter, 2005). In terms of neuromuscular efficiency a greater amount of mechanical work would therefore be required for a given plyometric action. Muscular co-contraction has been shown to decrease with age, suggesting that older children were able to display a greater neuromuscular efficiency (Lambertz et al., 2003). Conversely, it has been stated that muscle co-contraction ratios are not different between children and adults (Oliver and Smith, 2010; Russell, Croce, Swartz and Decoster, 2007; Kellis and Unnithan, 1999) thereby questioning the performance benefits of co-contraction during plyometric activity. Furthermore, it has been suggested that both children and adults typically utilize reciprocal inhibition to enhance stiffness as hopping frequency increases (Oliver and Smith, 2010), which would imply that co-contraction may not be a contributing factor to the overall age-related developments in plyometric ability.

It remains unclear as to the exact cause of the age-related changes in neural regulation, however research has indicated that alterations in the sensitivity of muscle spindles and Golgi tendon organs may be a plausible explanation (Grossett et al., 2007; Kubo et al., 2001; Lin et al., 1997). Muscle spindles and Golgi tendon organs, are two sensory proprioceptors present within the muscle-tendon complex, and these respond to both changes in length and tension, respectively. Both receptors are responsible for the protective mechanism that also plays a key role in successful plyometric performance. As tension, or rate of change in length, approaches a level that threatens the integrity of the muscle-tendon unit, both sensory receptors inhibit agonist activation and facilitate the antagonist musculature, thereby inducing a stretch reflex response. Research has indicated that the number, size, and sensitivity of Golgi tendon organ complexes decrease with age, and are considerably diminished by the time of adulthood (Ovalle, 1987). Similarly, it has been shown that children's muscle-tendon units are more susceptible to yielding during ground contact, suggesting an under-developed elastic quality inherent to the muscle structure, meaning that force is not transmitted effectively to the muscle spindles, resulting in a dampened stretch reflex response, and reduced muscle-tendon stiffness (Grosset et al., 2007).

The available literature would therefore suggest a natural development in the plyometric ability of children with age. It is suggested that, as a result of growth and maturation, children experience developments in feedforward anticipatory mechanisms that promote pre-activation to enhance joint stability, and a reduction in muscular co-contraction (Oliver and Smith, 2010). Additionally, children have been shown to increase rate of torque development (Grosset, Mora, Lambertz and Perot, 2005), muscle fibre twitch speed (Lin et al., 1997), and stiffness of the muscle-tendon unit (Grosset et al., 2007) as they become older. It must also be noted that as a result of growth and maturation, children will enhance their force-producing capabilities with increases in muscle cross-sectional area (Kanehisa, Ikegawa, Tsunoda and Fukunaga, 1994), however children will need to work against this additional muscle mass during plyometric activity. Additional structural changes that may influence plyometric ability include alterations in muscle and fascicle length (O'Brien, Reeves, Baltzopoulos, Jones, and Maganaris, 2010; Kubo et al., 2001), and modifications in muscle pennation angle (Binzoni et al., 2001). Both of these structural characteristics have previously been linked with increased muscular force output (Kawakami, Abe and Fukunaga, 1993; Willems and Huijing, 1994). It would appear from the literature, that plyometric ability improves naturally as a consequence of both neural and structural adaptations resulting from growth and maturational processes, and that this development is non-linear in nature.

Sprinting and Plyometric Training in Youths

The previous sections have discussed some of the issues associated with explosive performance in youths, especially highlighting the factors which determine sprint and plyometric performance and how they may be affected by development up to the age of adolescence. This final section will discuss the impact of structured physical training on sprinting and plyometric ability.

Studies with youths have shown that sprint and plyometric activity can be effectively employed as training modes (Chaouachi et al., 2008; Kotzaminidis, 2006) and also that both aspects of performance can be improved with appropriate training (Venturelli, Bishop and Pettene, 2008; Meylan and Malatesta, 2009). Both sprinting and plyometric activities are frequently seen in casual play as well as in sports activity. Anecdotally, the use of plyometrics in youths has sometimes been deemed inappropriate owing to the largely-erroneous concern that this form of exercise in training may be injurious. However, provided that plyometric drills are introduced gradually into training, the risk of injuries from these activities is low. Therefore the concerns about the safety of plyometrics in youths are gradually being reduced and the current view amongst researchers is that plyometrics are a safe and effective training mode to develop physical abilities in young athletes (Faigenbaum et al., 2009; Faigenbaum and Chu, 2007).

Regarding the training programmes that have used plyometric exercises as an intervention in youths, improvements have been reported for: rebound jump height (Meylan and Malatesta, 2009); agility and power (Thomas, French and Hayes, 2009); vertical jump performance (Sankey, 2008; Faigenbaum et al., 2007); running velocity (Kotzamanidis, 2006) and rate of force development (Matavulj, Kukolj, Ugarkovic, Tihanyi, and Jaric, 2001). The aforementioned studies have achieved performance adaptations following plyometric training programmes ranging in duration from six (Thomas, et al., 2009; Faigenbaum et al., 2007; Matavulj et al., 2001) to ten weeks (Kotzamanidis, 2006). The age range of the male participants in these training studies was from around 11 years (Diallo, Doré, Duche, and Van Praagh, 2001; Kotzaminidis, 2006) up to around 17 years (Thomas et al., 2009), thus spanning the period from pre-pubescence to adolescence, suggesting that plyometrics training may be suited to a range of age groups. No studies have yet systematically investigated the effect of age on the development of plyometric ability, although such studies would be a valuable addition to the literature given that notions of 'windows of opportunity' or critical periods for the development of certain fitness components have previously been proposed and debated (Balyi and Hamilton, 2004; Ford et al., 2011)

Very few studies have reported the use of sprint training as an intervention for the development of speed or power in youths. Training programmes using short sprints of between 10 and 30m have been shown to elicit improvements in short-sprint performance in both pre-pubescent and pubescent children (Venturelli et al., 2008; Chaouachi et al., 2008, respectively). Interestingly, the study of Venturelli et al. (2008) showed that the gains in sprint speed were not accompanied by improvements in squat or countermovement jump performance. These findings may suggest that the adaptations from sprint training are more specific to the sprint action itself when compared to those achieved from the use of plyometric training. However, conflicting findings have been shown, with Kotzamanidis (2003) observing that a short-sprint programme led to increases in sprint speed as well as squat jump performance. The literature is unclear as to which mechanisms may support the development of performance seen with the participants after these sprint training programmes.

Mechanistically it is likely that the performance adaptations gained from sprint and plyometrics training programmes are linked to neural plasticity especially prior to the onset of puberty. In adults it has previously been suggested that performance gains are a result of neural development, specifically from increased rate of force development, motor unit co-ordination, firing frequency and excitability, and a decrease in presynaptic inhibition and inhibitory neural pathways (Aagard, 2003). In youths, the specific mechanisms underpinning performance adaptations following exposure to plyometric training include: improvements in motor unit recruitment patterns and firing frequencies (Thomas et al., 2009); increased muscle force and rate of force development within the leg extensors (Matavulj et al., 2001); greater joint stiffness and elastic energy recoil (Kubo et al., 2007); earlier and increased activation of the stretch reflexes (Bosco, Vitasalo, Komi, and Luhtanen, 1982); and desensitization of the Golgi Tendon Organs, enabling a greater stretch of the elastic component of the muscle (Hutton and Atwater, 1992).

Given the wide range of neuromuscular factors that contribute to the performance of both plyometric and sprinting activity, it is difficult to speculate whether training at particular periods of development will have the greatest effectiveness. Although the literature is somewhat more developed in other areas of fitness (Ford et al., 2011), few studies have so far investigated the effects of a given training stimulus on the development of sprinting or plyometric performance. Hughes et al. (2011) employed a short training programme using a mixture of sprint and plyometric drills and found that boys aged 12 and 15 years had significant gains in sprint performance that were not seen in boys aged 11, 13 or 14 years. There were no significant differences in squat or countermovement jump performances in any groups (Hughes et al., 2011). However, more extensive research will be needed before a consensus can be reached about the issue of comparative effectiveness of training through different stages of development.

Concluding Comments

The literature shows that appropriate training is effective at enhancing the performance of plyometric and sprint activities in youths. The mechanisms which explain the training-induced performance gains are unclear and consequently, it is currently difficult to tailor certain activities to fit particular stages of development. However, coaches and educators are encouraged to adopt a logical and progressive approach to the development of sprinting and plyometric activities (Lloyd, Oliver and Meyers, 2011c; Faigenbaum, 2006; Faigenbaum and Chu, 2007). In keeping with the general principles of training planning, it is imperative that coaches consider and monitor the intensity, volume, frequency, repetition velocity and recovery of a training prescription to ensure optimal athletic development. As with any other aspect of physical performance, the use of sprinting and plyometric activities in training should be increased gradually and the nature of the activity should be tailored towards the capabilities of the participants.

Because the performance of sprinting and plyometric activities is highly dependent on neural factors their use in training should be considered as movement skill development.

Early development of movement patterns is likely to be a precursor to enhanced performance capacities in adulthood (Bengtsson et al., 2005). Given that the training to enhance sprinting and plyometric abilities in youths is effective and that these activities are fundamental to so many other activities, it should be considered both safe and beneficial for youths to include sprint and plyometric activities in their physical training.

References

Aagaard, P. (2003). Training-induced changes in neural function. *Exercise and Sport Sciences Reviews, 31* (2), 61-67.

Balyi, I., and Hamilton, A. (2004). *Long-term athlete development: trainability in children and adolescents. Windows of opportunity. Optimal trainability.* Victoria BC: National Coaching Institute British Colombia and advanced training and performance Ltd.

Bengtsson, S.L., Nagy, Z., Skare, S., Forsman, L., Forssberg, H., and Ullen, F. (2005). Extensive piano practising has regionally specific effects of white matter development. *Nature neuroscience, 8* (9), 1148-1150.

Beunen, G., and Malina, R. M. (1988). Growth and physical performance relative to the timing of the adolescent spurt. *Exercise and Sport Sciences Reviews, 16*, 503-540.

Binzoni, T., Bianchi, S., Hanquinet, S., Kaelin, A., Sayegh, Y., Dumont, M. and Jéquier, S. (2001). Human gastrocnemius medialis pennation angle as a function of age: from newborn to the elderly. *Journal of Physiological Anthropology and Applied Human Science, 20* (5), 293-298.

Bobbert MF, Gerritsen KGM, Litjens MCA, and Van Soest AJV. (1996). Why is countermovement jump height greater than squat jump height? *Medicine and Science in Sports and Exercise, 28,* 1402–1412.

Borms, J. (1986). The child and exercise: an overview. *Journal of Sports Sciences, 4* (1), 3-20.

Bosco, C, Vitasalo, J.T., Komi, P.V., and Luhtanen, P. (1982). Potentiation during stretch-shortening cycle exercise. *Acta Physiologica Scandinavica, 114,* 557–565.

Castagna, C., D'Ottavio, S., and Abt, G. (2003). Activity profile of young soccer players during actual match play. *Journal of Strength and Conditioning Research, 17* (4), 775-780.

Cavagna GA, Dusman B, and Margaria R. (1968). Positive work done by a previously stretched muscle. *Journal of Applied Physiology, 24*, 21– 32.

Chaouachi, A., Chamari, K., Wong, P., Castagna, C., Chaouachi, M., Moussa-Chamari, I., and Behm, D.G. (2008). Stretch and sprint training reduces stretch-induced sprint performance deficits in 13- to 15-year-old youth. *European Journal of Applied Physiology. 104*: 515-522.

Croce, R.V., Russell, P.J., Swartz, E.E. and Decoster, L.C. (2004). Knee muscular response strategies differ by developmental level but not gender during jump landing. *Electromyography and Clinical Neurophysiology, 44*, 339–48.

Doré, E., Martin, R., Ratel, S., Duche, P. Bedu, M., and Van Praagh, E. (2005). Gender differences in peak muscle performance during growth. *International Journal of Sports Medicine, 26*, 274-280.

Diallo, O., Doré, E., Duche, P., and Van Praagh, E. (2001). Effects of plyometric training followed by a reduced training programme on physical performance in prepubescent soccer players. *Journal of Sports Medicine and Physical Fitness, 41*, 342-348.

Faigenbaum, A.D. (2006). Plyometrics for kids – facts and fallacies. *Performance Training Journal, 5,* 13-16.

Faigenbaum, A.D. and Chu, D.A. (2007). *Plyometric training for children and adolescents.* ACSM Current Comment. Accessed from www.acsm.org on February 13th 2011.

Faigenbaum, A.D., Kraemer, W.J., Blimkie, C.J., Jeffreys, I., Micheli, L.J., Nitka, M. and Rowland, T.W. (2009). Youth resistance training: updated position statement paper from the National Strength and Conditioning Association. *Journal of Strength and Conditioning Research, 23* (5), S60-S79.

Faigenbaum, A.D., McFarland, J.E., Keiper, F.B., Tevlin, W., Ratamess, N.A., Kang, J. and Hoffman, J.R. (2007). Effects of a short-term plyometric and resistance training program on fitness in boys age 12 to 15 years. *Journal of Sports Science and Medicine, 6*, 519-525.

Ford, P., De Ste Croix, M., Lloyd, R., Meyers, R., Moosavi, M. and Oliver, J. (2011). The Long-Term Athlete Development model: Physiological evidence and application. *Journal of Sports Sciences, 29* (4), 389-402.

Frost, G., Dowling, J., Dyson, K., and Bar-Or, O. (1997). Cocontraction in three age groups of children during treadmill locomotion. *Journal of Electromyography and Kinesiology, 7* (3), 179-186.

Gerodimos, V., Zafeiridis, A., Perkos, S., Dipla, K., Manou, V. and Kellis, S. (2008). The contribution of stretch-shortening cycle and arm-swing to vertical jumping performance in children, adolescents, and adult basketball players. *Pediatric Exercise Science, 20*, 379-389.

Glaister, M. (2005). Multiple sprint work: physiological responses, mechanisms of fatigue and the influence of aerobic fitness. *Sports Medicine, 35* (9), 757-777.

Grosset, J.F., Mora, I., Lambertz, D. and Perot, C. (2005). Age-related changes in twitch properties of plantar flexor muscles in prepubertal children. *Pediatric Research, 58*, 966-970.

Grosset, J. F., Mora, I., Lambertz, D., and Perot, C. (2007). Changes in stretch reflexes and muscle stiffness with age in prepubescent children. *Journal of Applied Physiology, 102* (6), 2352-2360.

Harrison, A.J. and Gaffney, S. (2001). Motor development and gender effects on stretch-shortening cycle performance. *Journal of Science and Medicine in Sport, 4* (4), 406-415.

Hasegawa, H., Yamauchi, T., and Kraemer, W. J. (2007). Foot strike patterns of runners at the 15-km point during an elite-level half marathon. *Journal of Strength and Conditioning Research, 21* (3), 888-893.

Hay, J. G. (1993). *The biomechanics of sports techniques.* Englewood Cliffs, N.J.: Prentice-Hall.

Horita, T., Komi, P.V., Nicol, C. and Kyrolainen, H. (2002). Interaction between pre-landing activities and stiffness regulation of the knee joint musculoskeletal system in the drop jump: implications to performance. *European Journal of Applied Physiology, 88*, 76-84.

Hortobágyi, T. and DeVita, P. (2000). Muscle pre- and coactivity during downward stepping are associated with leg stiffness in aging. *Journal of Electromyography and Kinesiology, 10,* 117-126.

Hughes, M.G., Archer, M., Stembridge, M., Meyers, R., Oliver, J., Smith, P., O'Donoghue, P., Cronin, J., and Sephton, A. (2010). The influence of development and training on sprint speed in 11-16-year old boys. *Proceedings of the International Conference of Physical Education and Sports Science*, Singapore. May 2010.

Hunter, J. P., Marshall, R. N., and McNair, P. J. (2004). Interaction of step length and step rate during sprint running. *Medicine and Science in Sports and Exercise, 36* (2), 261-271.

Hutton, R.S. and Atwater, S.W. (1992). Acute and chronic adaptations of muscle proprioceptors in response to increased use. *Sports Medicine, 14*, 406-421.

Isaacs, L.D. (1998). Comparison of the Vertec and just Jump systems for measuring height of vertical jump by young children. *Perceptual and Motor Skills, 86*, 659-663.

Kanehisa, H., Ikegawa, S., Tsunoda, N. and Fukunaga, T. (1994). Strength and cross-sectional area of knee extensor muscles in children. *European Journal of Applied Physiology and Occupational Physiology, 68* (5), 402-405.

Kawakami, Y., Abe, T. and Fukunaga, T. (1993). Muscle-fiber pennation angles are greater in hypertrophied than in normal muscles. *Journal of Applied Physiology, 74*, 2740–2744.

Kellis, E. and Unnithan, V.B. (1999). Co-activation of vastus lateralis and biceps femoris muscles in pubertal children and adults. *European Journal of Applied Physiology, 79*, 504-511.

Komi, P.V. (2000). Stretch-shortening cycle: a powerful model to study normal and fatigued muscle. *Journal of Biomechanics, 33* (10), 1197-1206.

Komi, P. V., and Bosco, C. (1978). Utilization of elastic energy in jumping and its relation to skeletal muscle fiber composition in man. In E. Asmussen and K. Jorgensen (Eds.), *Biomechanics VI-A* (pp. 79-85). Baltimore, MD: University Park Press.

Komi, P.V. and Gollhoffer, A. (1997). Stretch reflex can have an important role in force enhancement during SSC-exercise. *Journal of Applied Biomechanics, 33,* 1197-1206.

Kotzmanidis, C. (2003). The effect of sprint training on running performance and vertical jumping in preadolescent boys. *Journal of Human Movement Studies, 44*, 225-240.

Kotzamanidis, C. (2006). Effect of plyometric training on running performance and vertical jumping in prepubertal boys. *Journal of Strength and Conditioning Research, 20* (2), 441-445.

Kubo, K., Kanehisa, H. and Fukunaga, T. (2001). Is passive stiffness in human muscles related to the elasticity of tendon structures. *European Journal of Applied Physiology, 85*, 226-232.

Kubo, K., Kanehisa, H., and Fukunaga, T. (2003). Gender differences in the viscoelastic properties of tendon structures. *European Journal of Applied Physiology, 88* (6), 520-526.

Kubo, K, Morimoto, M, Komuro, T, Tsunoda, N, Kanehisa, H, and Fukunaga, T. (2007). Influences of tendon stiffness, joint stiffness, and electromyographic activity on jump performances using single joint. *European Journal of Applied Physiology, 99*, 235–243.

Lambertz, D., Mora, I., Grosset, J. F., and Perot, C. (2003). Evaluation of musculotendinous stiffness in prepubertal children and adults, taking into account muscle activity. *Journal of Applied Physiology, 95* (1), 64-72.

Lazaridis, S., Bassa, E., Patikas, D., Giakas, G., Gollhofer, A. and Kotzamanidis, C. (2010). Neuromuscular differences between prepubescent boys and adult men during drop jump. *European Journal of Applied Physiology, 110* (1), 67-74.

Lin, J.P., Brown, J.K. and Walsh, E.G. (1997). Soleus muscle length, stretch-reflex excitability, and the contractile properties of muscle in children and adults: a study of the functional joint angle. *Developmental Medicine and Child Neurology, 39*, 469-480.

Lloyd, R.S., Oliver, J.L., Hughes, M.G. and Williams, C.A. (2009). Reliability and validity of field-based measures of leg stiffness and reactive strength in youths. *Journal of Sports Sciences, 27*, 1565-1573.

Lloyd, R.S., Oliver, J.L., Hughes, M.G. and Williams, C.A. (2011a). Specificity of test selection for the appropriate assessment of different measures of stretch-shortening cycle function in children. *Journal of Sports Medicine and Physical Fitness*, (in press).

Lloyd, R.S., Oliver, J.L., Hughes, M.G. and Williams, C.A. (2011b). The influence of chronological age on periods of accelerated adaptation of stretch-shortening cycle performance in pre- and post-pubescent boys. *Journal of Strength and Conditioning Research*, (in press).

Lloyd, R.S., Oliver, J.L. and Meyers, R.W. (2011c). The natural development and trainability of plyometric ability during childhood. *Strength and Conditioning Journal,* (in press).

Malina, R. M. (1969). Quantification of fat, muscle and bone in man. *Clinical Orthopaedics and Related Research, 65*, 9-38.

Malina, R. M., Bouchard, C., and Bar-Or, O. (2004). *Growth, maturation, and physical activity* (2nd ed.). Champaign, Ill: Human Kinetics.

Matavulj, D., Kukolj, M., Ugarkovic, D., Tihanyi, J. and Jaric, S. (2001). Effects of plyometric training on jumping performance in junior basketball players. *Journal of Sports Medicine and Physical Fitness, 41*, 159-164.

McMahon, T.A. and Cheng, G.C. (1990). The mechanics of running: how does stiffness couple with speed? *Journal of Biomechanics, 23*, 65-78.

McClymont, D. (2005). Use of the Reactive Strength Index (RSI) as an indicator of plyometric training conditions. In: *Science and Football V*; The Proceedings of the 5th World Congress on Science and Football. Reily, T, Cabri, J, and Araújo, D, eds. Routledge, 408-416.

Meyers, R., Oliver, J., Hughes, M.G., Stembridge, M. and Cronin. J. (2010). The influence of maturation status on maximal sprint speed characteristics in boys. *Proceedings of the International Conference of Physical Education and Sports Science*, Singapore. May 2010.

Meylan, C. and Malatesta, D. (2009). Effects of in-season plyometric training within soccer practice on explosive actions of young players. *Journal of Strength and Conditioning Research, 23* (9), 2605-2613.

Mirwald, R. L., Baxter-Jones, A. D., Bailey, D. A., and Beunen, G. P. (2002). An assessment of maturity from anthropometric measurements. *Medicine and Science in Sports and Exercise, 34* (4), 689-694.

Morris, A. M., Williams, J. M., Atwater, A. E., and Wilmore, J. H. (1982). Age and sex differences in motor performance of 3 through 6 year old children. *Research Quarterly for Exercise and Sport, 53* (3), 214-221.

Naughton, G., Farpour-Lambert, N. J., Carlson, J., Bradney, M., and van Praagh, E. (2000). Physiological issues surrounding the performance of adolescent athletes. *Sports Medicine, 30*, 309-325.

Nesser, T. W., Latin, R. W., Berg, K., and Prentice, E. (1996). Physiological determinants of 40-meter sprint performance in young male athletes. *Journal of Strength and Conditioning Research, 10* (4), 263-267.

Nicol, C., Avela, J. and Komi, P.V. (2006). The stretch-shortening cycle: A model to study naturally occurring neuromuscular fatigue. *Sports Medicine, 36* (11), 977-999.

Novacheck, T. F. (1998). The biomechanics of running. *Gait Posture, 7* (1), 77-95.

O'Brien, T.D., Reeves, N.D., Baltzopoulos, V., Jones, D.A. and Maganaris, C.N. (2010). Muscle-tendon structure and dimensions in adults and children. *Journal of Anatomy, 216* (5), 631-642.

Oliver, J.L., and Smith, P.M. (2010). Neural control of leg stiffness during hopping in boys and men. *Journal of Electromyography and Kinesiology, 20*, 973-979.

Ovalle, W.K. (1987). The human muscle-tendon junction. A morphological study during normal growth and maturity. *Anatomy and Embryology (Berlin), 176*, 281-294.

Ozmun, J. C., Mikesky, A. E., and Surburg, P. R. (1994). Neuromuscular adaptations following prepubescent strength training. *Medicine and Science in Sports and Exercise, 26* (4), 510-514.

Papaiakovou, G., Giannakos, A., Michailidis, C., Patikas, D., Bassa, E. and Kalopisis, V. (2009). The effect of chronological age and gender on the development of sprint performance during childhood and puberty. *Journal of Strength and Conditioning Research, 23* (9), 2568-2573.

Philippaerts, R. M., Vaeyens, R., Janssens, M., Van Renterghem, B., Matthys, D. and Craen, R. (2006). The relationship between peak height velocity and physical performance in youth soccer players. *Journal of Sports Sciences, 24* (3), 221-230.

Potach, D.H., and Chu, D.A. (2008). Plyometric Training. In: *Essentials of Strength Training and Conditioning*. Baechle, T.R., and Earle, R.W., eds. Champaign, IL, Human Kinetics, 413-456.

Ratel, S., Bedu, M., Hennegrave, A., Doré, E., and Duché, P. (2002). Effects of age and recovery duration on peak power output during repeated cycling sprints. *International Journal of Sports Medicine, 23*, 397-402.

Rimmer, E., and Sleivert, G. (2000). Effects of a plyometrics intervention program on sprint performance. *Journal of Strength and Conditioning Research, 14* (3), 295-301.

Russell, P.J., Croce, R.V., Swartz, E.E. and Decoster, L.C. (2007). Knee-muscle activation during landings: development and gender comparisons. *Medicine and Science in Sports and Exercise, 39* (1), 159-169.

Sankey, S.P. (2008). Effects of two plyometric training programmes of different intensity on vertical jump performance in high school athletes. *Serbian Journal of Sports Sciences, 2* (4), 123-130.

Schepens, B., Willems, P. A., and Cavagna, G. A. (1998). The mechanics of running in children. *Journal of Physiology, 509 (Pt 3)*, 927-940.

Schmidtbleicher, D. (1992). Training for power events. In *Strength and Power in Sport*, pp. 381-395. Oxford, England: Blackwell Scientific Publications.

Szczesny, S. and Coudert, J. (1993). Changes in running speed and endurance among girls during puberty. In Duquet, W and Day, A.P. (Ed.), *Kinanthropometry IV* (pp. 268-284). London: Chapman Hall.

Taylor, J. (2003). Basketball: Applying Time Motion Data to Conditioning. *Strength and Conditioning Journal, 25* (2), 57-64.

Thomas, K., French, D. and Hayes, P.R. (2009). The effect of plyometric training techniques on muscular power and agility in youth soccer players. *Journal of Strength and Conditioning Research, 23* (1), 332-335.

Van Ingen Schenau, G.J., Bobbert, M.F. and de Haan, A. (1997). Mechanics and energetics of the stretch-shortening cycle: a stimulating discussion. *Journal of Applied Biomechanics, 13*, 484-496.

Van Praagh, E. and Doré, E. (2002). Short-term muscle power during growth and maturation. *Sports Medicine, 32*, 701-728.

Venturelli, M., Bishop, D., and Pettene, L (2008). Sprint training in preadolescent soccer players. *International Journal of Sports Physiology and Performance, 3*, 558-562.

Viru, A., Loko, J., Harro, M., Volver, A., Laaneots, L., and Viru, M. (1999). Critical periods in the development of performance capacity during childhood and adolescence. *European Journal of Physical Education, 4* (1), 75 - 119.

Volver, A. and Viru., A. (1997). Motor development related to sexual maturation in 11- to 14-year-old girls. *Biology of Sport, 14*, 205-211.

Walshe, A.D., Wilson, G.J., and Ettema, G.J.C. (1998). Stretch-shorten cycle compared with isometric preload: contributions to enhanced muscular performance. *Journal of Applied Physiology, 84*, 97–106.

Weyand, P. G., Sternlight, D. B., Bellizzi, M. J., and Wright, S. (2000). Faster top running speeds are achieved with greater ground forces not more rapid leg movements. *Journal of Applied Physiology, 89* (5), 1991-1999.

Willems, M.E.T. and Huijing, P.A. (1994). Heterogeneity of mean sarcomere length in different fibres: effects on length range of active force production in rat muscle. *European Journal of Applied Physiology, 68* (6), 489-496.

Winter, D.A. (2005). *Biomechanics and motor control of human movement* – 3rd ed., John Wiley and Sons Inc., New York.

In: Reviews in Pediatric Exercise Science
Editor: Michael Duncan, pp. 217-240
ISBN: 978-1-61470-978-7

Chapter XIV

Methods of Monitoring Training in Adolescent Soccer Players

Matt Rains[1], Mark Noon[2] and Doug Thake[1]
[1] Coventry University, UK.
[2] Coventry University, UK and Coventry City Football Club, Coventry, UK.

Adolescents in Soccer, 'It's Not Fair!'

The football playing adolescents of today are our stars of tomorrow. Adolescence is a transitional phase of physical and mental development, generally occurring between puberty and adulthood, often characterised as beginning and ending with the teenage stage (ages 13-19; Kent, 1998). During this time physical, physiological and psychological features, essential for success in soccer, alter with growth and evolve at varying rates (Williams and Reilly, 2000). Thus adolescents, even within the same age group, often train with and compete against peers at different stages of development. This could be considered an unfair playing field, particularly in relation to talent identification where greater physical maturity and hence higher physical power are often favourable compared to less physically developed players (Brewer *et al*,. 1995). For example, at the start of the 2010-11 season height and weight within an under-14 elite academy squad varied by 22 cm and 25 kg respectively (tallest player 174 cm and 64 kg compared to shortest player 150 cm and 39 kg). Although an age gap of almost one year could exist within the same player group and account for a proportion of this difference these players were born at the end of September and November, respectively, within the same year. Were these players of similar stature and mass when originally selected for the academy? What if, once selected, an individual's growth rate lags in comparison to their peers? Will the potential talent of the smaller player now be obscured due to relative biological/developmental immaturity? Do coaches really mistake talent for early maturation? There is, indeed, a known bias towards continuing to select older and therefore bigger children within association football (Simmons and Paull, 2001). In reality the exclusion of developmentally 'younger' age matched players is potentially costly for professional teams.

Thus the construct of attempting to prescribe age appropriate training as well as establish 'normal' age appropriate performance test scores for specific player groups is inherently floored. The ideal focus should be on developing a performance management strategy to facilitate and optimise individual player development within a squad environment. Player responses to training (during and recovery from) alongside physical performance tests are key tools that can be applied within an appropriate framework to help optimise an adolescents football development. The following chapter outlines the rationale for and current methods used within an elite youth academy environment (an English Championship club) to monitor the training.

The Trainability of Adolescents

Training programmes are often designed based on a player's chronological age and do not take into account a player's biological/developmental age or the number or years the player has specialised in playing football (training age). Ideally aspects of an individual player's conditioning programme should be differentiated and prescribed on the basis of biological/developmental age however, this can be problematic in squad training. One possible solution is to categorise age groups into several sub-groups based on levels of maturation. A straight forward and inexpensive method to non-invasively determine biological age, is to regularly measure height (every 3 months). This enables the determination of Peak Height Velocity (PHV), the maximum rate of growth in stature. When the rate of growth is known training, competition and recovery programmes can then be adjusted according to the tempo of growth (Balyi and Way, 2005). For example, as outlined within the training to train stage (usually 12-16 years old, ±2 years) of the Long Term Athlete Development (LTAD) model (Balyi and Hamilton, 1999), a window of optimal trainability exists for aerobic system at the onset of PHV, whereas that for maximal strength training is after PHV. These components are thus based on developmental age. However, within this model, the trainability of speed, skill and flexibility are based on chronological age. Therefore it is also important for the coach to account for the impact of growth on skill. Accordingly an understanding of this can be developed through adding measures of sitting height and arm span every 3 months after the onset of PHV to determine what part of the body is growing and at what rate. After the "Training to Train" stage players (usually aged 16-18) enter the "Training to Compete Stage" (Balyi *et al.,* 2006). In this phase of development fitness programs, recovery programs, psychological preparation and technical development are incorporated to the training programme. Although many governing bodies have adopted the LTAD model set out by Istvan Bayli the guidelines should be interpreted with caution as empirical evidence on the model is lacking.

All training programmes are implemented through a periodised training plan. During each training macro-cycle the key technical, tactical, physical and psychological aspects are integrated. In the "Training to Compete" stage, these factors are incorporated into the demands of the fixture schedule and the development of each individual. In each macro-cycle different areas are prioritised. For example, in pre-season a large focus is on physical preparation and as the season progresses a greater emphasis is put on technical and tactical development. Throughout the competition phase the athletic development program is integrated into the technical and tactical program. Physical characteristics such as endurance, speed, maximum strength and agility are prioritised at various points throughout the year Each macro cycle lasts ~6 weeks (Figure 1) and the effectiveness of the macro-cycles are assessed using a battery of tests and monitoring tools to which the periodised plan is altered accordingly.

	July	Aug	Sept	Oct	Nov	Dec	Jan	Feb	Mar	Apr	May	Jun
Phase	Pre Season		Competition			Br eak	Competition			Maintenance / Rest		
Cycle	General	Specific	Early Season 1	Early Season 2	Mid Season 1		Mid season 2	Late Season	End of Season	Maintenance / Rest		

Figure 1. An example of an elite soccer team's periodised training programme (Noon, unpublished data).

Monitoring Adolescent Soccer Players

Player progress is monitored by an interdisciplinary support network comprised of physiotherapists, strength and conditioning coaches, sport scientists, and football coaches. Measurements conducted are height, weight, body fat and flexibility screenings, analysis of players functional movement capabilities via a system called Motion Assimilation Performance in Sport (MAPS) (Tierney and Knight, unpublished data), muscle function (hamstring : quadriceps ratio via isokinetic dynamometry; Coombs and Garbutt, 2002) various physical performance tests such as speed, countermovement jump, agility (T-test) and the Yo-Yo Intermittent Recovery Test (Bansgbo, 1993). Other important areas include monitoring training load, perceptions of player recovery by means of a Recovery Questionnaire (Taylor and Thake, unpublished data) and identifying training status via a Heart Rate Interval Monitoring System (HIMS) (Lamberts *et al,*. 2004) and a reactive strength index (RSI) (Hore, 2003).

Height, Weight and Flexibility Screening

Player height and weight are measured once per month to identify trends in growth and the onset of PHV (Table 1). Players who have grown >2cm in 3 months are highlighted, regular stretching is reiterated and coaches may be advised to reduce the players training load to reduce injury risk. Due to the sudden growth of bones, tendons, ligaments and muscles resulting in coordination changes during PHV flexibility monitoring is important. The risk of Severs (heel injury) and Osgoods Schlatters (knee injury) may be increased during this time which can cause long term absence from participation therefore monitoring player growth is of high importance.

Table 1. Stature and seasonal growth of elite under-14 soccer players

Subject	September Growth (cm)	October Growth (cm)	November Growth (cm)	December Growth (cm)	January Growth (cm)	February Growth (cm)	Total Seasonal Growth (cm)	Previous 3 month growth (cm)
1	165.6	No Result	167.1	167.5	168.3	169.4	3.8	2.3
2	170.5	173.0	171.5	172.0	173.0	173.6	3.1	2.1
3	No Result	158.1	159.1	158.2	159.8	161.1	3.0	2.0
4	No Result	150.6	No Result	152.1	152.4	153.4	2.8	2.0
5	145.5	146.6	147.2	147.5	148.4	149.0	3.5	1.8
6	158.0	No Result	158.8	158.9	159.4	160.5	2.5	1.7
7	No Result	No Result	156.6	156.5	157.5	158.0	1.4	1.4
8	No Result	178.1	No Result	179.2	179.7	179.7	1.6	1.1
9	173.4	173.5	173.8	174.5	174.5	174.8	1.4	1.0
10	147.0	147.5	148.5	148.6	148.6	149.1	2.1	0.6
11	147.5	147.7	149.0	149.0	149.7	150.0	2.5	1.0
12	166.5	No Result	168.6	168.0	No Result	169.5	4.0	0.9

Accordingly, all players undergo a flexibility screening once per month assessing the lower limbs, including the hip flexors, quadriceps, hamstrings and gastrocnemius (Table 2 to 3). Flexibility is important in soccer as match-play requires a combination of coordinated movements including reaching, bending, leaning and twisting in activities such as a slide tackle or reaching to control a pass, therefore increasing the range of motion available at a joint can help performance and reduce injury risk. Players undertaking strength training along with soccer training must ensure they perform static stretching after each session as strength training has been shown to inhibit flexibility in adolescent soccer players (Christou *et al.* 2006). Inadequate flexibility increases injury risk, and stretching exercises must be emphasised when strength training is undertaken as flexibility is already compromised by maturation status. The results of the flexibility screening inform individual static stretching programmes to increase the length of specific muscles (compare Table 2 to Table 3 for the benefit of a 3 month intervention).

Furthermore, to monitor the effects of training and dietary intervention on body composition, under-18 squad players have body fat percentage estimated once per month. Excess weight has an adverse effect upon locomotion and soccer-specific actions such as jumping to contest aerial possession of the ball, whilst lean muscle mass is important for the production of speed, strength and power, and for injury prevention. Ideally, all age groups should have body composition measured as an educational tool to inform players about their dietary needs.

Table 2. Flexibility scores of elite under-14 football players pre flexibility training (R=right, L=left; light grey = pass, dark grey = borderline, and black = fail)

Subject	Hamstrings		Quadriceps		Groins		Hip Flexors		Gastrocnemius	
	Right	Left	R	L	R	L	R	L	R	L
1										
2										
3										
4										
5										
6										
7										
8										
9										
10										
11										
12										

Table 3. Flexibility scores of elite under-14 football players post flexibility training (R=right, L=left; light grey = pass, dark grey = borderline, and black = fail)

Subject	Hamstrings		Quadriceps		Groins		Hip Flexors		Gastrocnemius	
	Right	Left	R	L	R	L	R	L	R	L
1										
2										
3										
4										
5										
6										
7										
8										
9										
10										
11										
12										

Performance and Developmental Testing

Introduction

Players undertake a battery of performance tests to enable monitoring and evaluation of training stress and adaptation over a macro-cycle. In addition, physical testing data can be used to track a player's development over time and highlight possible injury risk further informing the training process. Between the ages of 11-14 performance test scores increase due to growth and maturation (Mirkov et al., 2010), consequently early maturers are likely to excel in physical performance tests because of physical development advantage. Therefore, when analysing such data an individual's biological age needs to be considered as maturation levels between players aged 11-17 (17 is the age the maturation process is expected to last approximately) can vary by as much as 2 years (Table 4) (Helsen et al., 2000). Regular testing intervals are used ~4 times per year in under 9's to under-16's squads and ~6 times per year in under-18 squads. All test results inform individual developmental training programmes. Of particular importance to the coach is ensuring increases in performance are transferred onto the pitch to improve game specific attributes such as speed, agility, power and endurance.

Demands

These aspects have relevance to game situations (e.g. tackling, jumping, kicking, turning and changing pace) and speed, power and agility have been shown to discriminate between elite young players and sub-elite ones (Reilly *et al.,* 2000; Mirkov *et al.,* 2010). Analysis of under-12 to under-16's elite youth soccer matches reveal on average 3.6% (0.3-8.8%) of total match time is spent sprinting (Harley *et al.,* 2010). Although this makes up a small proportion of the total distance covered, high-intensity runs may have implications on the outcome of a match, for example accelerating away from an opponent is required for an attacking opportunity. Agility has high relevance to match-play as rapid and whole body changes in direction in response to an opponent's actions or to outwit an opponent are frequently needed. Power can be measured by a countermovement jump (CMJ) and has relevance in soccer for when attempting to out jump an opponent to head the ball. Furthermore, the ability to repeatedly perform intense exercise and recover quickly in between bursts is an important characteristic of an elite player's make-up. Elite youth soccer players can cover up to 7672 m in a competitive game (Harley *et al.,* 2010) comprised of motions such as walking, jogging, and sprinting indicating the importance of high soccer specific endurance capacity.

How We Test and Why

Players are tested for power using a countermovement jump (CMJ), speed over 5, 15 and 30m and agility via a t-test. All tests are performed in a controlled environment using electronic equipment. The agility t-test and sprint tests are performed from a stationary start however, a more realistic representation of sprint and agility performance may be obtained using a flying start (walk, jog or stride), since few movements are commenced from a stationary start during a match. A further limitation of testing agility using the t-test is the test does not hold any perceptual or decision making components, these aspects are relevant in soccer as changes of direction and speed are often performed in response to an opponent's actions (Young, James, and Montgomery, 2002). Consequently a reactive agility test with a soccer specific stimulus would be more applicable. Soccer specific endurance capacity is tested by the Yo-Yo Intermittent Recovery Test (Bangsbo, 1994) which consists of 20m shuttle runs at rapidly increasing speeds interspersed with 10 second periods of active recovery. Such a test can also help inform individual training programmes. A player demonstrating a reduction in performance on this test could require additional training stimuli to keep their fitness levels high, ensuring they can compete at match intensity when selected this may also be the case for regular non-starters. Conversely, training emphasis could shift to another important variable that needs improving for players showing improved performance. This test can also be utilised when injured players are returning to training to determine how much reversibility has occurred in their fitness levels. If players are put straight back into training the physiological load could be too high for them to tolerate and cause re-injury halting their recovery further. Recent training intensity should be reviewed and a baseline score established for the player to achieve on the test before returning to training. Players in the under-14, 15, 16, and 18 categories undertake this test, however it is not suitable for younger players as their aerobic capabilities do not fully develop until the onset of PHV.

Whilst measuring these aspects in a controlled environment informs the coach on the effectiveness of the training programme, measuring their effect in a match environment is less straight forward. One rationale for improving a player's speed is to get to the ball in a faster time than an opponent, but if speed has improved in the performance tests does this transfer to the pitch? This type of physical data could be provided by through a combination of notational analysis, ProZone® or Global Positioning Systems (GPS) and could help determine this but in some elite academies this type of software is not feasible.

Table 4. Average anthropometric and physical test values for each age group in adolescent elite academy soccer players

	Height (cm)	Weight (kg)	Body Composition (%)	CMJ (cm)	5m Sprint (secs)	15m Sprint (secs)	30m Sprint (secs)	Yo-Yo Intermittent Recovery Test (m)
Under 13's	162 ± 7	50.4 ± 7.8		40.33 ± 7.85	1.23 ± 0.07	2.78 ± 0.16	4.89 ± 0.33	
Under 14's	163.6 ± 10.5	51.8 ± 10.6		39.32 ± 5.91	1.24 ± 0.04	2.67 ± 0.09	4.56 ± 0.20	
Under 15's	176.5 ± 4.6	62.4 ± 5.7		43.03 ± 5.85	1.15 ± 0.12	2.54 ± 0.18	4.44 ± 0.25	2680
Under 16's	178.4 ± 6.6	65.0 ± 5.8		42.97 ± 3.08	1.12 ± 0.07	2.54 ± 0.08	4.37 ± 0.09	3000
Under 18's	180.4 ± 6.5	73.8 ± 6.6	11.5 ± 1.4	45.79 ± 5.04	1.17 ± 0.08	2.58 ± 0.09	4.42 ± 0.13	3640

Maturation

The modern day professional soccer player is fast, strong and agile and the coach should look to improve these aspects in adolescent soccer players to help them reach the elite level. After the onset of PHV players should be introduced to a periodised strength training programme, which has also been shown to improve vertical jump height, agility, and running speed (Christou *et al.,* 2006), highlighting the importance of such programmes for match-specific actions. A significant relationship has also been observed between one repetition maximum (1RM) and 10m sprint time, 30m sprint time, 10m shuttle run and jumping height providing further evidence an increase in strength will benefit performance (Wisløff *et al.,* 2004). Further to this on pitch specific speed training can be incorporated into the weekly training programme consisting of explosive-strength sport-specific exercises to improve speed in young elite soccer players (Mujika, Santisteban, and Castagna, 2009). These sessions should be conducted 1-2 times per week over a 7 week period. Agility training is already incorporated into the training programme due to the continual changes in direction associated with soccer training drills as a result agility improves by soccer training alone (Christou *et al.,* 2006).

Injury Risk

Strength and conditioning is not based solely on performance it can also play a major role in reducing and identifying injury risk which can be assessed by isokinetic dynamometry where force production during eccentric and concentric phases of the hamstring and quadriceps is measured to identify muscle strength imbalances. Due to the activities common in soccer including rapid turns, accelerations and decelerations (Bangsbo, 1994) the hamstring muscle undergoes frequent eccentric contractions, where the contracting muscle is lengthened and this has been linked to hamstring muscle strains (Kujala *et al,*. 1997). Muscles undergo eccentric contractions whenever they act as brakes to slow down a movement causing microscopic damage to muscle fibres, if the eccentric contractions continue, the microscopic areas of damage may provide a point of weakness from which a major tear may arise (Brockett, Morgan, and Proske 2001). A study concluded that hamstring strains were associated with a low hamstring-to-quadriceps ratio of peak torque on the injured side (Orchard *et al.,* 1997). Additionally, an under-18 age group demonstrated a significant move away from functional hamstring quadriceps equality when compared to the under-13 age group and also the under-12 age group on the dominant limb (Forbes *et al.,* 2009). To counteract this, specific eccentric hamstring exercises such as Nordic Hamstring Curls should be implemented to increase hamstring strength and reduce injury risk.

To further reduce injury risk and improve movement efficiency, all players within the academy are required to undertake a movement screening 3 times per season, called Motion Assimilation Performance for Sport (MAPS) (Tierney and Knight, unpublished data). MAPS is formulated from analysis of the most common functional movements that occur in competitive youth soccer matches, movements highlighted are the lunge, squat, jump, linear single leg jump and land, lateral cut and lateral cut-cut back. These movements make up a battery of repeatable tests to assess a player's efficiency of movement. Each screening is video recorded and analysed post assessment, performance in each movement is rated (1-6) and an individual training programme is implemented to correct poor movement and stability patterns therefore reducing the risk of injury and improving test score, with a view to improving overall on pitch performance.

Conclusion

A variety of attributes are required to perform at the elite level, therefore when preparing an adolescent to play at the highest level a periodised strength and conditioning training programme incorporating strength, power, and endurance is of high importance as not only can it benefit performance but also prevent injury risk. A common error in training adolescents is the prescription of 'watered down' adult training regimes. Training programmes should be prescribed for an individual taking into account biological age of the player and optimising the use of the "open windows" occurring around PHV.

The Holistic Training Process

The basic principle of training is that breakdown (training) is followed by recovery (rest) resulting in a supercompensation and improved performance. If the balance between training and recovery is disrupted negative consequences on performance occur (Nederhof *et al.,* 2008). If these outcomes are reversed within a short period of time, the state is called functional overreaching, however if the recovery period takes longer than desired, the state is referred to as non-functional overreaching (Budgett, 1998; Nederhof *et al.,* 2008). Thus, recovery is a key determinant of adaptation. However, the coach's attention is often focused on monitoring load and stimulus without a real consideration of the level of recovery.

Monitoring Training Load

Various methods are used to quantify the training stimulus such as heart rate monitoring (Achten, and Jeukendrup, 2003), training impulses (TRIMPS) (Stagno, Thatcher, and Van Someren, 2007) and session-RPE (rating of perceived exertion; Foster *et al.,* 1996). Although these methods either measure or estimate the physiological stress (internal training load) imposed on the player, the context of the response is limited if it cannot be considered in relation to the actual physical activity conducted (external training load; e.g., 4v4, 4x4 minutes of small sided games; SSG's). Monitoring the external training load is of equal importance because each player will perform different amounts of work and react to the training stimulus differently even though the training prescription for each player is the same, as evidenced by players with superior fitness levels not increasing their physiological capacity in SSG's due to an insufficient training stimulus (Hoff *et al.,* 2002). Conversely, players with lower fitness levels may be overstressed during team-based training sessions leading to increased fatigue and potential non-functional overreaching. However team based training is a necessity in soccer to aid tactical development and acquire positional-relationships. Additionally training can elicit higher than expected heart rates and RPE scores for a given player when under recovered, injured or ill. In isolation these responses can be misinterpreted as the player undertaking a high volume and intensity of work rather than the physiological strain of less work being greater. An RPE takes into account the external training load as well as the internal load, as perception of physical effort can be affected by a player's psychological state, an under-recovered player may perceive the exercise intensity within a given session to be harder than that of a player who is optimally recovered. Additionally, an individual with life stresses or lack of sleep could find the training prescription harder to tolerate consequently increasing their subjective psychological stress. The external training load experienced by a player can further be quantified by them wearing portable GPS's. This, for example, has made the evaluation and monitoring of the demands in SSG's more accessible, reliable and accurate (Portas *et al.,* 2011). Indeed, GPS technology provides a practical method for recording time-motion characteristics (such as distance, speed, and frequency of sprints) during all forms of soccer training (Hill-Haas *et al.,* 2009). The coach can then quantify total distance covered and its components in training and competitive environments, and where appropriate use in conjunction with heart rate data.

Heart Rate Monitoring

Measuring heart rate is a relatively cheap and easy dependable method. The rationale for heart rate measurement is based on the principle that a linear relationship exists between heart rate and oxygen consumption over a wide range of steady-state submaximal workloads (Astrand, and Rodahl, 1986). This relationship holds when the exercise is discontinuous (Bangsbo, 1994). Heart rate has been shown to be a valid method of monitoring training intensity when soccer drills or SSG's are of sufficient duration, for example, >3 minutes (Little, and Williams, 2007). Whereas heart rate monitoring in short, intense drills such as a 2v2 SSG with 2 minute work periods underestimates the intensity of the drill because the adaptation of the circulatory system is incomplete and heart rate lags behind.

Many other factors influence the relationship between work load and heart rate such as state of training, environmental conditions, exercise duration, hydration status, altitude and medication however, if these are controlled the reliability and accuracy of measuring internal load improves (Achten, and Jeukendrup, 2003). A further limitation to heart rate monitoring is if the transmitter has a technical failure during the exercise bout the measurement is lost. It is also important the players adhere to wearing their heart rate monitors in each training session although some players report irritation from them during exercise. Within the under-18 youth squad the internal training load is monitored via this method and analysed on a daily basis. All players are provided with an individual heart rate monitor that is required to be worn during all on pitch training sessions. The high intensity minutes (minutes spent above 85% heart rate max during exercise) and a training impulse (TRIMP) are extracted from the data.

Training Impulse (TRIMP)

Various methods to quantify a TRIMP have been proposed including calculating the components of training into a single figure (Banister *et al.,* 1991) or accumulating the minutes spent in defined heart rate zones and multiplying it by a weighting factor (i.e., 50-60% = 1, 60-70% = 2, 70-80% = 3, 80-90% = 4 and 90-100% = 5 of HR_{max}), with the computed sum of all zones giving an arbitrary unit for the training session (Foster *et al.,* 2001). However, these methods are limited as the mean exercise heart rate in intermittent sports fails to reflect the variation in exercise intensity and heart rate zones do not reflect physiological responses to exercise above the lactate threshold (Stagno, Thatcher, and Van Someren, 2007).

The TRIMP has been modified ($TRIMP_{MOD}$) to quantify the in-season training load of field hockey players by individualising the heart rate zones based on physiological responses to laboratory tests (Stagno, Thatcher, and Van Someren, 2007). To do this 5 HR zones were established based on when the players reached their lactate threshold and the onset of blood lactate accumulation (OBLA), defined as blood lactate concentrations of 1.5 and 4 $mmol^{-1}$ respectively (Usaj, and Starc 1996; see Table 5). $TRIMP_{MOD}$ was calculated by multiplying the weighting factor by the time spent in the respective heart rate zone with the total $TRIMP_{MOD}$ being the sum of all heart rate zones (Table 5). Using this method Stagno, Thatcher, and Van Someren (2007) were able to accurately estimate the field hockey player's metabolic stress in training. Clearly calculating a TRIMP is appealing as training intensity within a given session is quantified into a single figure. However a limitation of applying heart rate zones in this manner is that within each zone the lowest and highest heart rate are weighted the same despite a difference in the physiological load. Also when heart rates fluctuate around a zonal boarder a 1% variation will change the zone weighting factor, thereby increasing or decreasing the calculated load.

Table 5. $TRIMP_{MOD}$ heart rate zones, corresponding weighting factors and training description (Stagno, Thatcher and Van Someren 2007)

Zone	Percentage Maximal Heart Rate (%)	Weighting	Training Type
5	93-100	5.16	Maximal Training
4	86-92	3.61	OBLA Training
3	79-85	2.54	Steady-State Training
2	72-78	1.71	Lactate Threshold Training
1	65-71	1.25	Moderate Activity

The $TRIMP_{MOD}$ heart rate zones and multiplication factors are now applied to quantify the training load in academy soccer players. However, the usefulness of using normative pre-determined heart rate zones is limited as anaerobic threshold varies between individuals, even those with equal aerobic power. Consequently the metabolic stress experienced by players is different even when exercising at the same percentage of maximal heart rate. With appropriate resource available each player's lactate threshold should be measured, as noted above, to improve the accuracy of $TRIMP_{MOD}$ to quantifying exercise intensity. Furthermore lactate threshold is sensitive to changes in training, with the onset occurring at higher running speeds during a graded exercise test following a training intervention in soccer players (Helgerud, et al., 2001), and thus would need to be regularly tested. Individualising the $TRIMP_{MOD}$ would enable a more accurate analysis of a player's physiological response to training.

Session RPE

A cost effective, non invasive method of quantifying the combined effect of internal and external exercise intensity is to collect RPE from players. This requires the player to inherently estimate exercise intensity through the physiological stress their bodies experience during exercise (Borg, 1982). A variation of this method is the session RPE, which is a global rating of the overall difficulty of the exercise bout obtained 30 minutes after the cessation of training by asking the player "how hard was your training session?", this unit is then multiplied by training duration (minutes) to calculate session load (Foster et al., 1996). When collecting the data the player is shown the RPE scale with verbal anchors (Table 6) and it is explained that a global rating of the entire training is required using whatever cues they feel appropriate (Foster et al., 2001). By delaying securing the session RPE rating for 30 minutes particularly difficult or easy drills towards the end of training session will not dominate the player's rating (Foster et al., 2001).

Table 6. The category rating of perceived exertion (RPE) scale (used by Foster *et al.,* 1996)

Rating	Descriptor
	Rest
1	Very, Very Easy
2	Easy
3	Moderate
4	Somewhat Hard
5	Hard
6	-
7	Very Hard
8	-
9	-
10	Maximal

In addition coaches can provide an RPE score for each training session (coach RPE). Doing this provides the coach with valuable feedback to use when reflecting on their training prescription in relation to the players perception of effort. Players appear to more regularly overestimate than underestimate training session intensity compared to the coach's rating (Rains, Noon, and Thake, unpublished data; Figure 2). Furthermore it is evident that position specific differences exist in how the exercise intensity is perceived indicating that the type of training session prescribed impacts differently on each playing position due to the individual activity profile of each position. For example, a training session designed to work on wide and flank play, will elicit a greater perception of effort on the wingers and full backs because the emphasis and the coaching will be focused on these areas.

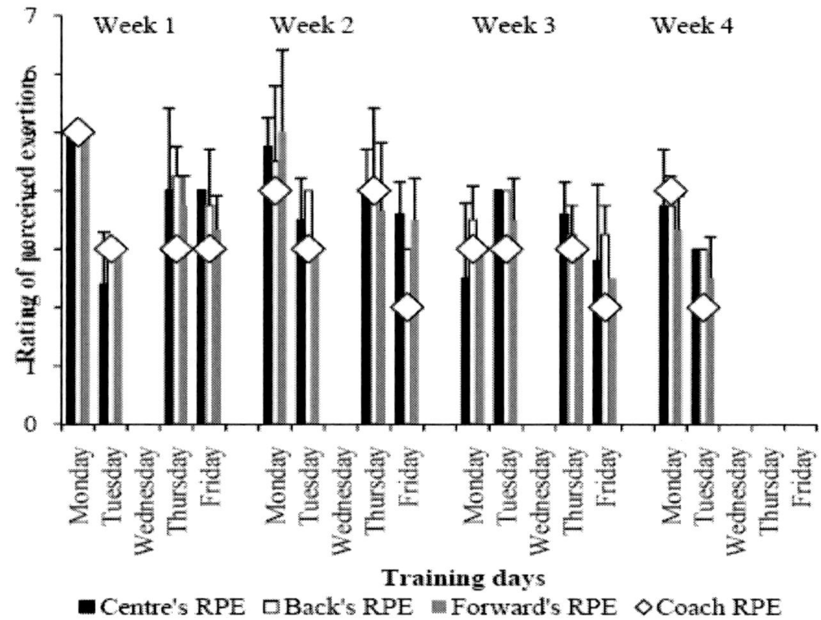

Figure2. Ratings of perceived exertion (RPE) for each positional group (Centre's, Back's and Forward's; mean±SD) and the coach RPE for each training session (Rains, Noon and Thake, unpublished data).

Recovery Time

Inadequate recovery time between training and competition causes a homeostatic imbalance and players will not be able to perform at their optimal level (Onkenttä and Hassmén, 1998). Consequently, coaches may taper training intensity and duration in the run up to a competitive match to provide adequate recovery time and less physiological stress (Figure 3). It is important to note from a monitoring perspective that it is not solely the training stimulus that causes stress. Young elite footballers have a multitude of other stressors to balance such as team selection, attempting to secure a contract and relationships to name a few. Furthermore level of recovery is influenced by a multitude of factors including sleep, nutrition and relaxation. A battery of measures using a holistic and individual approach is vital to prescribe optimal training stimuli and ensure recovery from the possible stressors required and add armour to the coach on making informed decisions on training methods. There are several possible performance, biochemical, immunological and psychological markers that may identify a risk of non functional overreaching (Gleeson, 2002). However, a European College of Sport Science consensus statement reported there is no definitive marker of non functional overreaching (Meeusen *et al.,* 2006). Therefore, monitoring player training status can be achieved by a battery of indicators such as the HIMS (Lamberts *et al.,* 2004), and RSI (Hore 2003), in addition to measures of immune function, subjective questionnaires and training load.

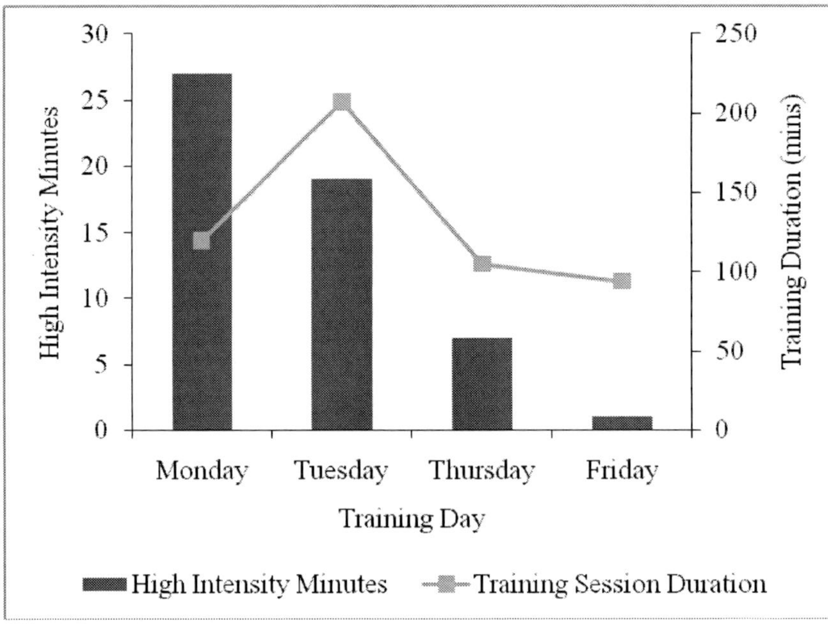

Figure 3. Training intensity and training session duration for one week in an elite academy football player. High intensity minutes = time spent exercising above 85% of maximum heart rate.

Heart Rate Recovery

On a weekly basis heart rate recovery is evaluated to further explore how the player is coping with and recovering from training and match play. A submaximal heart rate shuttle test, known as HIMS, comprising 4 stages of increasing intensity interspersed with recovery periods (Lamberts et al., 2004) is currently used. Players are required to run between two lines that are 20m apart. The pace of running within each of the four stages ($8.4 km.h^{-1}$, $9.6 km.h^{-1}$, and $12.0 km.h^{-1}$, respectively) is set by a pre-recorded auditory signal. Each stage lasts 2 minutes followed by rest for 1 minute after each of the three stages and two minutes after the fourth stage. Therefore, the total duration of the test is 13 minutes and can replace the normal warm-up routine. Both the heart rate during exercise and the heart rate recovery, the rate at which heart rate decreases after moderate to heavy exercise, are then compared to previous HIMS responses. Heart rate at a fixed submaximal exercise intensity decreases as aerobic fitness improves, whereas an elevated heart rate at a fixed submaximal exercise intensity could indicate a state of overtraining or lack of conditioning (Jeukendrup and Van Diemen, 1998). It is known that heart rate recovery responds to acute changes in training load with recovery slowing slightly after increases in training load and improving when training load decreased (Borresen and Lambert, 2007). This test is submaximal so it can be administered frequently during different phases of training. Furthermore, the test is inexpensive, easy to administer so an entire squad can do the test simultaneously.

Subjective Assessments

When interpreted in context with data gathered on training load and training status, subjective recovery assessments contribute useful information to making decisions on individual training prescription, adding further to the coach's overview on how an individual is responding to the training load. Monitoring instruments can be used to assess an individual's mood, their need for recovery, and current life circumstances and are advantageous as they provide information quickly and are non-invasive. Various questionnaires used with athletes include the Profile of Mood States (POMS) (McNair, Lorr, and Dropplman, 1971), Recovery-Stress Questionnaire (RESTQ-Sport) (Kellmann 2002); Daily Analysis of Life Demands of Athletic (DALDA) (Halson *et al.,* 2002), and the 'perceived recovery status (PRS) scale' (Laurent *et al.,* 2010).

The POMS questionnaire measures mood state on a 65-item Likert questionnaire, rated on a scale of 1 (not at all) to 4 (extremely) and has been used to examine psychological responses to intense training loads (Morgan *et al.,* 1987; Morgan *et al.,* 1988; O'Connor, Morgan, and Raglin, 1991). Results suggest a dose-response relationship exists between training and mood. In particular, mood disturbance increases as training load intensifies, however, following reductions in training load, global mood disturbance returns to baseline (Morgan *et al.,* 1987; Morgan *et al.,* 1988; O'Connor, Morgan, and Raglin, 1991).

The RESTQ-Sport has been widely used in rowers (Kellmann and Günther 2000; Kellmann *et al.,* 2001; Maestu *et al.,* 2005; Maestu *et al.,* 2006) and recently rugby league players (King, Clark, and Kellmann, 2010) and elite adolescent soccer players (Brink *et al.,* 2010) to measure the frequency of current stress as well as the frequency of recovery-associated activities. The RESTQ-Sport is based on the hypothesis that an accumulation of stress in different areas of life, along with insufficient recovery possibilities, leads to a changed psychophysical state (Kellmann and Kallus, 2001). The questionnaire is made up of seventy-seven items consisting of twelve scales of general recovery-stress questions and an additional seven sport-specific scales (total = nineteen scales, 4 items per scale plus 1 warm-up item). Questions are answered on a Likert scale, values ranging from 0 (never) to 6 (always) indicating the frequency of their stress-and recovery-related activities during the previous 3 days/nights. The mean of each scale can range from 0 to 6, with high scores in the stress-associated activity scales reflecting intense subjective stress, whereas high scores in the recovery-orientated scales mirror plenty of recovery activities (e.g., social activities, vacation, sauna etc.). RESTQ-Sport appears to be sensitive to changes in training load. Increases in stress were seen in twelve national level male rowers during high volume training and stress decreased during the recovery period, an opposite effect was found on the recovery scales (Mäestu *et al.,* 2006). The RESTQ-Sport also identified injury and illness when administered monthly in a group of adolescent soccer players (Brink *et al.,* 2010). Results showed that physical stress was related to both injury and illness and psychosocial stress and recovery were related to the occurrence of illness.

The use of the POMS and RESTQ-Sport questionnaire in a soccer team on a day-to-day basis is unrealistic due to the large volume of questions and vast amounts of time would be spent filling in questionnaires and analysing the data. Also, the data would not be reported back to the coach in enough time to inform training prescription for the day which is a fundamental use of a daily questionnaire. Additionally, filling in long questionnaires will become monotonous for player's resulting in unreliable data.

All player's in the U18 squad are required to independently complete a short Recovery Questionnaire (Taylor and Thake, unpublished data; Figure 4) on arrival at training to provide an overview of their recovery status . A laminated A4 copy of the Recovery Questionnaire is pinned above their peg in the changing room and completed using a white board marker. This activity has now been embeded within the players' daily routine. All questions are answered on a Likert scale ranging from 3 (very good) to -3 (very poor) and take approximately 30 seconds in total to complete. Each question is scored the same, an above zero score indicates good recovery, a below zero score indictes poor recovery and a score of zero denotes normal recovery. The amount of hours sleep the player acquired the previous night is also recorded. The responses are collected before the commencement of training and reported to the coach to inform the training prescription for that day. The coach then evaluates the level of recovery of the squad and of individuals and training intensity is manipulated accordingly. Additionally, individual players can be withdrawn from training if recovery scores are extremely low. However, as the topics in the Recovery Questionnaire are generic and do not indicate the specific problem an interview between coach and player may be needed to establish the underlying issue (see case study below). Once the data have been stored on a computer each Recovery Questionnaire is wiped clean ready for use the next day. Individual responses to the questionnaire are tracked and analysed over time in conjunction with training load data to identify changes in recovery status. To monitor player responses to the questionnaire baseline levels are established for each player based on the way they regularly answer each question. Daily responses can then be compared to the individual's baseline measure and any reductions below the baseline can be highlighted and discussed with the coach.

	Very Good		Good	Normal	Poor		Very Poor
Level of motivation to train	3	2	1	0	-1	-2	-3
Quality of sleep	3	2	1	0	-1	-2	-3
Level of recovery	3	2	1	0	-1	-2	-3
Level of appetite	3	2	1	0	-1	-2	-3
Feelings of fatigue	3	2	1	0	-1	-2	-3
Feelings of stress	3	2	1	0	-1	-2	-3
Muscle soreness	3	2	1	0	-1	-2	-3

Figure 4. Recovery Questionnaire (Taylor and Thake, unpublished data).

It is important that players are aware of the rationale behind filling out the questionnaire. Accordingly the coach should explain that these measures are to help improve training methods to gain greater knowledge on how the individual is feeling prior to exercise. It is of equal importance that players are educated on how to answer the questions and how they should interpret them to provide reliable data. Responses to the questionnaire could be influenced by personality, fear of being replaced or showing weakness, or even player position. Interestingly forwards, commonly considered to have high self-esteem, consistently tend to return the highest or most positive scores (Figure 5). The fear of not being selected or substituted may result in players manipulating answers to the questionnaire so under-recovery may be, at least initially, less evident. Additionally, the Recovery Questionnaire should be administered pre-training each day and ideally at the same time, although this is not always possible due to sporadic training times.

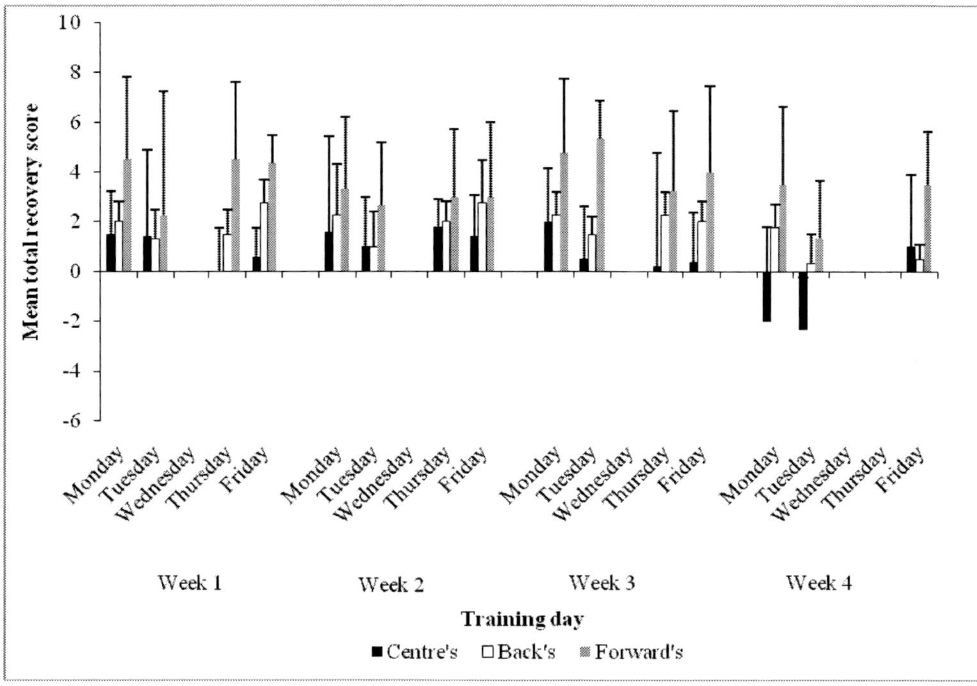

Figure 5. Recovery Questionnaire score (mean±SD) for each positional group (Centre's, Back's and Forward's) on each training day of a four week period (Rains, Noon, and Thake, unpublished data).

Immunological Testing

Suppressed immune function and the risk of upper respiratory tract infection (URTI) has been linked to under-recovery and non functional overreaching (Kingsbury, 1998). It is currently unclear whether suppressed immune function is a key factor in the onset of non functional overreaching although it is accepted that an increase in stress as a result of intense training is a factor influencing the increased risk of URTI (Meeusen *et al.,* 2006). The J-shaped curve shows the relationship between exercise and immunity where at high exercise intensities and high training loads the risk of infection increases (Nieman ,1994).

Salivary IgA (S-IgA) is considered the first line of defence against pathogens and monitoring this marker of mucosal immunity may help identify the risk of URTI in athletes (Gleeson and Pyne, 2000). Given mucosal measures of immunity are non invasive and simple to administer they are often used as a marker of immune function in athletes. Much of the research in this area has been carried out in individual sports and no longitudinal research has been published on football players to date. A longitudinal study in American football players over a 12 month period reported a decrease in S-IgA and an increase in URTI in periods of intensified training (Fahlman and Engles, 2005). Further to this an investigation into S-IgA and URTI over a 12 month period in Americas Cup Sailors and reported players with a relative S-IgA <40% of the healthy baseline had a 48% chance of contracting a URTI in the following 3 weeks (Neville *et al.* 2008). Therefore, although S-IgA may not predict every incidence of URTI it may have real value as a monitoring tool. Unfortunately given the financial implications and expertise needed for S-IgA analysis it may not be possible to gain access to measures of mucosal immunity. Another practical issue to consider is the time it takes the analysis in the laboratory. If the sample takes several days or even several hours to analyse it could be suggested that the measure becomes redundant as the player will have already trained therefore it could be argued immediate feedback is necessary interestingly, a simple questionnaire has been found to be highly correlated with levels of S-IgA (Neville *et al.,* 2008). The athletes were asked 'how rested do you feel?' and on a 3 point scale a) worse than normal b) normal c) better than normal. Athletes who reported to be better than normal had a relative S-IgA above baseline whereas when the athlete perceived to be worse than normal the relative S-IgA was below baseline. This further supports the use of a simple subjective assessment in a practical setting and may be of real value from a practical perspective when trying to identify risk of URTI in soccer players.

Case Study

On the day of the Yo-Yo Intermittent Recovery Test Player A reported inadequate recovery on the Recovery Questionnaire (Table 7). He complained of feeling unwell and tired but wished to train, which the coach allowed. He achieved a distance of 2680 m on the Yo-Yo Test. In the previous Yo-Yo Test (3 months before), this player achieved a distance of 3760 m and his responses to the corresponding Recovery Questionnaire had indicated adequate recovery. The decrease in Yo-Yo test performance could not be attributed to a lower level of fitness as he had completed 94% of game time for the U18 squad and 96% of all training sessions between the first and second test indicating that a reduction in fitness was an unlikely cause. In this instance the result of the Recovery Questionnaire, indicating that Player A had not recovered properly alongside self-reporting feeling unwell corresponded with a reduction in physical performance (Table 7). Consequently, Player A was given 2 days off training and did not participate in the weekends match and instructed to stay at home to ensure a full recovery and reduce the risk of the illness spreading amongst the squad. When Player A returned to training 4 days later his recovery scores had rebounded back to normal indicating a full recovery (Table 7).

Conclusion

Further investigation into Player A's internal training load responses and the squads mean internal physiological response in the 15 preceding training days before the onset of illness and the Yo-Yo Intermittent Recovery Test do not explain the underlying reason behind Player A's consistent perception of feeling fatigued (Figure 6).

However, it is apparent that Player A was struggling to tolerate the demands of training and a heavy fixture list. Having completed 94% of all game time adds increased unmeasured stress to the additional prescribed training load and is likely to have contributed to the subsequent illness. Further analysis of external training load data (e.g., distance covered or RPE scores in training and matches) in conjunction with immunological markers or a HIMS test to evaluate HRR at the beginning of each training week could have predicted illness. This type of scenario reveals that a holistic approach involving a combination of physical, physiological, subjective and immunological information is required for the coach to build a clear picture on how a player is developing and coping with training and competition to inform the training process and improve player performance.

Table 7. Player A's subjective responses to the Recovery Questionnaire on the day of the Yo-Yo Intermittent Recovery Test and subsequent test results

	Hours Sleep	Motivation	Sleep Quality	Recovery	Appetite	Fatigue	Stress	Yo-Yo Test Score (m)
06/10/2010	8	2	0	0	0	0	0	2680
04/01/2011	9	1	0	-1	0	-1	0	3760
10/01/2011	9	2	0	0	0	0	0	N/A

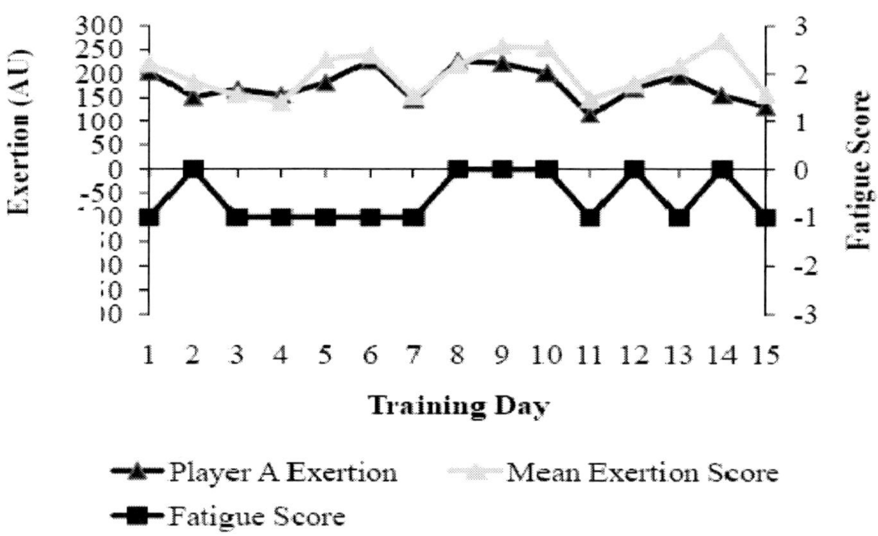

Figure 6. Player A's fatigue rating scores and exertion scores in comparison to the teams mean exertion score (exertion calculated from TRIMPMOD) for the 15 previous training days before the Yo-Yo Intermittent Recovery Test on 04/01/2011 (Rains, Noon, and Thake 2011).

The Future

Providing the level of support outlined here and beyond within an academy environment is challenging but essential to promote player development. There is pressure for English academies to produce elite home-grown players for club and country due to UEFA's ruling where each professional squad of 25 players has to contain 8 'locally' trained players who have been involved in the English Academy system for a minimum of 3 years whilst under the age of 21 (Johnson, Doherty, and Freemont, 2009). Furthermore, from the 2012-2013 season the Premier League are aiming to implement an Elite Player Performance Plan which will split each elite academy into four categories of excellence with a view to start producing more technically gifted English players. The new system will allow player and coach contact time to treble (current academy set-up is approximately 3,760 training hours), with the aim of reaching 10,000 hours and 10 years of deliberate practice by the time players turn 21 years old. Under such guidelines young athletes would have participated in adequate training to reach the highest level of performance by the time they are young adults. Furthermore current players are most likely to be the managers and coaches of future generations thus the application of science in football will continue to be embedded within the professional game.

Conclusion

For the coach, quantity of data is irrelevant, evaluation and action upon the data is vital. Monitoring an adolescents training is a complex process. The 'Holy Grail' for coaches is to quantify training load into a single number, however, a number of factors need to be taken into account, such as the internal and external training load and the player's recovery status which can be monitored through psychological, immunological and physiological markers. The coach should apply all resources at their disposal to manage individual players at their specific stage of physical development and on their training status to ensure player's are receiving optimal training stimuli both individually and within squad based training.

Factors such as, level of maturation, biological age and rate of growth (PHV) should determine the focus of a players training within a periodised cycle. Implementing simple tests to determine an individual's level of maturation can inform coaching staff of what to expect of the player at their particular stage of development and inform the training process so more individualised training programme can be integrated. Therefore, let's push towards 'making it fair' for our adolescent football players and make sure that their rate of growth and maturation do not ultimately determine their chances of progression into the adult professional game.

References

Achten, J., and Jeukendrup, A. E. (2003). 'Heart Rate Monitoring Applications and Limitations.' *Sports Medicine,* 33, (7) 517-538.

Astrand, P. and Rodahl, K. (1986). *Textbook of Work Physiology.* New York: McGraw Hill.

Balyi, I. and Hamilton (1999). North American Soccer - Overplayed and Underdeveloped. Long-term planning Part V. The Training to Perform Phase of Training. Performance Conditioning Soccer Lincoln NE 5, (4) 4.

Balyi, I. and Way, R. (2005). '*Canadian Sport for Life: LTAD Resource Paper.*' Canadian Sports Centres: Vancouver.

Bangsbo, J. (1994). *Fitness Training in Football – A Scientific Approach.* Baegsvard: H + O Storm.

Bannister, E. W. (1991). Modelling Athletic Performance. In H. J. Green, J. D. McDougal, and H. Wenger (Eds.), *Physiological Testing of Elite Athletes* (pp. 403 – 424). Champaign, IL: Human Kinetics.

Borg, G. A. (1982). 'Psychophysical Bases of Perceived Exertion.' *Medicine and Science inSports and Exercise,* 14, (5) 377-381.

Borresen, J. and Lambert, M. (2007). 'Changes in Heart Rate Recovery in Response to Acute Changes in Training Load.' *European Journal of Applied Physiology,* 101, 503-511.

Borresen, J. and Lambert, M. I. (2009). 'The Quantification of Training Load, the TrainingResponse and the Effect on Performance.' *Sports Medicine,* 39, (9) 779-795.

Brewer, J., Balsom, P., and Davis, J. (1995). 'Seasonal Birth Distribution Amongst European Soccer Players.' *Sports Exercise and Injury,* 1, 154-157.

Brink, M., Visscher, C., Arends, S., Zwerver, J., Post, W., and Lemmink, K. (2010). 'Monitoring Stress and Recovery: New Insights for the Prevention of Injuries and Illnesses in Elite Youth Soccer Players.' *British Journal of Sports Medicine,* 44, 809-815.

Brockett, C., Morgan, D., and Proske, U. (2001). 'Human Hamstring Muscles Adapt to Eccentric Exercise by Changing Optimum Length.' *Medicine and Science in Sports and Exercise,* 33, 783-790.

Budgett, R. (1998). 'Fatigue and Underperformance in Athletes: The Overtraining Syndrome.'*British Journal of Sports Medicine,* 32, (2) 107-110.

Christou, M., Smilios, I., Sotiropoulos, K., Volaklis, K., Pilianidis, T., and Tokmakidis, S. (2006). 'Effects of Resistance Training on the Physical Capacities of Adolescent Soccer Players.' *Journal of Strength and Conditioning Research,* 20, (4) 783-791.

Coombs, R. and Garbutt, G. (2002). 'Development in the Use of the Hamstring/Quadriceps Ratio for the Assessment of Muscle Balance.' *Journal of Science and Medicine in Sport,* 1, 56-52.

Fahlman, M. and Engles, H. (2005). 'Mucosal IgA and URTI in American College Football Players: A Year Longitudinal Study.' *Medicine and Science in Sports and Exercise,* 37, (3) 374-280.

Forbes, H., Sutcliffe, S., Lovell, A., McNaughton, L., and Siegler, J. (2009). 'Isokinetic Thigh Muscle Ratios in Youth Football: Effect of Age and Dominance.' *International Journal of Sports Medicine,*30, 602-606.

Foster, C., Florahaug, J. A., Franklin, J., Gottschall, L., Hrovatin, L. A., Parker, S., Doleshal,P., and Dodge, C. (2001). 'A New Approach to Monitoring Exercise Training.' *Journal of Strength and Conditioning Research,* 15, (1) 109-115.

Foster, C., Hector, R., Welsh, M., Schrager, M., Green, A., and Snyder A,. (1995). 'Effects of specific versus cross-training on running performance.' *European Journal of Applied Physiology and Occupational Physiology,*70, 367–372.

Daniels, I., Hector, A., Snyder, A., and Welsh, R. (1996). 'Athletic Performance in Relation to Training Load.' *Wisconsin Medical Journal,* 95, 370-373.

Gleeson, M. (2002). 'Biochemical and Immunological Markers of Over-training.' *Journal of Sports Science and Medicine,* 1, 31-41.

Gleeson, M. and Pyne, D. (2000). 'Exercise Effects on Mucosal Immunity.' *Immunology and Cell Biology,* 78, 536-544.

Halson, S., Bridge, M., Meeusen, R., Busschaert, B., Gleeson, M., Jones, D., and Jeukendrup, A. (2002). 'Time Course of Performance Changes and Fatigue Markers During Intensified Training in Trained Cyclists.' *Journal of Applied Physiology,* 93 (3), 947-956.

Harley, J., Barnes, C., Portas, M., Lovell, R., Barrett, S., Paul, D., and Weston, M. (2010). 'Motion Analysis of Match-Play in Elite U12 to U16 Age-Group Soccer Players.' *Journal of Sports Sciences,* 28, (13) 1391-1397.

Helgerud, J., Engen, L., Wisløff, U., and Hoff, J. (2001). 'Aerobic Endurance Training Improves Soccer Performance.' *Medicine and Science in Sports and Exercise,* 33, (11) 1925-1931.

Helson, W., Hodges, N., Van Winckel, J., and Starkes, J. (2000). 'The Roles of Talent, Physical Precocity and Practice in the Development of Soccer Expertise.' *Journal of Sports Sciences,* 18, 727-736.

Hill-Haas, S., Roswell, G., Dawson, B., Coutts, A. (2009). 'Acute Physiological Responses and Time-Motion Characteristics of Two Small-Sided Training Regimes in Youth Soccer Players.' *Journal of Strength and Conditioning Research,* 23, (1) 111-115.

Hoff, J., Wisloff, U., Engen, L. C., Kemi, O. J., and Helgerud, J. (2002). 'Soccer SpecificAerobic Endurance Training.' *British Journal of Sports Medicine,* 36, (3) 218-221.

Hore (2003) 'Use of the Reactive Strength Index (RSI) as a Plyometric Monitoring Tool.'

Jeukendrup, A. and Van Diemen, A. (1998). 'Heart Rate Monitoring During Training and Competition in Cyclists.' *Journal of Sports Sciences,* 16, S91-S99.

Johnson, A., Doherty, P., and Freemont, A. (2009). 'Investigation of Growth, Development, and Factors Associated with Injury in Elite Schoolboy Footballers: A Prospective Study.' *British Medical Journal.*

Kellman, M., Altenburg, D., Lormes, W., and Steinacker, J. (2001). 'Assessing Stress and Recovery During Preparation for the World Championships in Rowing.' *The Sport Psychologist,* 15, 151-167.

Kellmann, M. (2002). *Enhancing Recovery: Preventing Underperformance in Athletes.* Champaign, Illinois: Human Kinetics.

Kellmann, M. and Günther, K. (2000). 'Changes in Stress and Recovery in Elite Rowers during Preparation for the Olympic Games.' *Medicine and Science in Sports and Exercise,* 32, (3) 676-683.

Kellmann, M. and Kallus W. (2001). '*Recovery Stress Questionnaire for Athletes: User Manual.*' Human Kinetics; Champaign, IL.

Kent, M (1998). *Oxford Dictionary of Sports Science and Medicine.* Second Edition. Oxford University Press: Oxford UK.

Kenttä, G., and Hassmén, P. (1998). 'Overtraining and Recovery A Conceptual Model.'*Sports Medicine,* 26, (1) 1-16.

King, D., Clark, T., and Kellmann, M. (2010). 'Changes in Stress and Recovery as a Result of Participating in a Premier Rugby League Representative Competition.' *International Journal of Sport Science and Coaching,* 6, (2) 223-237.

Kingsbury, K., Kay, L. and Hjelm (1998). 'Contrasting Amino Acid Patterns in Elite Athletes: Association with Fatigue and Infection.' *British Journal of Sports Medicine,* 32, 25-33.

Kujala, M., Orava, S., and Jarvinen, M. (1997). 'Hamstring Injuries: Current Trends in Treatment and Prevention.' *Sports Medicine,* 23, 397-404.

Lambert, M., and Borresen, J. (2006) 'A Theoretical Basis of Monitoring Fatigue: A Practical Approach for Coaches.' *International Journal of Sports Science and Coaching,* 1, (4) 371-388.

Lamberts, R., Lemmink, K., Durandt, J., and Lambert, M. (2004). 'Variation in Heart Rate during Submaximal Exercise: Implications for Monitoring Training.' *Journal of Strength and Conditioning Research,* 18, (3) 641-645.

Little, T., and Williams, A. G. (2007). 'Measures of Exercise Intensity during Soccer TrainingDrills with Professional Soccer Players.' *Journal of Strength and ConditioningResearch,* 21, (2) 367-371.

Mäestu, J., Jürimäe, J., and Jürimäe, T. (2005). 'Monitoring of Performance and Training in Rowing.' *Sports Medicine,* 35, (7) 597-617.

Mäestu, J., Jürimäe, J., Krregipuu, K., and Jürimäe, T. (2006). 'Changes in Perceived Stress and Recovery During Heavy Training in Highly Trained Male Rowers.' *The Sport Psychologist,* 20, 24-39.

McNair, D., Lorr, M., and Droppleman L. (1971). *Manual for the Profile of Mood States.* San Diego: Educational and Industrial Testing Services.

Meeusen, R., Duclos, M., Gleeson, M., Rietjens, G., Steinacker, J., and Urhausen, A. (2006). 'Prevention, Diagnosis and Treatment of the Overtraining Syndrome.' *European Journal of Sport Sciences,* 6, (1) 1-14.

Mirkov, D., Kukolj, M., Ugarkovic, D., Koprivica V., and Jaric, S. (2010). 'Development of Anthropometric and Physical Performance Profiles of Young Elite Male Soccer Players: A Longitudinal Study.' *Journal of Strength and Conditioning Research,* 24, (10) 2677-2682.

Morgan, W., Brown, D., Raglin, O'Connor, P., and Ellickson, K. (1987). 'Psychological Monitoring of Overtraining and Staleness.' *British Journal of Sports Medicine,* 21, 107-114.

Morgan, W., Costill, D., Flynn, M., Raglin, J., and O'Connor, P. (1988). 'Mood Disturbance Following Increased Training in Swimmers.' *Medicine and Science in Sports and Exercise,* 20, 408-414.

Mujika, I., Santisteban, J., and Castagna, C. (2009). 'In-Season Effect of Short-Term Sprint and Power Training Programs on Elite Junior Soccer Players.' *Journal of Strength and Conditioning Research,* 23, (9) 2581-2587.

Nederhof, E., Zwerver, J., Brink, M., Meeusen, R., and Lemmink, K. (2008). 'Different Diagnostic Tools in Nonfunctional Overreaching.' *Int. J. Sports Med.* 29, 590-297.

Neville, V., Gleeson, M., and Folland, J. (2008). 'Salivary IgA as a Risk Factor for Upper Respiratory Infections in Elite Professional Athletes.' *Medicine and Science in Sports and Exercise,* 40, (7) 1228-1236.

Nieman, D. (1994). 'Exercise, Infection, and Immunity.' *International Journal of Sports Medicine,* 15, S131-S141.

Noon, M. '*A Periodised Training Cycle for Elite Youth Soccer Players.*' Unpublished Manuscript, Coventry University.

O'Connor, P., Morgan, W., and Raglin J. (1991). 'Psychobiological Effects of 3 Days Increased Training in Female and Male Swimmers.' *Medicine and Science in Sports and Exercise,* 23, 1055-1061.

Orchard, J., Marsden, J., Lord, S., and Garlick, D. (1997). 'Preseason Hamstring Muscle Weakness Associated with Hamstring Muscle Injury in Australian Footballers.' *American Journal of Sports Medicine*, 81-85.

Portas, M., Harley, J., Barnes, C., and Rush, C. (2011). 'The Validity and Reliability of 1-Hz and 5-Hz Global Positioning Systems for Linear, Multidirectional, and Soccer-Specific Activities.' *International Journal of Sports Physiology and Performance,* 5, 448-458.

Rains, M., Noon, M., and Thake, D. '*Perceptions of Recovery and Physiological Responses to Training over an Annual Season in Elite Youth Soccer Players.*' Unpublished Maunscript, Coventry University.

Reilly, T., Williams, A., Nevill, A., and Franks, A. (2000). 'A Multidisciplinary Approach to Talent Identification in Soccer.' *Journal of Sports Sciences,* 18, 695-702.

Simmons, C. and Paull, G. (2001). 'Season-of-Birth Bias in Association Football.' *Journal of Sports Sciences,* 19, 677-686.

Stagno, K. M., Thatcher, R., and Van Somermen, K. A. (2007) 'A Modified TRIMP toQuantify the In-Season Training Load of Team Sport Players.' *Journal of Sports Sciences,* 25, (6) 629-634.

Taylor, R. and Thake, D. '*Recovery Questionnaire.*' Unpublished Manuscript, Coventry University .

Tierney, P. and Knight, R. '*Motion Assimilation for Performance in Sport.*' Unpublished Manuscript, Coventry University.

Usaj, A., and Starc, V. (1996). 'Blood pH and Lactate Kinetics in the Assessment of Running Endurance.' *International Journal of Sports Medicine,* 17, 34-40.

Williams, A. and Reilly, T. (2000). 'Talent Identification and Development in Soccer.' *Journal of Sports Sciences,* 18, 657-667.

Wisløff, U., Castagna, C., Helgerud, J., Jones, R., and Hoff, J. (2004). 'Strong Correlation of Maximal Squat Strength with Sprint Performance and Vertical Jump Height in Elite Soccer Players.' *British Journal of Sports Medicine,* 38, 285-288.

Young, W., James, R., and Montgomery I. (2002). 'Is Muscle Power Related to Running Speed with Changes of Direction?' *Journal of Sports Medicine and Physical Fitness,* 43, 282-288.

Index

A

abuse, 194
academic performance, x, xv, 13, 37, 40, 63, 97, 98, 99, 102, 108, 111, 113
academic success, 100
accelerometers, 17, 75, 84, 135, 137, 139, 140, 153, 154
access, xi, 6, 14, 33, 36, 38, 68, 69, 71, 73, 75, 76, 84, 195, 234
accessibility, 86
accounting, 3, 137
accumulation of blood, xi, 28
achievement test, 102
active transport, xi, 14, 79, 143
activity level, x, xi, xiv, 3, 7, 13, 14, 21, 25, 45, 70, 72, 73, 74, 76, 79, 84, 85, 97, 99, 117, 126, 134, 136, 145, 192
acupuncture, 172, 179
adaptation, 183, 204, 213, 222, 225, 226
adaptations, 207, 208, 209, 212, 214
ADHD, 105, 112
adipose, 51
adipose tissue, 51
adiposity, xvii, 25, 73, 84, 91, 92, 120, 126, 145, 157
adjustment, 21, 134, 177
administrators, xv, 33, 36, 98
adolescent boys, 50, 51, 90, 93, 204
adolescent female, 31
adult obesity, 70, 73
adult onset diabetes, xii, 28
adulthood, ix, x, xii, xiii, xvii, xx, 1, 9, 14, 17, 18, 21, 22, 23, 28, 44, 61, 67, 82, 125, 150, 201, 204, 207, 210, 217
adverse effects, 55
advertisements, 70
aerobic capacity, 145, 166
aerobic exercise, 100, 101, 102, 109
aesthetic, 91
aesthetics, 92
aetiology, 51
Africa, 40
African Americans, 150
African-American, 160
aggressive behavior, 4
agility, 208, 215, 219, 222, 224
agonist, 206, 207
alcohol use, 85
alienation, 18, 19, 22
alters, 182
ambulatory electrocardiographic monitoring, 158
amenorrhea, 92
American Heart Association, 30
American Psychological Association, 95
amplitude, 101, 102, 108
Amsterdam Growth Study, x, 13
anatomy, 31
androgen, 204
androgens, 4
angina, xii, 28
anhydrase, 170
ankles, 187
anorexia, xiv, 87, 88, 89, 92, 93, 94, 193
anorexia nervosa, xiv, 88, 89, 92, 93, 94
ANS, xvii, 147, 152
anxiety, 149
aptitude, 70
arithmetic, 102
arrest, 18, 19, 20, 21
arteries, xi, 27
artery, xi, 28
assessment, xiv, xix, 8, 11, 21, 59, 87, 88, 89, 94, 102, 103, 118, 119, 135, 137, 140, 141, 153, 181, 186, 190, 193, 194, 195, 213, 224, 234
assets, 80
asthenia, 105

asymmetry, 105
asymptomatic, 188
atherosclerosis, xi, 27, 40, 142
atherosclerotic plaque, xii, 28, 33
athletes, ix, xix, 153, 155, 164, 168, 169, 178, 181, 183, 184, 185, 188, 189, 190, 193, 194, 195, 196, 197, 198, 208, 213, 214, 231, 233, 236
attachment, 182, 189
Australian pre-school aged children, ix, 1
authority, 37
autism, 101
automaticity, 112
autonomic activity, xvii, 147, 151, 160
autonomic nervous system, 158, 159
avoidance, xii, 28, 29, 192
awareness, xii, 28, 29, 33, 36, 163, 170, 195

B

Bangladesh, 127
barriers, 6, 16, 40, 52, 142
base, ix, x, 1, 7, 13, 14, 16, 154
behaviors, xiv, 3, 39, 40, 62, 87, 91
Belgium, 8
bending, 220
beneficial effect, 6, 47, 53, 56, 151, 152
benefits, ix, x, xi, xiii, xiv, xvi, xvii, 1, 4, 13, 14, 16, 44, 47, 48, 49, 51, 52, 59, 63, 67, 97, 98, 100, 101, 102, 105, 108, 111, 116, 118, 125, 172, 195, 205, 207
benign, 194, 197
beverages, 47
bias, xiii, 44, 99, 102, 106, 107, 217
biceps femoris, 212
biomechanics, xix, 34, 181, 184, 211, 214
Black students, 133
Blacks, 129, 130, 131
bleeding, 187
blood, xi, xii, 27, 28, 32, 34, 47, 48, 49, 51, 56, 57, 58, 59, 60, 62, 63, 64, 143, 144, 145, 172, 227
blood flow, xi, xii, 27, 28, 172
blood pressure, 32, 63, 143, 144, 145
blood supply, xii, 28
BMI, x, 14, 35, 45, 46, 47, 48, 49, 51, 52, 59, 69, 70, 81, 90, 92, 93, 113, 120, 128, 143, 151, 187, 191
body composition, xvii, 9, 44, 63, 123, 125, 133, 154, 220
body dissatisfaction, 90, 91, 92, 93, 96
body fat, xiv, 31, 32, 35, 46, 60, 64, 72, 87, 91, 128, 129, 143, 145, 156, 174, 219, 220
body image, xiv, 19, 87, 88, 89, 90, 91, 92, 93, 94, 95
body mass index, ix, 1, 24, 35, 45, 59, 60, 64, 85, 90, 120, 122
body shape, 88, 89, 90, 91, 93, 94
body size, xiv, 87, 89, 91, 140, 173, 204
body tissues., xii, 28
body weight, xiv, 49, 53, 59, 61, 63, 65, 80, 87, 90, 91, 93, 95, 129, 154, 166
bonds, 10
bone, ix, xix, 1, 2, 45, 181, 182, 183, 185, 188, 189, 190, 193, 213
bone growth, 182, 185, 189
bone health, ix, 1, 2
bones, xiii, 67, 182, 183, 219
bounds, xiv, 97
bradycardia, 156
brain, xv, 4, 53, 57, 62, 97, 98, 101, 105, 106, 110, 113
brain-derived neurotrophic factor (BDNF), xv, 98
Brazil, 91, 93
breakdown, xix, 6, 181, 225
breathing, 148, 153
breathing rate, 149
Britain, 26
building blocks, 118
bulimia, xiv, 87, 88, 89, 92, 93, 94
bulimia nervosa, xiv, 88, 89, 92
burn, 171, 175
Butcher, 116, 122

C

calcium, 44, 45, 48, 59, 64
calibration, 158
calorimetry, 129, 131, 135, 136, 137
cancer, xiv, 65, 97
capillary, 34
capsule, 182
carbohydrate, 45, 47, 48, 49, 50, 51, 55, 61, 62, 64, 65
carbohydrates, 48, 52, 60
cardiac output, 173
cardiovascular disease, ix, xi, xii, xiv, xvii, 1, 9, 27, 28, 29, 30, 32, 33, 34, 35, 36, 37, 38, 39, 40, 97, 125, 142, 157
cardiovascular disorders, xviii, 147
cardiovascular physiology, 34
cardiovascular risk, 29, 31, 35, 40, 49, 51, 52, 142, 143, 144, 145, 151
cardiovascular system, 34, 151
Caribbean, xvii, 125, 126, 130, 132, 144, 157
cartilage, 182, 190
cartilaginous, 182, 189
case studies, xix, 181

case study, 11, 171, 184, 186, 190, 232
Caucasian population, 150
Caucasians, 129, 150
causal relationship, 99
causality, 45, 47, 52, 151
CDC, 175
central nervous system, 57, 168, 185
central obesity, 144
cerebellum, 103, 111, 113
cerebral palsy, 169, 172, 177, 178, 179, 180
challenges, xii, 22, 23, 29, 35, 38, 100, 163, 183, 193
chaos, 23
Chicago, 81
child athletes, 175
child development, 4, 5, 9, 10
childcare, 2, 11
cholesterol, xii, xvii, 28, 46, 47, 63, 125
chronic diseases, xiii, 67, 116
chronic illness, 73
chronic obstructive pulmonary disease, xii, 28
cigarette smoking, 29
circadian rhythm, xviii, 148
circadian rhythms, xviii, 148
circulation, 51
City, 31, 217
clarity, xiii, 43
classes, xi, 14, 15, 18, 25, 29, 74, 84, 93, 107, 118
classification, 5, 101, 102
classroom, xi, xii, xv, 3, 8, 14, 29, 30, 31, 33, 34, 36, 40, 53, 98, 108
classroom activity, 8
classroom environment, 108
classroom teacher, 33, 34
classroom teachers, 33
climate, 167, 178, 179
clinical application, 175
clinical diagnosis, 190
clinical disorders, 100, 101, 109
clothing, xviii, 19, 161, 162, 179
clustering, 9
coaches, xix, 181, 185, 189, 194, 195, 209, 217, 219, 228, 229, 236
cognition, 60, 63, 113, 140
cognitive ability, 37
cognitive development, 12, 117
cognitive dimension, 15
cognitive function, xiii, xvi, 43, 45, 52, 53, 54, 55, 56, 57, 58, 59, 60, 62, 63, 98, 100, 101, 105, 108
cognitive performance, 58, 60, 61, 65, 101
cognitive process, 62, 101, 153
cognitive processing, 101
cognitive skills, 103, 109
collisions, 184
Colombia, 210
combined effect, 228
commercial, 69, 103
commercials, 71
communication, 93
communities, 4, 6, 30, 33, 35, 71, 73, 79, 80, 81, 144
community, 4, 6, 10, 16, 17, 24, 29, 32, 33, 35, 39, 40, 41, 70, 73, 80, 83, 118, 150, 159, 197
competition, 183, 184, 185, 193, 218, 229, 235
complement, 169
complex carbohydrates, 47
complexity, 4
compliance, 77, 131, 160
complications, xviii, 147, 185, 186, 195
composition, xiii, 24, 43, 44, 45, 47, 52, 53, 55, 57, 59, 62, 86, 128, 129, 131, 133, 212, 220
comprehension, 103, 109
compression, 186
compulsory education, 17, 19
computation, 100
computer, 72, 80, 232
conception, 68
conceptual model, 22
concordance, 91
concussion, 185, 186, 198
conditioning, 188, 190, 192, 194, 195, 196, 218, 219, 224, 225, 230
conference, 155
confounders, 46, 107
confounding variables, 46, 99, 107
congestive heart failure, xii, 28
Congress, 38, 213
connectivity, 73
consensus, 124, 186, 209, 229
construction, 40, 90
consumers, 45, 46, 47
consumption, xii, xiii, 28, 29, 31, 32, 43, 44, 45, 46, 47, 48, 49, 51, 52, 53, 54, 55, 56, 57, 58, 59, 60, 62, 63, 64, 65, 142
consumption patterns, 63
contact time, 205, 206, 236
Continental, 139
control condition, 54
control group, 34, 99, 103, 104, 106, 107, 108, 173
controlled trials, 47, 49, 190
controversial, 91
controversies, 60
cooling, xviii, 161, 170, 174, 177, 178
coordination, 122, 190, 195, 206, 219
COPD, 40
coronary artery disease, 39, 158
coronary heart disease, x, 13, 142, 144, 154, 159
correlation, 91, 119, 128, 160

correlations, 69, 105
cortex, 106
cost, xi, 7, 27, 32, 35, 48, 63, 75, 153, 179, 228
cost effectiveness, 7
Costa Rica, 82
country of origin, 126
covering, 171
CPT, 53
creativity, 5
critical period, xii, 28, 118, 208
criticism, 16, 88, 104
cross sectional study, 142
cross-sectional study, 54, 81, 157
cues, 228
cure, 194
curriculum, 8, 19, 20, 22, 26, 29, 30, 31, 32, 33, 34, 36, 37, 38, 100, 110, 116
CVD, xvii, 125, 126
cycles, xviii, 148, 219
cycling, 62, 72, 85, 140, 177, 179, 188, 214
Cyprus, 82
Czech Republic, 91

D

dance, 119
danger, 6, 18
data collection, 75, 99, 130, 132, 133, 140, 141, 183
database, 34, 126
death rate, xi, xvii, 27, 125, 163
deaths, xi, 27, 163, 176
decision makers, 30
decreased quality of life, xi, 27
defence, 233
deficiency, 46
deficit, xiii, 46, 67, 101, 102, 103, 105, 112, 122
demographic data, 102
Denmark, 137
dependent variable, 104
deposits, 19
depth, 141
desensitization, 209
designers, 34
detection, 143
developing countries, xiv, 87
developmental change, 137
developmental dyslexia, 102
developmental milestones, 194
deviation, 204
diabetes, xi, xiv, xvii, 27, 44, 48, 51, 81, 97, 125, 143, 144, 150, 183
diamonds, 167
diaphysis, 182
diastolic blood pressure, xvii, 125
dichotomy, 53
diet, xi, xii, 14, 28, 29, 30, 31, 32, 44, 48, 49, 58, 59, 61, 62, 64, 81, 82, 112, 143, 158
dietary fat, 31
dietary intake, 29, 82
dieting, 19
direct measure, 8
direct observation, 7
disability, 172, 183, 190
disclosure, 108
discomfort, 192
disease rate, 35
diseases, xi, xiv, 14, 74, 97
dislocation, 197
disorder, 94, 105, 122
displacement, 121, 205
disposable income, 16
disruptive behaviours, 101
dissatisfaction, xiv, 87, 88, 89, 90, 91, 92, 93, 95, 96
dissatisfaction among women, xiv, 87
distress, 90
distribution, xviii, 46, 104, 136, 148
DOI, 9, 11
dosage, 108, 109, 190
dose-response relationship, xiv, 97, 231
drawing, xv, 97
drug treatment, 169
dyslexia, 102, 103, 105, 106, 110, 111, 112, 113

E

East Asia, 131
eating disorders, xiv, 87, 88, 89, 92, 93, 95, 96
economic evaluation, 11
economic status, 68, 99, 106, 110, 112, 113
ectodermal dysplasia, 169
editors, 95
education, ix, x, xv, 1, 2, 8, 13, 16, 17, 18, 19, 20, 21, 23, 24, 30, 31, 33, 34, 35, 36, 37, 39, 40, 46, 98, 110, 117
educational attainment, xv, 98
educators, 37, 117, 209
effusion, 185
electrocardiogram, 149, 156
electrolyte, 175
electromagnetic, 149
elementary school, 29, 30, 33, 34, 35, 36, 37, 38, 39, 62, 84
emergency, 162, 163, 178
employees, 74
encouragement, 73
endocrine, 150

endocrine disorders, 150
endurance, 64, 152, 153, 158, 166, 167, 169, 171, 175, 177, 195, 214, 219, 222, 223, 225
energy, 5, 31, 46, 48, 50, 55, 56, 57, 58, 65, 76, 77, 116, 126, 134, 136, 138, 139, 140, 143, 151, 153, 154, 159, 205, 209, 212
energy expenditure, 5, 31, 46, 77, 126, 134, 136, 138, 139, 140, 143, 153, 154
enforcement, 195
England, xv, 5, 10, 11, 16, 23, 25, 38, 79, 97, 98, 106, 109, 112, 122, 144, 146, 184, 186, 188, 214
environment, xix, 3, 4, 6, 10, 11, 12, 16, 17, 31, 36, 38, 68, 69, 70, 71, 72, 75, 76, 77, 78, 80, 81, 82, 83, 84, 85, 161, 162, 171, 174, 175, 177, 218, 222, 223, 235
environmental change, 81
environmental conditions, 37, 162, 163, 166, 167, 226
environmental factors, xiv, 32, 67, 119, 142
environmental influences, 3, 71, 138
environmental stress, 163, 174
environmental stresses, 163
environmental temperatures, 163, 164, 165, 166, 176
environmental variables, xiv, 67
enzyme, 204
enzymes, 170
epidemic, 81, 150
epidemiology, 22, 197, 199
epiphyses, 182, 183
epiphysis, 182
episodic memory, 56, 64
equality, 224
equipment, 2, 8, 103, 149, 189, 222
ERPs, 101
Estonia, 137
ethnic background, xvii, 126, 135, 139, 142
ethnic groups, xvii, 92, 125, 126, 127, 130, 131, 133, 140, 141, 142, 143
ethnic minority, 82, 126
ethnicity, xvii, 69, 78, 80, 83, 91, 96, 121, 125, 126, 128, 129, 132, 138, 140, 141, 142, 143, 144, 150, 156
EU, 128, 131, 132
Europe, 65, 90, 139, 143
European Union, 9
event-related potential, 101
excitability, 209, 213
exclusion, 100, 217
exercise participation, 22
exercise performance, xviii, xix, xx, 64, 161, 162, 166, 167, 169, 176, 177, 179, 201
exertion, 111, 171, 225, 228, 229, 235
experimental design, 203
expertise, 234
exposure, xii, 28, 107, 149, 162, 163, 175, 176, 178, 183, 184, 185, 209
extensor, 206, 212
eye movement, 103

F

facilitators, 34
factor analysis, 94
families, xi, 2, 4, 11, 14, 31, 33, 85, 90, 169
family hardship, xi, 27
fascia, 189
fast food, 69, 73, 85
fasting, xvii, 57, 63, 92, 125, 143, 145
fasting glucose, 145
fat, 19, 31, 32, 35, 46, 47, 48, 49, 50, 51, 52, 59, 62, 65, 89, 90, 95, 120, 128, 129, 133, 134, 136, 137, 139, 143, 151, 174, 213
fat intake, 48
fear, xiv, 88, 107, 232
fears, xv, 4, 6, 98
feelings, 14, 15, 18, 187
fever, 193
fiber, 59, 60, 212
financial, xi, 18, 27, 234
fires, 72
first aid, 185, 193
flank, 228
flaws, 104, 109
flexibility, 2, 5, 100, 185, 190, 194, 218, 219, 220, 221
flexor, 189, 211, 220
flight, 202
fluctuations, xvii, 147
fluid, xviii, 161, 175
fluid balance, 175
food, xiv, 23, 29, 30, 32, 37, 46, 48, 51, 62, 64, 65, 68, 69, 71, 73, 74, 81, 82, 83, 88, 89, 92
food intake, 32, 51, 62, 65
football, xx, 75, 76, 83, 119, 162, 184, 185, 191, 197, 217, 218, 219, 221, 230, 233, 236
Football, 80, 197, 198, 213, 217, 236, 237, 240
football injuries, 197
footwear, 189
force, 105, 183, 202, 205, 206, 207, 208, 209, 212, 215, 224
Ford, 204, 208, 209, 211
forebrain, xvi, 98
formal education, 33
formation, 17, 19, 37, 205
foundations, 117
fractures, xix, 181, 184, 185, 199

fragments, 190
freedom, 5
frontal lobe, 56
fructose, 48
fruits, 48
fundamental movement skills (FMS), xvi, 115, 117, 121

G

gait, 202
gastrocnemius, 187, 192, 210, 220
gel, 190, 199
gender differences, 4, 25, 119, 120, 132, 144, 145, 150, 182
gender effects, 211
gene pool, xiv, 67
general knowledge, 32
genetic factors, xiv, 67
geometry, 120
Germany, 8, 123
gestation, 182
gifted, 236
gland, 170, 171
glucose, 47, 48, 49, 51, 53, 56, 57, 58, 60, 62, 63, 64, 65, 143, 150
glucose regulation, 53, 57, 58
glucose tolerance, 62, 143, 150
GLUT, 64
glycaemic index (GI), xiii, 43
glycogen, 46, 51, 65
GPS, 75, 76, 77, 78, 79, 80, 83, 84, 85, 223, 226
grades, xv, 30, 33, 36, 98, 99, 101, 186
graffiti, 70
Greece, 62, 90
group work, 4
grouping, 104, 135, 136
growth, xii, xv, xx, 28, 53, 98, 110, 123, 140, 149, 182, 183, 186, 188, 190, 191, 194, 203, 207, 210, 214, 215, 217, 218, 219, 220, 222, 236
growth factor, 110
growth rate, 217
growth spurt, 182, 183, 186, 188, 191, 194
guardian, 37
guidance, 8, 24
guidelines, ix, xv, 1, 2, 11, 16, 25, 36, 39, 74, 78, 97, 116, 124, 151, 218, 236
gymnastics, 119, 184, 185, 189, 198
gymnasts, 196

H

hair, 88
hamstring, 187, 192, 195, 219, 224
harmful effects, 30
healing, 183, 186, 187, 192, 195
health care, xi, xii, 27, 28, 35, 162
health care system, xii, 28, 35
health condition, 44
health education, xii, 28, 35, 36, 37, 38, 39
health effects, 83
health information, 33
health insurance, xi, 27
health practitioners, 20
health problems, 71, 150
health promotion, 29, 32, 35, 39, 40
health status, x, xii, 14, 28, 38, 90
heart attack, xi, 28
heart disease, xi, 27
heart failure, xii, 28, 152
heart rate, xvii, 76, 77, 80, 99, 102, 128, 130, 133, 134, 135, 137, 139, 147, 149, 153, 155, 156, 157, 158, 159, 160, 171, 173, 225, 226, 227, 230
Heart Rate Variability (HRV), xvii, 147
heat illness, 162, 163
heat loss, xix, 161, 164
heat stroke, 163
height, xiii, 35, 40, 43, 88, 120, 182, 188, 194, 203, 205, 206, 208, 210, 212, 214, 217, 218, 219, 224
hemisphere, 105
heredity, xii, 28
heterogeneity, 105
high frequency (HF), xviii, 148
high school, 22, 24, 31, 65, 91, 99, 155, 162, 184, 185, 196, 198, 214
hippocampus, xv, 98, 108
Hispanics, 130, 131, 134, 140
history, 190, 193, 199
homes, 68, 73, 76
homework, xi, 14
Hong Kong, 39
House, xviii, 161, 177
hub, 110
human, xvi, 5, 10, 12, 75, 77, 88, 90, 98, 140, 153, 175, 178, 179, 182, 205, 206, 212, 214, 215
human development, 182
human right, 10
human rights, 10
humidity, 162, 171, 173, 174
Hunter, 135, 143, 144, 145, 202, 212
hyperactivity, 105
hyperglycaemia, 49, 61

hypertension, x, xi, xii, xvii, 14, 27, 28, 125, 144, 150
hyperthermia, 170, 171, 173, 174, 175, 177, 178
hypertrophy, xii, 28
hypothesis, 101, 102, 103, 105, 106, 112, 118, 122, 231

I

ice pack, 191
ideal, xi, xiv, 7, 14, 87, 88, 89, 90, 92, 218
ideals, xiv, 87, 90
identification, ix, 217
iliopsoas, 192
illiteracy, 33
image, xiv, 19, 24, 87, 88, 89, 90, 91, 92, 94, 95, 96
images, xiv, 87
imagination, 4, 5
imbalances, 108, 224
immersion, 174, 176
immune function, 229, 233
immunity, 233
impairments, 103, 106, 175
improvements, ix, xvi, 1, 37, 54, 98, 99, 100, 102, 103, 104, 106, 107, 108, 152, 202, 203, 204, 208, 209
impulses, 225
incidence, xix, 61, 93, 144, 170, 181, 183, 184, 189, 190, 194, 197, 198, 234
income, xv, 31, 69, 70, 71, 79, 82, 98
independent variable, 104
India, 127
Indians, 129, 132, 139, 146
individual character, 101
individual characteristics, 101
individual development, 222
individuals, xi, xv, xviii, xx, 16, 27, 32, 36, 52, 63, 69, 70, 75, 77, 84, 89, 90, 97, 102, 103, 106, 147, 148, 150, 151, 152, 155, 164, 182, 183, 201, 227, 232
inertia, 182
infancy, ix, 1, 4, 5
infants, xx, 2, 9, 201
infarction, 28, 157
infection, 190, 233
inflammation, 110
inflammatory disease, 193
information processing, 56, 105
information processing speed, 105
infrastructure, 2
ingestion, xviii, 48, 61, 64, 161, 177
inhibition, 109, 170, 207, 209
injuries, xix, xx, 163, 164, 174, 178, 181, 182, 183, 184, 185, 186, 188, 189, 191, 193, 194, 195, 196, 197, 198, 199, 208
injury, xviii, xix, 6, 161, 162, 163, 169, 171, 177, 181, 183, 184, 185, 186, 187, 188, 189, 193, 194, 195, 196, 197, 198, 206, 219, 220, 222, 223, 224, 225, 231
injury prevention, 162, 195, 220
insertion, 189
insulin, xvii, 44, 49, 51, 58, 61, 63, 64, 65, 125, 126, 143, 144, 145
insulin resistance, xvii, 51, 61, 126, 144, 145
insulin sensitivity, 44, 49, 51, 64
integration, 37
integrity, 207
intellectual disabilities, 177
intelligence, 102
interface, 172
interference, 149
internal consistency, 20, 89
internal validity, 104
internalization, 90
internalizing, 33
intervention, xi, xii, 6, 7, 8, 9, 10, 14, 28, 29, 30, 31, 32, 33, 34, 35, 37, 38, 39, 40, 41, 59, 84, 102, 103, 104, 106, 107, 108, 109, 124, 152, 154, 195, 197, 208, 214, 220, 227
intervention strategies, xii, 28, 30, 35
intrinsic motivation, 22
inversion, 187
investment, 6
iron, 44
isolation, 18, 205, 226
Israel, 86
issues, 4, 6, 11, 20, 22, 23, 25, 32, 38, 46, 60, 77, 100, 121, 142, 143, 145, 206, 208, 213
Italy, 35, 90

J

Japan, 163, 176, 177
joint damage, 185
joints, xiii, 67, 193
Jordan, 102, 107, 108, 109, 111, 157
Judo, 195, 199
jumping, 211, 212, 213, 220, 224

K

Keynes, 22
kill, 36, 37
knees, 183

L

laboratory tests, 227
lack of control, 104
lactate level, 204
landings, 184, 214
latency, 101, 103
later life, xi, 14, 65
laxatives, xiv, 88, 92
lead, xii, 17, 28, 29, 31, 32, 35, 37, 38, 46, 51, 90, 99, 100, 121, 149, 151, 182, 196
lean body mass, 129
learning, xv, 5, 34, 36, 37, 38, 57, 97, 98, 99, 101, 102, 103, 106, 108, 117, 118, 195, 203
learning difficulties, 102, 103, 106, 109
learning efficiency, 99
learning process, 37, 38
legs, 88, 91, 172
leisure, xi, 4, 14, 16, 74, 82, 174, 175
leisure time, xi, 14, 16, 74, 174, 175
lesions, 186
level of education, 106
life course, x, 14, 22
life expectancy, x, xi, 13, 27
lifestyle changes, 33
lifestyle decisions, 38
ligament, 182, 183, 185, 187, 188, 195, 198
light, 8, 132, 160, 162, 164, 195, 221
limb stiffness, 206
lipid oxidation, 63
lipids, 59
lipolysis, 51
literacy, xv, 34, 97, 98, 102, 103, 105, 106, 109, 110, 112, 117
liver, 51, 150
liver disease, 150
living conditions, xiii, 44
local government, 80
location information, 75
locomotor, 117, 119, 120, 121
longitudinal study, 25, 82, 92, 94, 107, 157, 199, 233
love, 17
low-density lipoprotein, 47
lumbar spine, xix, 181
lying, 182

M

machinery, 205
Mackintosh, 157
macronutrients, 61, 82
magnitude, 35, 99, 107, 149
magnocellular deficit, 102
majority, xvi, 4, 6, 7, 48, 76, 91, 100, 109, 116, 121, 203
malaise, 193
malignancy, 193
mammals, 5
man, 111, 154, 158, 176, 179, 212, 213
management, 94, 117, 119, 143, 185, 186, 187, 188, 189, 190, 192, 195, 196, 199, 218
manipulation, xiii, 44, 47, 51, 117
mapping, 83
masculinity, 19
mass, xviii, 19, 62, 74, 120, 128, 129, 131, 133, 134, 136, 137, 139, 143, 149, 151, 161, 166, 172, 182, 183, 184, 205, 217
materials, 30, 34
mathematics, 40, 100, 103, 107, 108
matter, 12, 82
maturation process, 222
measurement, 11, 20, 25, 30, 58, 63, 71, 75, 83, 84, 104, 121, 124, 140, 144, 145, 148, 149, 159, 183, 226
measurements, xiii, 34, 44, 57, 70, 75, 124, 149, 156, 158, 159, 213
media, xiv, 11, 68, 87, 90
medial epicondyle, 189
medical, xi, xix, 27, 181, 184
medication, 169, 190, 226
medicine, 84, 155, 196
mellitus, xvii, 125, 143
membership, 25
memory, xvi, 52, 53, 54, 55, 56, 57, 60, 65, 98
menarche, 91
mental development, xx, 217
mental health, x, xiii, 13, 67
mental retardation, 101
messages, 33, 34, 36, 85, 89, 90
meta-analysis, 59, 100, 142
Metabolic, 59, 60, 62, 80, 81, 177
metabolic changes, 49, 53, 61
metabolic disease risk, xvii, 49, 125
metabolic syndrome, 49, 124, 143
metabolism, 49, 53, 62, 178
meter, 214
methodology, 36, 93, 135, 136
micronutrients, 47
military, xviii, 161
Ministry of Education, 34
minorities, xvii, 69, 71, 125, 142
mixing, 103
modelling, 33
models, 3, 73, 175, 202
moderate activity, 130, 131, 140

modifications, 207
modules, 34
monosaccharide, 48
Moon, 32, 40
morbid fear of gaining weight,, xiv, 88
morbidity, xiv, 88
mortality, xiv, xvii, xviii, 88, 125, 142, 147, 155, 157, 163, 175, 176
mortality rate, xvii, 125
motivation, 25, 102, 106, 118, 140
motor control, 215
motor skill development, ix, 1
motor skills, 117, 121, 122, 123, 124
MRI, 185
MTI, 131
multi-ethnic, 127
multimedia, 34
multiple regression, 107
multiple regression analysis, 107
multiple sclerosis, 169, 178
multiple-choice questions, 33
multiplication, 227
muscle mass, 164, 183, 204, 207, 220
muscle performance, 210
muscle strain, 224
muscle strength, 2, 188, 224
muscles, 173, 183, 193, 211, 212, 219, 220
musculoskeletal system, xix, 181, 211
myocardial infarction, xi, 28, 152, 155
myocardial ischemia, 157
myocardium, xii, 28, 157
myositis, 186

N

naming, 102, 103, 105, 106, 108, 112
national curricula, x, 13
National Health Service, xv, 97
navigation system, 84
negative attitudes, 17, 18, 21
negative consequences, 225
neglect, 194
negotiating, 4
nerve, xvii, 147, 159
nervous system, 158, 159, 160
neural development, 209
neural function, 210
neural network, 102
neural networks, 102
neuroimaging, 102
neuromotor, 117
neurons, xv, 98
neuroscience, 210
New England, 24, 82, 142
New Zealand, 16, 84, 127, 131, 195
next generation, 25
non-clinical population, 89
North America, 21, 127, 139, 160, 236
Norway, 137, 195
nursing, xi, 27
nursing home, xi, 27
nutrient, 31, 44, 45, 46, 47, 48, 59, 60, 63, 64
nutrients, 51, 57, 60
nutrition, 2, 29, 30, 31, 32, 33, 36, 37, 44, 48, 52, 73, 81, 83, 229
nutritional status, xiv, 37, 44, 47, 57, 63, 87, 88, 91, 92

O

obesity prevention, 8, 12
obstacles, 16
occlusion, 172
oculomotor, 106
oesophageal, 164
officials, 31, 37
omission, xiii, 44, 47, 52, 53, 54, 58
open spaces, 12
operations, xviii, 161
opportunities, xvi, 2, 6, 16, 18, 25, 32, 70, 71, 74, 93, 115
organ, 207
organs, 207
ossicles, 190
ossification, 182
osteoarthritis, 151
osteoporosis, x, 13, 65
overtraining, 230
overweight, ix, x, xii, xiii, xiv, xvi, 1, 6, 9, 11, 14, 16, 22, 23, 28, 31, 32, 40, 46, 51, 52, 61, 63, 67, 68, 71, 72, 78, 81, 82, 87, 88, 89, 90, 91, 92, 113, 115, 122, 128, 145, 156, 159
overweight adults, x, 14, 72
ox, xii, 28
oxidation, 51, 52, 61, 64
oxygen, 129, 134, 135, 137, 139, 142, 164, 166, 167, 173, 226
oxygen consumption, 134, 135, 137, 142, 164, 166, 173, 226

P

pain, xii, xix, 28, 181, 183, 186, 187, 188, 190, 191, 193, 194, 195, 197
Pakistan, 95, 127

palpation, 187, 191
parallel, 5, 75, 107
paralysis, 173
parasympathetic activity, 150, 151, 152
parasympathetic nervous system, xviii, 148
parental involvement, 7, 31
parental support, 112
parenting, 8, 9, 79, 106
parents, x, xv, xix, 2, 3, 4, 6, 9, 13, 22, 24, 31, 32, 36, 37, 70, 72, 73, 74, 77, 81, 85, 93, 98, 104, 106, 181, 185, 187, 189, 191, 192, 193, 194, 195
participants, 18, 29, 32, 37, 53, 54, 56, 70, 75, 76, 77, 84, 99, 101, 103, 104, 106, 127, 134, 136, 152, 164, 166, 167, 168, 171, 172, 184, 195, 197, 206, 208, 209
patellar tendon, 189, 195
pathogenesis, 189
pathogens, 233
pathology, 183, 193
pathways, 209
peer assessment, 118
peer review, 7
pelvis, 182
PEP, 40
peptide, 143
percentile, 90
peripheral nervous system, 170
permission, 3, 165
personal computers, xi, 14
personality, 22, 38, 94, 232
pH, 240
phonological deficit, 102, 111
physical education, x, xi, xii, xv, 7, 13, 14, 16, 17, 18, 19, 20, 21, 22, 23, 24, 25, 26, 28, 29, 31, 33, 36, 40, 84, 98, 110, 111, 122, 123
physical environment, 6, 68, 75
physical exercise, 92, 153, 154, 158, 170
physical fitness, x, 13, 23, 29, 31, 36, 72, 117, 123, 135, 137, 139, 140, 141, 142, 143, 144, 145, 154, 155
physical health, xiii, 6, 29, 34, 43
physical inactivity, 7, 32, 68, 72, 100
physical structure, 68
physical therapist, 199
physical therapy, 199
physics, 178
Physiological, 60, 108, 111, 176, 179, 180, 210, 211, 213, 214, 237, 238, 240
physiological factors, 162
physiological mechanisms, xviii, 140, 148
physiology, xix, 31, 34, 181, 182, 188
piano, 210
pilot study, 38, 61, 63, 175
pitch, 222, 223, 224, 225, 226
placebo, 104, 106
plaque, xi, 27
plasticity, xvi, 98, 110, 113, 209
platform, xiii, 44
playing, xv, xx, 5, 6, 11, 70, 72, 74, 85, 98, 123, 187, 189, 191, 194, 217, 218, 228
plethysmography, 121
Poland, 20
policy, 6, 80, 81, 83
population, x, xi, xviii, xix, 2, 6, 7, 9, 20, 27, 35, 54, 64, 84, 85, 90, 99, 100, 108, 109, 126, 127, 142, 143, 148, 150, 151, 153, 155, 156, 159, 162, 163, 165, 166, 169, 172, 174, 183, 198
population group, 20, 109
Portugal, 137
positive attitudes, x, 13, 16, 17, 18, 19, 20, 21, 33, 38
positive correlation, 69
positive relationship, 47, 99
postural control, 119
potato, 48
poverty, 32, 86
preadolescents, 155
pregnancy, xv, 82, 98
prejudice, 90
preparation, 18, 36, 48, 218
preschool, 85, 90, 120, 123, 144, 155
preschool children, 90, 123, 144, 155
pre-school children, ix, x, xvi, 1, 2, 3, 4, 7, 8, 9, 10, 11, 61
pre-school children, 116
prevention, ix, xi, xii, xix, 1, 6, 11, 14, 28, 29, 33, 34, 35, 36, 38, 39, 40, 41, 65, 95, 142, 162, 181, 198
primary school, xii, 18, 22, 23, 24, 25, 28, 32, 37, 39, 74, 75, 76, 108, 110, 111, 116, 117, 118, 121, 122, 124
primate, 11
principles, 34, 190, 196, 209
prior knowledge, 38
professionals, xix, 3, 33, 93, 181, 193
profit, 102
prognosis, 192, 198
programming, 31, 32, 33, 36
project, 30, 75, 79, 80, 85
promotion of positive attitudes, x, 13
protection, ix, 1, 39, 40, 157, 186
proteins, 108
psychological stress, 226
psychological welfare, ix, 1
psychology, 23
psychosocial stress, 231
pubertal development, 19

puberty, xix, xx, 19, 53, 60, 91, 119, 128, 141, 182, 183, 209, 214, 217
public health, xvi, 2, 24, 30, 37, 39, 44, 76, 82, 116, 142, 157
public schools, 31

Q

quadriceps, 192, 219, 220, 224
qualitative research, 17, 144
quality of life, xi, 27
quantification, 20
questioning, 207
questionnaire, 20, 24, 30, 31, 32, 40, 89, 94, 95, 107, 152, 194, 231, 232, 234

R

race, xii, 28, 69, 71, 80, 83, 126, 128, 142, 150, 159
racial differences, xviii, 147
racial minorities, 70
racism, 142
reactivity, 159
reading, xv, 7, 98, 102, 103, 104, 105, 106, 107, 108, 109, 111
reading comprehension, 102, 109
reading difficulties, 103, 104, 105, 106, 111
reading skills, 102
real time, 83
reality, 92, 217
reasoning, 37
recall, 56
reception, 6
receptors, 49, 207
recognition, xi, xii, 14, 28
recommendations, x, xi, 2, 14, 16, 74, 132, 141, 146, 153, 156, 162
recovery, xix, 64, 173, 176, 178, 181, 185, 209, 214, 218, 219, 223, 225, 229, 230, 231, 232, 233, 234, 236
recreation, 69, 70, 71, 72
recreational, 4, 36, 68, 73, 118, 183, 198
rectal temperature, 165, 167, 168, 169, 171, 173, 174
recurrence, 196
reflexes, 102, 106, 107, 108, 109, 205, 209, 211
regression, 101, 194
rehabilitation, xix, 181, 186, 188
reinforcement, 72, 118
relaxation, 229
relevance, xvi, 9, 44, 45, 98, 193, 222
reliability, 20, 21, 89, 95, 105, 141, 148, 149, 152, 153, 155, 158, 159, 178, 226
relief, 187
repetitions, 189
replication, 107
requirements, 36, 186
researchers, xiv, 7, 20, 21, 29, 31, 32, 33, 34, 35, 36, 37, 68, 74, 87, 88, 100, 104, 107, 117, 119, 150, 205, 208
resistance, 211
resources, 22, 69, 101, 197, 236
respiration, 148
response, 20, 30, 34, 49, 51, 53, 89, 99, 101, 102, 149, 155, 157, 172, 182, 183, 186, 206, 207, 210, 212, 222, 223, 225, 227, 234
response time, 53, 206
responsiveness, 151
restaurants, 69, 73
restrictions, 99
retardation, 101
rhythm, xvii, 147
riboflavin, 44
risk factors, xii, 9, 28, 30, 31, 32, 35, 36, 38, 39, 41, 46, 47, 79, 80, 93, 142, 145, 151, 154, 159, 197, 198
risk profile, x, 13
risks, xiv, 70, 97, 99, 189, 195, 197
room temperature, 171
root, xviii, 148
routes, 75
routines, 184
Royal Society, 25, 60, 82, 145
rugby, 118, 119, 184, 185, 195, 197, 198, 231
rules, 5, 68, 195
rural areas, 72, 91

S

SA node, xvii, xviii, 147, 148
safety, x, 2, 6, 9, 40, 69, 70, 72, 82, 142, 168, 208
saturated fat, xii, 28, 29, 45
Scandinavia, 176
scar tissue, 170, 171, 195
school support, 103
science, ix, xii, 28, 29, 32, 34, 40, 144, 236
scoliosis, 182, 189
scope, ix, 174
search terms, 7, 126
seasonal growth, 220
secondary schools, 19, 24
secondary sexual characteristics, xiii, 43
secretion, 142, 144
sedentary behavior, ix, x, 2, 7
sedentary lifestyle, x, 14, 29
segregation, 71

self-efficacy, 29, 118
self-esteem, 10, 92, 189, 232
sensation, 89, 171
sensitivity, 30, 142, 144, 156, 171, 207
sepsis, 193
serum, 29, 47, 204
services, xi, 2, 27, 188
SES, 99
sex, xii, 9, 18, 24, 28, 55, 78, 93, 158, 159, 197, 213
sex differences, 158, 213
shape, xiv, 19, 25, 34, 37, 38, 87, 88, 93, 95, 183
shin splints, 189
shock, 190
shoot, 188
short-term memory, 62
showing, 35, 57, 68, 121, 223, 232
siblings, x, 2
side effects, 169, 170
signal transduction, 113
signalling, 51
signals, 77
signs, 106, 170, 190, 193
silhouette, 89, 91, 92
Sinai, 84
Singapore, 163, 179, 212, 213
sinoatrial node, xvii, 147
skeletal muscle, 51, 153, 178, 179, 212
skeleton, 182, 183, 189
skin, 170, 171, 172, 173, 174, 175, 176, 177, 179, 180
smoking, xii, 23, 28, 30, 31, 33, 40
snacking, 46, 61
SNS, 151
soccer, xx, 184, 185, 198, 210, 211, 213, 214, 215, 217, 219, 220, 222, 223, 224, 225, 226, 227, 231, 234
social activities, 231
social behavior, 4, 6
social benefits, 3, 16
social class, 93
social development, ix, 1
social exclusion, xv, 16, 97
social justice, 79
social learning, 38
social psychology, x, 13, 14
social relations, 4, 6
social relationships, 4, 6
social structure, 68
socialization, 4, 119
society, xi, xiv, xv, 27, 87, 97, 155
socioeconomic status, 47, 73, 80, 83, 96
sodium, 48
software, 223
solution, 6, 30, 81, 218
South Asia, xvii, 125, 126, 130, 131, 132, 138, 139, 140, 142, 144, 145
Spain, 36, 39
spastic, 172
spatial location, 77
spatial memory, xv, 53, 55, 98
special education, xv, 98, 110
special educational needs (SEN), xv, 98
specialists, 116, 117
species, 174
spelling, 102, 106, 107, 108
spending, 4, 68, 135
spinal cord, 164, 169, 172, 178
spinal cord injury, 164, 169, 172, 178
spondylolisthesis, xix, 181
sprains, xix, 181, 186
Spring, 24, 85
Sprint, 202, 215, 223, 239, 240
Sri Lanka, 138
stability, 103, 188, 192, 206, 207, 225
staffing, 36
stakeholders, 29, 33
standard deviation, xviii, 148, 203
stars, xx, 217
stasis, 187, 188
state, xx, 2, 6, 8, 30, 36, 49, 51, 74, 91, 111, 116, 157, 158, 182, 225, 226, 230, 231
states, 4, 18, 20, 33, 36, 162, 194
statistics, xvi, 16, 40, 104, 106, 110, 115, 145
stigmatized, 89
stimulus, 95, 101, 209, 223, 225, 229
stomach, 88
storage, 65
strength training, 190, 214, 218, 220, 224
stress, xii, 28, 31, 33, 63, 157, 169, 170, 171, 175, 176, 177, 179, 182, 187, 189, 198, 222, 225, 227, 228, 229, 231, 233, 234
stressors, 189, 229
stretching, 101, 103, 190, 192, 195, 196, 205, 219, 220
stroke, 40, 64, 145, 149, 177, 179
stroke volume, 149
structural changes, 204, 207
structural characteristics, 207
structure, 20, 30, 33, 71, 105, 207, 214
style, 5, 31
subgroups, xix, 138, 162
substance use, 45
substrate, 49, 61, 64, 65
sucrose, 48
supervision, 104
surface area, xviii, 161, 164, 170, 171, 180, 204

surveillance, xix, 182, 183, 197
survival, xv, 98
sweat, xviii, 153, 161, 170, 171, 173, 174, 178
swelling, 186, 190, 191
Switzerland, 8
symbolic activity, 5
symmetry, 105
sympathetic nervous system, 151, 154
symptoms, 93, 95, 96, 105, 170, 178, 179, 185, 189, 190, 192, 193, 194
synaptic plasticity, 113
syndrome, xix, 70, 181, 182, 189, 190, 192, 194, 197, 198

T

talent, ix, 217
target, 35, 52, 53, 71, 99, 103, 170
target population, 99
teacher training, 18
teachers, ix, 2, 3, 15, 18, 19, 20, 22, 31, 34, 36, 70, 90, 107, 119, 185
team sports, 18
teams, 217, 235
techniques, xviii, 20, 40, 83, 120, 161, 195, 211, 215
technology, 81, 118, 226
teens, 182
television viewing, 9, 32, 74
temperature, xviii, xix, 161, 162, 163, 164, 165, 166, 167, 168, 170, 171, 172, 173, 174, 175, 176, 177, 178, 179, 180
tempo, 218
tendon, 182, 189, 190, 196, 204, 207, 212, 214
tendons, 198, 219
tennis elbow, 195
tension, 190, 207
test scores, 34, 145, 218, 222
testing, 24, 29, 30, 129, 137, 177, 192, 193, 205, 206, 222, 223
testosterone, 204
test-retest reliability, 20, 148
therapist, 190
therapy, 38, 103, 152, 159, 173, 177, 188
thermoregulation, xviii, xix, 161, 162, 165, 169, 174, 176, 178
threats, 5
tibia, 189, 192
time constraints, 18, 118
time frame, 34
tissue, xix, 120, 129, 170, 181, 182, 185, 186, 187, 195, 196
TLR, 106
tobacco, xii, 28, 29, 45, 70, 81
tonic, xvii, 106, 147
total cholesterol, 29
total energy, 45, 52, 55, 56, 57, 58, 74, 134, 136, 138
toys, 5, 90
trajectory, 32
transformation, 204
transition period, 61
translocation, 2
transparency, 107
transport, 71, 72, 73, 77, 78, 79, 80, 81
transportation, 69, 72
trauma, 185, 190
treatment, 6, 11, 37, 61, 64, 89, 95, 103, 104, 106, 107, 108, 169, 170, 175, 178, 186, 190, 192, 193, 195, 196, 198
trial, 7, 8, 11, 26, 39, 56, 62, 64, 65, 105, 109, 111, 174, 186, 188, 198
triangulation, 21
tuition, xv, 98, 99, 106
tumours, 190
Turkey, 19
type 1 diabetes, 64, 160
type 2 diabetes, xvii, 62, 125, 145, 183
type 2 diabetes mellitus, xvii, 125

U

UK, ix, xv, xvi, xix, 1, 2, 6, 9, 11, 13, 16, 35, 43, 67, 97, 98, 109, 112, 115, 116, 125, 127, 129, 134, 143, 146, 147, 161, 181, 194, 201, 217, 238
uniform, 19
United, ix, xi, xvi, 1, 4, 8, 11, 16, 24, 27, 29, 36, 41, 63, 78, 90, 94, 110, 115, 136, 144, 162, 163, 175, 176, 196
United Kingdom, ix, xvi, 1, 8, 16, 115
United Nations, 4, 11
United States, xi, 24, 27, 29, 36, 41, 63, 78, 90, 110, 136, 144, 162, 163, 175, 176, 196
upper respiratory tract, 233
urban, 39, 72, 76, 77, 79, 80, 81, 82, 85, 91, 95
urban areas, 79, 91
urban population, 82
USA, 8, 30, 111

V

valgus, 183, 189
validation, 60, 94, 109, 118
variables, x, xiv, xvi, 14, 50, 55, 58, 67, 71, 116, 119, 120, 140, 141, 153, 154, 202
variations, 54, 69, 80, 153, 184, 190, 198, 205
vasoconstriction, 172

vasodilation, 176
vasodilator, 176
vastus lateralis, 212
vegetables, 68, 69
vegetation, 76
velocity, xiii, 43, 75, 172, 202, 203, 208, 209, 214
venue, 30
Verbal IQ, 107
video games, 70, 74, 151
video gaming, xvi, 115, 116
videos, 72
viscoelastic properties, 212
visco-elastic properties, 204
visual attention, 53, 55
vitamins, 44, 47
volleyball, 184
vomiting, xiv, 88

W

wages, xv, 98
waking, xi, 14, 193
Wales, 184, 201
walking, 2, 59, 69, 70, 72, 73, 75, 76, 78, 83, 84, 85, 101, 123, 173, 177, 179, 202, 222
war, 194
Washington, 39
watching television, xi, xvi, 14, 74, 115, 186
water, 128, 129, 134, 136, 138, 169, 170, 173, 174, 175, 176, 177, 180
weakness, xix, 181, 224, 232
weapons, 194
weight control, xiv, 88
weight gain, ix, 1, 19, 44, 45, 46, 48
weight loss, 46, 48, 90, 92, 157, 158, 178, 193
weight reduction, 62, 90, 91
weight status, xvii, 46, 60, 71, 116, 119, 120, 121, 123, 142, 151
welfare, ix, 1
well-being, xii, 16, 21, 22, 28, 52, 123, 159
western culture, 89
Western Europe, ix, 1, 2
white matter, 210
WHO, xvii, 100, 125, 146
windows, 70, 208, 225
Wisconsin, 237
withdrawal, 118, 151
workers, xi, 27, 29, 30, 33, 36
working memory, 53, 54, 55, 56, 100, 104
workload, 129, 139, 185
World Health Organisation, xiv, 80, 84, 97, 113
worldwide, xi, xiii, 27, 67, 122
worry, xiv, 70, 87, 193
wrestling, 4, 184

X

x-rays, 190

Y

Yale University, 25
yield, 141, 175
young adults, 38, 60, 85, 142, 154, 157, 177, 198, 236
young people, x, xi, xiii, xiv, xv, xix, 2, 10, 13, 14, 15, 16, 17, 18, 19, 20, 21, 22, 24, 26, 36, 43, 44, 45, 46, 47, 48, 49, 50, 52, 53, 57, 58, 59, 61, 67, 71, 74, 85, 97, 98, 121, 134, 136, 157, 177, 181, 182, 183
young women, 19
youth populations, xi, 14

Z

zinc, 44